£146.00

NLM   WE
Class   725
Mark: YOU
L.G.I.

D1493484

MICROSURGERY OF THE CERVICAL SPINE

Microsurgery of the Cervical Spine

Paul H. Young, M.D.
Director
Microsurgery and Brain Research Institute
Assistant Clinical Professor
Departments of Anatomy-Neurobiology and Neurosurgery
St. Louis University School of Medicine
St. Louis, Missouri

with contributions by:
Wolfhard Caspar
Margaret H. Cooper
Haynes Louis Harkey
Paul C. McCormick
Bennett M. Stein
Vernon L. Yaeger
Paul A. Young

Raven Press 🦅 New York

Raven Press, 1185 Avenue of the Americas, New York, New York 10036

© 1991 by Raven Press, Ltd. All rights reserved. This book is protected by copyright. No part of it may be reproduced, stored in a retrieval system, or transmitted, in any form or by any means, electronic, mechanical, photocopying, recording, or otherwise, without the prior written permission of the publisher.

Made in the United States of America

Library of Congress Cataloging in Publication Data

Young, Paul H. (Paul Henry), 1950–
    Microsurgery of the cervical spine / author, Paul H. Young.
        p.   cm.
    Includes bibliographical references and index.
    ISBN 0-88167-799-X
    1. Vertebrae, Cervical—Surgery.   2. Microsurgery.   I. Title.
    [DNLM: 1. Cervical Vertebrae—surgery.   2. Microsurgery.
    3. Spinal Diseases—surgery.   WE 725 Y75m]
    RD533.Y68   1991
    617,4′82059—dc20
    DNLM/DLC
    for Library of Congress   91-18632
                                                                        CIP

The material contained in this volume was submitted as previously unpublished material, except in the instances in which some of the illustrative material was derived.

Great care has been taken to maintain the accuracy of the information contained in the volume. However, neither Raven Press nor the editors can be held responsible for errors or for any consequences arising from the use of the information contained herein.

Materials appearing in this book prepared by individuals as part of their official duties as U.S. Government employees are not covered by the above-mentioned copyright.

With admiration to my children—Julie, Jennifer, Jason, and Jacqueline, whose accomplishments at such young ages far exceed my expectations and encourage me to expand my own horizons. With gratitude to Jean B., whose patience and understanding has provided me with the courage and strength to open new doors. With thanks to my wife, Mary Ann, and my family, friends, associates, and partners; without your willing support, this work would not have been possible.

Contents

Contributing Authors

Wolfhard Caspar, M.D. *Oberarts, Department of Neurosurgery, University of Saarland, Homburg/Saar, Germany*

Margaret H. Cooper, Ph.D. *Associate Professor, Departments of Anatomy–Neurobiology and Otolaryngology–Head and Neck Surgery, St. Louis University School of Medicine, 3635 Vista Street, St. Louis, Missouri, 63110-0250*

Haynes Louis Harkey, M.D. *Assistant Professor of Neurosurgery, University of Mississippi Medical Center, 2500 North State Street, Jackson, Mississippi 39216*

Paul C. McCormick, M.D. *Assistant Professor of Neurosurgery, Columbia Presbyterian Medical Center, 710 West 168th Street, New York, New York 10032*

Bennett M. Stein, M.D. *Byron Stookey Professor and Chairman, Department of Neurosurgery, Columbia Presbyterian Medical Center, 710 West 168th Street, New York, New York 10032*

Vernon L. Yaeger, Ph.D. *Professor of Anatomy, Department of Anatomy–Neurobiology, St. Louis University School of Medicine, 3635 Vista Street, St. Louis, Missouri, 63110-0250*

Paul A. Young, Ph.D. *Chairman and Professor, Department of Anatomy–Neurobiology, St. Louis University School of Medicine, 3635 Vista Street, St. Louis, Missouri, 63110-0250*

Paul H. Young, M.D. *Director, Microsurgery and Brain Research Institute, Assistant Clinical Professor, Departments of Anatomy–Neurobiology and Neurosurgery, St. Louis University School of Medicine, 3635 Vista Street, St. Louis, Missouri, 63110-0250*

Preface

There has been an explosion of interest in microsurgical approaches to the lumbar spine over the past decade. The standard lumbar laminectomy-discectomy has given way to the microdiscectomy; the decompressive total laminectomy, partial facetectomy, and foraminotomy is now commonly performed as the microlaminoplasty and facetoplasty. The smaller, more precise operative approach paying meticulous attention to anatomical integrity is the rule; reduced postoperative morbidity with shorter hospital stay and fewer operative casualties is the reward.

The traditional operative approaches to the cervical spine have included high risk of spinal cord injury. To many cervical spine surgeons, postoperative quadriplegia is as bad a complication as death; neither complication is ever tolerable, particularly during disc surgery. The advantages of microscopic technique in spine surgery, which include better illumination, magnification, and clear stereoscopic vision, permit the precise and meticulous anatomical dissection that is essential in minimizing these dreaded complications.

Microsurgery of the cervical spine encompasses a variety of pathological processes and operative approaches. As more lumbar microsurgeons perform microsurgery of the cervical spine, the spectrum of techniques should be examined. This book redefines established microsurgical approaches for use during cervical spine surgery. This should ultimately lead to a reduction of postoperative morbidity in cervical spine patients. If even a single postoperative quadriplegia is prevented, my energies will have been very well spent.

Paul H. Young, M.D.

Acknowledgments

I would like to extend my appreciation to those who always make me look good: my entire office staff, especially my secretary, Rona, and my brother, Steve. My thanks also go to Jill Witterschein for spending hours proofreading and typing the manuscript many times over. I would also like to thank Larry Clifford and Julie Young for the excellent illustrations.

CHAPTER 1

Surgical Anatomy of the Cervical Spine and Surrounding Structures

Vernon L. Yeager and Margaret H. Cooper

The *neck* is the region of the body that connects the head and thorax. It is surrounded by skin and *superficial fascia* (tela subcutanea). This layer largely contains fat and areolar tissue, and is continuous around the entire body. In the neck region, this layer also contains the platysma muscle (a muscle of facial expression), the external jugular vein, and the cutaneous sensory nerves. Throughout the neck, all fascias internal or deep to the superficial fascia are considered *deep fascia*.

The structures deep to the superficial fascia are compartmentalized by sleeves of deep fascia and interfascial spaces, which tend to separate tissues into groups of structures. In this discussion, the term "fascia" will be used for a sheet or layer of condensed fibroelastic connective tissue and the term "interfascial space" will be used for very loose connective tissue between fascias (with the understanding that the space is a potential space). An insight into how the fascias are formed will be helpful in understanding the compartmentalization of the neck.

When nerves, blood vessels, bones, muscles, and other organs are first formed, they are surrounded by mesenchyme. As they grow and move relative to adjacent structures, lines of force are set up in the mesenchyme, causing it to condense. The pulsation of the vessels and the contraction of muscles cause the formation of an adventitia around blood vessels and an epimysium around muscles. Thus, each structure has its own protective *minor fascia*.

When a group of structures move during embryological development as a unit with respect to adjacent structures, they develop a *major fascia* which surrounds them. These major fascias anatomically compartmentalize the neck (Fig. 1). For example, the common carotid artery, internal jugular vein and vagus nerve move up or down as a group; similarly, the viscera of the neck (esophagus, trachea, etc.) move as a group. Each group of tissue is thereby compartmentalized within a major fascia.

To allow this movement, some mesenchymal tissue between major fascias remains very loose, thus forming an *interfascial space*. All the fascias and interfascial spaces develop from early mesenchyme, and, therefore, they are all continuous. The degree of relative movement determines the eventual strength of the fascias and the looseness of the interfascial spaces. Vessels and nerves passing through major fascias and interfascial spaces have their own minor fascias and will tend to join major fascias together.

Diagrams of major fascias are usually oversimplified, and diagrams from different sources vary because each author's interpretation of what he/she has observed differs. Major fascias that are easily identified at one level may be difficult to identify at other levels, as in the case of the carotid sheath. In addition, as fascias directly cross bone or cartilage, they typically fuse to the periosteum or perichondrium.

GENERAL ORGANIZATION OF THE NECK

Figures 1–5 refer to the general organization of the neck.

Immediately deep to the superficial fascia is the *outer investing layer of deep fascia*. This is the out-

1

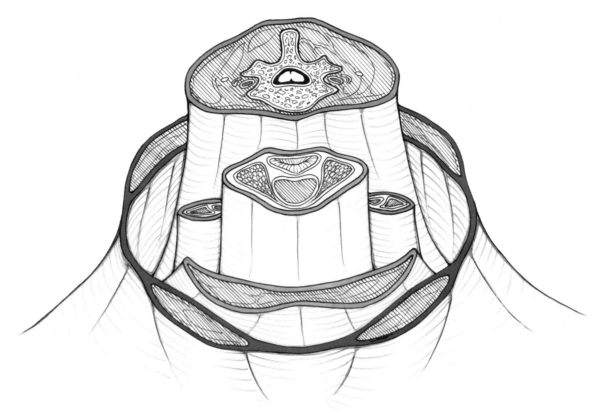

FIG. 1. Compartmentalization of the neck by deep fascia, outer investing layer of deep fascia, middle cervical fascia, visceral fascia, carotid sheath, and prevertebral fascia.

ermost sleeve of fascia that splits to enclose the sternocleidomastoid and trapezius muscles, and surrounds all other sleeves of fascia in the neck. The most anterior compartment within the outer investing layer is surrounded by the *middle cervical* fascia, enclosing the infrahyoid or strap muscles. The middle cervical fascia is sometimes called the "fascia of the infrahyoid muscles." The *visceral fascia* lies behind the middle fascia and surrounds the visceral organs of the neck, such as the thyroid gland, larynx, trachea, pharynx, and esophagus. Immediately lateral to the visceral compartment is the *carotid sheath*. This is the only paired compartment of the neck. It contains the carotid artery, internal jugular vein, and vagus nerve. Posterior to the visceral compartment and the carotid sheaths is the *prevertebral fascia*. The cervical spine and the associated muscles are surrounded by the prevertebral fascia. The deep fascia fuses to the periosteum, where parts of the vertebrae such as the spinous and transverse processes are not covered by muscles.

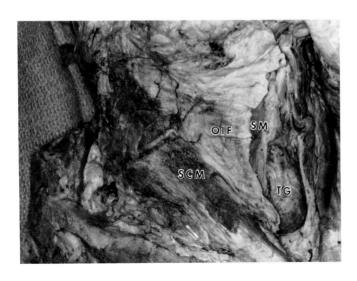

FIG. 2. The outer investing layer of deep fascia (OIF) covers the anterior triangle of the neck and encloses the sternocleidomastoid muscle (SCM), strap muscles (SM), and thyroid gland (TG).

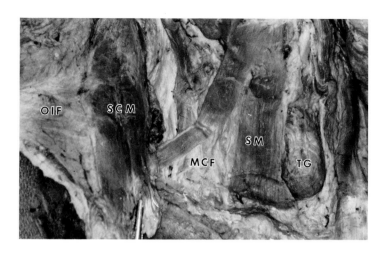

FIG. 3. The outer investing layer of deep fascia (OIF) has been reflected with the sternocleidomastoid muscle (SCM) to expose the middle cervical fascia (MCF), strap muscles (SM), and thyroid gland (TG).

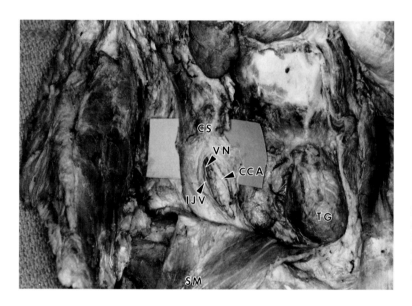

FIG. 4. The carotid sheath (CS) has been separated from the visceral and prevertebral fascia by blue paper and has been opened to show the common carotid artery (CCA), internal jugular vein (IJV), and vagus nerve (VN). The strap muscles (SM) and their middle cervical fascia have been reflected inferiorly. TG, thyroid gland.

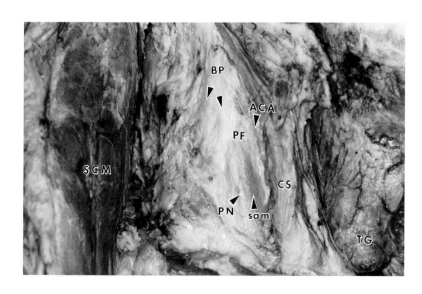

FIG. 5. The prevertebral fascia (PF) can be seen between the carotid sheath (CS) and sternocleidomastoid muscle (SCM) covering the anterior scalene muscle (sam) and upper portion of the brachial plexus (BP). The phrenic nerve (PN) and ascending cervical artery (ACA) lie on the scalenus anterior muscle. TG, thyroid gland.

The fascial compartments are traversed by nerves and blood vessels. The external carotid artery has branches that leave the carotid sheath to supply structures in the visceral, middle cervical, and outer investing layers of fascia. Cranial nerves supply visceral structures and muscles within the outer investing layer of fascia. The *glossopharyngeal nerve* passes between the internal and external carotid arteries, gives pharyngeal branches to the pharyngeal plexus, and supplies the stylopharyngeous muscle as it crosses its external surface to enter the tongue deep to the hyoglossus muscle. The right *vagus nerve* gives off the *recurrent laryngeal nerve*, which leaves the lower end of the carotid sheath and enters the visceral fascia. When there is an aberrrant right subclavian artery, the recurrent laryngeal nerve goes directly from the carotid sheath to the visceral fascia at or above the level of the sixth cervical vertebra. The *accessory nerve* passes adjacent to the internal jugular vein, usually anterior to it, to supply the sternocleidomastoid and trapezius muscles. The *hypoglossal nerve* passes superficial to both internal and external carotid arteries, hooks under the occipital artery, and enters the tongue between the mylohyoid and hyoglossus muscles. Cervical nerves leave the prevertebral fascia to innervate muscles in the middle cervical and outer investing fascias or pierce the outer investing fascia to supply the skin of the neck.

In summary, the neck is surrounded by skin and superficial fascia and is compartmentalized by sleeves of deep fascia. The outermost sleeve of deep fascia is the *outer investing layer*, which encloses all other sleeves. The middle cervical fascia contains the strap muscles and is located between the outer investing layer of deep fascia and the visceral fascia. The *visceral fascia* contains the visceral structures of the neck and lies anterior to the prevertebral fascia. The *carotid sheath* contains the major neurovascular bundle connecting the thorax and head. It is located immediately lateral to the visceral fascia and anterior to the prevertebral fascia. The *prevertebral fascia* surrounds the cervical spine and associated muscles. There are *interfascial spaces* separating these major fascias. Most structures tend to remain in their fascias, but nerves and blood vessels frequently violate them. The interfascial spaces between these major fascias are good surgical routes, as long as the nerves and vessels that cross the planes are anticipated.

The important fascia layers of the neck are the *outer investing layer of deep fascia*, the *middle cervical fascia*, the *carotid sheath*, the *visceral fascia*, and the *prevertebral fascia*.

OUTER INVESTING LAYER OF DEEP FASCIA

The trapezius and sternocleidomastoid muscles act on the pectoral girdle moving relative to the other structures in the neck (Figs. 1–3). They are enclosed within the *outer investing layer of fascia*, which covers their superficial and deep surfaces as it surrounds the entire neck. Laterally the fascia between the adjacent borders of these muscles forms a roof for the posterior triangle of the neck, and anteriorly the fascia connecting the medial borders of the sternocleidomastoid muscles forms a roof over the anterior triangles. Surrounding its contained muscular attachments, the outer investing layer of deep fascia fuses to the skull at the external occipital protuberance, superior nuchal line, mastoid process, parotid fascia, and lower border of the mandible above and to the sternum, clavicle, acromion process, and spine of the scapula below. It passes superficial to the digastric muscle, splitting to surround the submandibular gland before fusing to the mandible and the parotid fascia. Immediately above the sternum, it splits into superficial and deep layers, which fuse to the anterior and posterior surfaces of the sternum. This fascia invests all the other major fascias and is pierced by cutaneous nerves, external jugular vein, and the numerous small vessels.

MIDDLE CERVICAL FASCIA AND ITS CONTENTS

The strap or infrahyoid muscles act as a group and cause the development of the *middle cervical fascia* (sometimes called the "fascia of the strap" or "infrahyoid muscles") (Figs. 1 and 3). The middle cervical fascia lies directly anterior to the visceral compartment and is the most anterior of the fascias inside the outer investing layer of deep fascia. The middle cervical fascia encloses the strap muscles from their origins on the sternum, sternoclavicular joint, and the scapula to their insertions on the thyroid cartilage and hyoid bone. The middle cervical fascia fuses to the visceral fascia at the insertion of the muscles. A thickening of fascia behind the sternocleidomastoid muscle forms a pulley for the intermediate tendon of the omohyoid muscle. The infrahyoid or strap muscles are innervated by cervical nerves (C1–C3) which form the ansa cervicalis. They exit the prevertebral fascia, pass through or lie in the carotid sheath, and enter the middle cervical fascia.

CAROTID SHEATH AND ITS CONTENTS

The *carotid sheath* surrounds the *carotid artery, internal jugular vein,* and *vagus nerve* (Figs. 1, 4, and 5). It is the only paired major fascia in the neck. The carotid sheath lies lateral to the visceral compartment and anterior to the cervical spine compartment, and is separated from them by interfascial spaces. In the supraclavicular region, the carotid sheath surrounds only the common carotid artery, internal jugular vein, and vagus nerve. At the level of the upper border of the thyroid cartilage, however, the carotid sheath is more complex due to the splitting of the common carotid into internal and external carotid arteries, the branching of the deep venous system, and the multiplicity of cranial nerves traveling in this region. The branches of the external carotid artery in the neck include the superior thyroid, lingual, facial, ascending pharyngeal, occipital, and posterior auricular arteries. The superior thyroid, lingual, and ascending pharyngeal arteries leave the carotid sheath and enter the visceral fascia. The facial, occipital, and posterior auricular arteries leave the carotid sheath and eventually pierce the outer investing layer of fascia as they proceed upward.

Approximately 0.5% ($\frac{1}{200}$) of individuals have a *non-recurrent (aberrant) laryngeal nerve* on the right. It leaves the vagus nerve and exits the carotid sheath at the level of the fifth or sixth cervical vertebra and goes directly towards the larynx. When this occurs, the right subclavian artery is the fourth branch of the aortic arch usually passes posterior to the esophagus.

The *superior laryngeal branch* of the vagus passes deep to both carotid arteries, leaves the carotid sheath and divides into internal and external branches to enter the visceral fascia. The *internal branch* (sensory) pierces the thyrohyoid membrane to innervate the mucosa lining the vestibule of the larynx. This initiates the cough reflex when it is stimulated. The *external branch* (motor) pierces the inferior pharyngeal constrictor to reach the cricothyroid muscle.

The *hypoglossal nerve* passes superficial to both carotid arteries and enters the visceral fascia to pass between the mylohyoid and hyoglossus muscles. The *glossopharyngeal nerve* and its pharyngeal and carotid sinus nerves pass between the carotid arteries. The main trunk of the glossopharyngeal nerve crosses the external surface of the stylopharyngeous muscle, supplies it, and enters the tongue deep to the hyoglossus.

The *cervical sympathetic chain* lies on the longus colli muscles along the posterior surface of the carotid sheath and extends from C2 to T1. The superior and middle cervical cardiac nerves from the sympathetic trunk may be found at the C5 or C6 level.

VISCERAL FASCIA AND ITS CONTENTS

The *visceral compartment* lies in the midline directly anterior to the vertebral compartment and behind the middle cervical fascia. It contains the *larynx, trachea, pharynx, esophagus,* and *thyroid gland,* and is surrounded by the visceral fascia (Figs. 1 and 4).

Below the C6 vertebra, the trachea and esophagus are immediately adjacent to each other, yet separated by their individual fascial sleeves within the visceral (pretracheal) fascia. The visceral fascia is simpler in the inferior region of the neck and becomes more com-

plicated as it ascends. Inferiorly, at the level of the jugular notch, the trachea and esophagus are the only visceral structures in this fascia. Above this level, the thyroid gland is intimately related to the trachea and larynx, and is also invested within the visceral fascia. The thyroid gland has two lobes and an isthmus. The isthmus of the thyroid gland typically crosses tracheal rings 2, 3, and 4, and the lobes project up to the oblique line of the thyroid cartilage under the sternothyroid muscle. At the base of the neck, the recurrent or inferior laryngeal nerve enters the visceral fascia and ascends in the groove between the trachea and esophagus (tracheoesophageal groove). More superiorly, the thyroid gland covers this groove and converts it into a triangular space, which at this level contains the nerve.

At the level of the sixth cervical vertebra, the larynx meets the trachea and the pharynx meets the esophagus. The inferior laryngeal vessels join the recurrent nerve, and together they enter the larynx posterior to the cricothyroid synovial joint. The sternothyroid muscle inserts on the oblique line causing a fusion of the middle cervical fascia and visceral fascia. The larynx is suspended from the hyoid bone by the thyrohyoid membrane. The rest of the strap muscles insert on the hyoid bone with a fusion of middle and visceral fascias.

Above the sixth cervical vertebra (C6), the digestive and respiratory systems are closely interrelated. The portion of the visceral fascia extending from the base of the skull posteriorly to the lower margin of the inferior pharyngeal constrictor muscle is called the "buccopharyngeal fascia." This fascia of the pharynx is continuous with the fascia of the buccinator muscle, across the pterygomandibular raphe. The retropharyngeal space lies between the prevertebral and visceral fascias at the level of the pharynx.

Above the level of the larynx, the visceral fascia becomes complex. It fuses to the facial bones, pharyngeal tubercle, medial pterygoid plate (hamulus), mandible, hyoid bone, and larynx. Anteriorly, the visceral fascia covers the thyrohyoid membrane and hyoid bone, as well as the digastric, stylohyoid, mylohyoid, and hyoglossus muscles. Laterally, a number of structures enter the visceral fascia, including the superior laryngeal nerves and vessels, the lingual vessels, stylopharyngeous and styloglossus muscles, hypoglossal nerve, duct and deep part of the submandibular gland, glossopharyngeal nerve, and lingual nerve. The submandibular gland is surrounded by the outer investing layer of deep fascia, which splits to enclose it; the deep part of the gland and duct pierce the visceral fascia to enter the mouth.

PREVERTEBRAL FASCIA AND ITS CONTENTS

The *prevertebral fascia,* contrary to its name, totally surrounds the cervical spine and muscles associated with it. Anteriorly (where the name fits), it covers the cervical spine, and the longus capitis and cervicis muscles (Figs. 1 and 5). The retropharyngeal space is anterior to the prevertebral fascia. Laterally, the fascia continues to the anterior and posterior tubercles of the transverse processes, covering the scalene muscles. Posteriorly, the levator scapulae and deep back muscles in the cervical region are covered. The prevertebral fascia from each side fuse to the ligamentum nuchae in the posterior midline.

Superiorly, the prevertebral fascia attaches to the external occipital protuberance of the skull, the superior nuchal line, and the mastoid process. It then passes medially, passing posterior to the jugular foramen, anterior to the occipital condyle, and posterior to the pharyngeal tubercle in the midline.

The prevertebral fascia continues into the thorax following the thoracic spine after fusion to the first rib. The contents of the prevertebral fascia include the cervical spine and assorted muscles and nerves.

CERVICAL SPINE IN ITS ENTIRETY

Simply stated, the cervical spine supports the head and allows it to be moved in respect to the trunk and limbs. Its three major functions are (a) to support the weight of the head, (b) to allow free and quick movement of the head and (c) to protect the spinal cord. There are seven cervical vertebrae encasing the cervical spinal cord, which gives origin to eight cervical nerves and the spinal part of the accessory nerve. The cervical spine, surrounded by its muscles and fascia, is located in the posterior part of the neck.

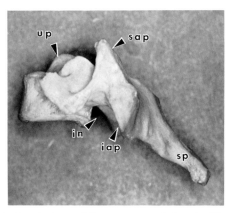

FIG. 7. Lateral view of the same vertebra in Fig. 6. The inferior intervertebral notch (in), uncal process (up), inferior (iap) and superior (sap) articular process, and spinous process (sp) are shown.

CERVICAL VERTEBRAE

The third through the sixth cervical vertebrae are considered *typical cervical vertebrae*. A typical cervical vertebra (Figs. 6–8) consists of a *body*, a *vertebral arch*, a *vertebral foramen*, a *spinous process*, paired *transverse processes*, paired *superior articular processes*, and paired *inferior articular processes*.

The *body* of a typical cervical vertebra (Figs. 6, 9 and 10) is relatively small and oval in shape, with the longest diameter running transversely. The superior and inferior surfaces are saddle shaped. The anterior

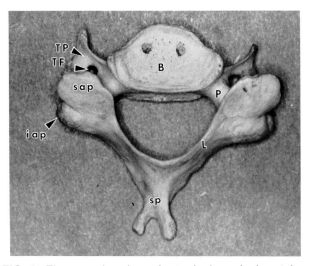

FIG. 6. The superior view of a typical cervical vertebra shows the following features: body (B), pedicle (P), lamina (L), transverse process (TP) with transverse foramen (TF), bifed spinous process (sp) and superior (sap), and inferior (iap) articular processes.

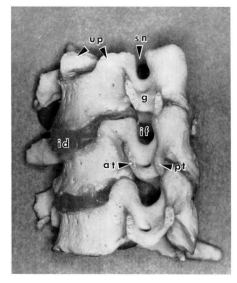

FIG. 8. Three typical vertebrae joined by artificial discs and articular cartilages. Note that the borders of the intervertebral disc (id) do not stay in the same plane. The anterior and posterior borders are inferior to the lateral borders. The uncal process (up), superior notch (sn), intervertebral foramen (if), anterior (at) and posterior (pt) tubercles of transverse process, and groove for spinal nerve (g) are shown.

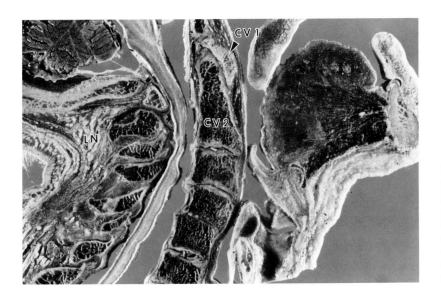

FIG. 9. Sagittal section through the cervical region showing the close relationship between the posterior wall of the pharynx and the bodies of the cervical vertebrae. Note that the irregularities of the posterior surface of the bodies have left their mark on the spinal cord. The ligamentum nuchae (LN), atlas (CV1), and axis (CV2) are shown.

and posterior margins of the superior surfaces are beveled downward, the anterior side more than the posterior side. The lateral surfaces project upwards. The supralateral margins of the vertebrae C3–C7 project sharply upward, conforming to small grooves in the inferolateral borders of the opposing vertebra, thereby

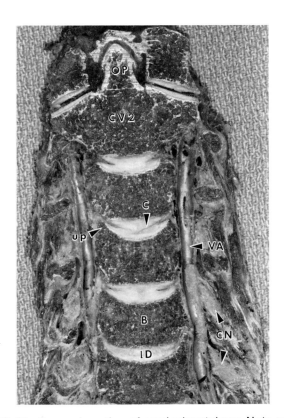

FIG. 10. Coronal section of cervical vertebrae. Note concavity of the upper surface of the typical vertebral body (B). Clefts (C) are seen in most intervertebral discs (ID), vertebral artery (VA), cervical nerves (CN), uncal process (up), and odontoid process (OP).

forming the uncovertebral joints (joints of Lushka). These joints that do not appear until the latter part of the first decade are filled by a small cleft of disc upon which some colloid has been deposited. As a result, they cannot be considered a true joint. Physiologically these joints act to limit lateral flexion, and clinically they serve as a barrier to the direct extrusion of disc material posterolaterally into the foramen.

A midsagittal section of the superior surface of the body of a typical cervical vertebra is convex, whereas in the coronal or frontal section it is concave (Figs. 9 and 10). The central area of the superior surface is flat. The inferior surface is opposite in shape to the superior surface so that the adjacent vertebra conform to each other.

The posterior surface of the body is flat, with numerous foramina for veins draining the hematopoietic tissue contained within the medullary spaces. There is a thin layer of compact bone on the surface of the body, with cancellous or spongy bone occupying the inside. The spongy bone consists primarily of horizontal and vertical trabecula surrounding medullary spaces. The trabeculae are arranged in recognizable patterns, corresponding to the direction of forces. This structure permits the vertebral body to accommodate tremendous compressive forces. The body grows in height by means of epiphyseal or growth plates of hyaline cartilage. The osseous epiphyses consist of a ring of bone along the periphery of the upper and lower surfaces. At maturity, the ring fuses to the body, but the growth plate persists centrally throughout life.

The *vertebral arch* consists of paired *pedicles* and *laminae*. The pedicles are short and nearly round in cross-section, and project posterolaterally from the bodies (Figs. 6, 7). The pedicles attach the vertebral arch to the posterior surface of the bodies of the vertebra in such a way as to form a notch superior and inferior to the pedicle. When two vertebrae are placed together, the notches contribute to the intervertebral foramen. The superior and inferior vertebral notches are not equal; the superior notch is larger, and the nerve lies in a notch adjacent to the underlying pedicle (Figs. 7 and 8). This is in contrast to the lumbar region, where the inferior notch is larger and the nerve lies against the pedicle above. At all cervical spine segments (except C8), the exiting nerve is named by the pedicle above which it exists and to which it is most clearly related. Thus, the C5 nerve is above and related to the pedicle of the C5 vertebra. The C7 nerve is above and related to the pedicle of the C7 vertebra. The C8 nerve exits below the pedicle of the C7 vertebra but above the T1 vertebra. In the thoracic and lumbar segments, the nerve root is named by the pedicle below which it exits.

The paired laminae join in the midline. A section through a lamina shows it to be oval in shape. The laminae are longer from side to side, narrower from above downwards, and thinner than in other regions of the spine (Fig. 6). The anterior surface of the lamina, which faces into the vertebral foramen, has a horizontal ridge extending from end to end. The ridge is at the junction of upper and middle thirds. This marks the highest attachment of the *ligamentum flavum*. The surface of the lamina below the ridge is rough for the bony attachment of the ligament. The upper border of the lamina may be similarly rough for the inferior attachment of the ligamentum flavum above. In the normal anatomical position, there is little space between the laminae of adjacent vertebrae. Extending the neck decreases the distance between laminae of adjacent vertebrae, whereas flexing the neck increases that distance.

The *superior and inferior articular processes* are located at the junction of pedicle and lamina. The inferior articular process of one vertebra and the superior articular process of the vertebra below form the bony posterior wall of the intervertebral foramen, except for cervical vertebrae 1 and 2.

The *pedicles* join the laminae, and together they form the *vertebral arch*. The body and vertebral arch form a triangular *vertebral foramen* with rounded angles (Fig. 6 and 12). The cervical spinal cord is larger than in the thoracic or lumbar regions and the vertebral canal is correspondingly large to house it. Normal sagittal diameters of the cervical spine are as follows: C1, 23 mm; C2, 20 mm; C3, 18 mm; C4, 17 mm; and C5–C7, 16 mm.

The *intervertebral foramina* are bounded rostrally and caudally by the pedicles, posteriorly by the facets, and anteriorly by the vertebral bodies and intervertebral discs. The intervertebral foramina align along the posterolateral angles of the vertebral canal. The cervical intervertebral foramina are relatively large (12 mm in height and 6 mm in width) to allow the cervical nerves through them. The foramina may be pathologically narrowed by disc protrusions, osteoarticular spurs projecting from the zygoapophyseal or uncovertebral articulations, or tumors arising from neural tissue or bone.

The *spinous process* is short and bifed. When cut in cross-section, it is shaped like an inverted V.

The *transverse processes* are more complex than in other regions. Each transverse process has two roots, one from the body and one from the junction of the pedicle and lamina (Fig. 6). The anterior root is the costal element, which ends as the anterior tubercle. Cervical vertebra C6 has a very prominent *anterior tubercle* (carotid tubercle) that can be used as a surgical landmark, since it protrudes anteriorly with respect to that of C7. The posterior root of the transverse process is the true transverse process, and it ends as the posterior tubercle. The *costotransverse lamella* connects the anterior and posterior roots near their

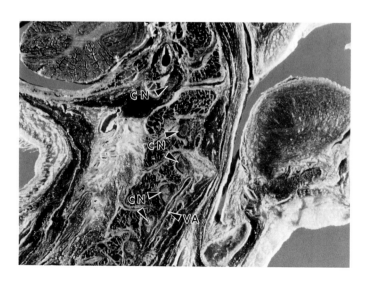

FIG. 11. Sagittal section through cervical region lateral to Fig. 9. The spinal nerves can be seen passing posterior to the vertebral artery (VA). CA, cervical nerves.

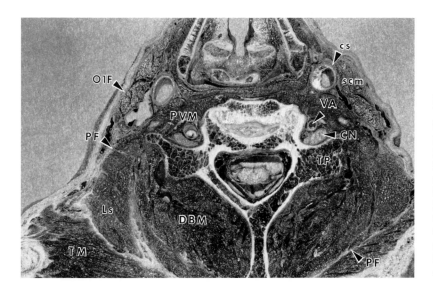

FIG. 12. Cross-section through the neck. The cervical nerve (CN) is passing behind the vertebral artery (VA). The foramen does not appear closed because the costal element and costotransverse lamella are not in the same plane as the true transverse process. The prevertebral fascia (PF) encloses the prevertebral muscles (PVM) and deep back muscles (DBM) from the midline anteriorly to the midline posteriorly. The transverse process (TP), sternocleidomastoid muscle (scm), levator scapulae muscle (Ls), trapezius muscle (TM), outer investing fascia (OIF), and carotid sheath (CS) are shown.

distal ends. It is concave above and attaches to the lower edge of the roots, thus forming a groove for the spinal nerve.

The *transverse foramen*, for passage of the vertebral artery and plexiform vertebral venous system, is located between the roots of the transverse process medial to the costotransverse lamella and lateral to the body of the vertebra. The *vertebral artery* is anterior to the spinal nerves as they curve around the artery posteromedial to anterolateral (Figs. 11 and 12). The vertebral arteries supply the contents of the posterior cranial fossa, the vertebrae and attached ligaments and muscles, the meninges, the spinal cord, the zygoapophyseal joints, the posterior root ganglion, and all proximal cervical nerve roots.

The *superior and inferior articular processes* are located at the junction of the pedicles and laminae, and together form the lateral mass. The lateral masses of typical cervical vertebrae are much smaller than those of the first two cervical vertebrae. The superior articular facet faces upwards and backwards, whereas the inferior articular facet faces downwards and forwards, thereby forming a shingled configuration inferiorly and posteriorly (Fig. 8). The cervical facet joints (zygoapophyseal joints) have synovial membranes and fibrous capsules that are more lax than at thoracic or lumbar levels to permit a gliding motion. When menisi are present, they are better developed than in other regions (1).

Cervical vertebrae 1, 2, and 7 are considered *atypical*, with the atlas or first cervical vertebra being the most atypical (Figs. 9 and 13). The atlas consists of: *anterior* and *posterior arches*, paired *lateral masses with superior and inferior articular processes*, and paired *transverse processes*.

It lacks a body since its embryonic anlage is fused to the axis or second cervical vertebra as the *dens* or *odontoid process*. The *anterior arch* is one-half the

length of the posterior arch and in the midline has an anterior tubercle facing anteriorly and an articular facet on its posterior surface for the dens. Laterally, the anterior arch attaches to the lateral mass. In the midline, the *posterior arch* has a posterior tubercle on its posterior surface but no spinous process. Laterally near its junction with the lateral mass, its upper surface is grooved for the vertebral artery, which passes from the first transverse foramen, around the posterior surface of the superior articular process, to enter the foramen magnum. As the vertebral artery and its surrounding venous plexus (suboccipital plexus) pass over the lateral posterior arch of C1, they pose a significant surgical hazard to approaches in this region. As previously noted, the vertebral foramen at C1 is

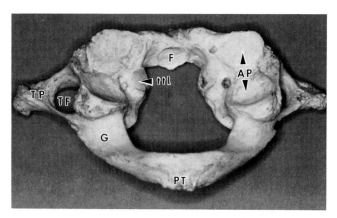

FIG. 13. Superior surface of atlas. Note that the suboccipital nerve will pass posterior to the articular processes. The transverse process (TP) with posterior tubercle and transverse foramen (TF) for vertebral artery are shown. Facet for odontoid process of CV2 (F) on anterior arch, tubercle for attachment of the transverse ligament (ttl), groove for vertebral artery and CN1 (suboccipital nerve) (G), posterior tubercle (PT), and superior articular process (AP) are also shown.

large since it contains the dens and its ligaments in addition to the medullary spinal cord.

The lateral masses connect the anterior and posterior arches, and have *articular* facets on their superior and inferior surfaces. The superior facet is concave to receive the occipital condyle, and the inferior facet is flat and articulates with the superior facet of the lateral mass of the axis (Fig. 10). The lateral surface of the lateral mass is much higher than the medial surface; therefore, the superior and inferior facets approach each other medially. The medial surfaces, marked by a tubercle for the attachment of the transverse ligament of the atlas, keeps the dens in contact with the anterior arch (Fig. 13). The lateral surface of the lateral mass has a transverse process attached to it. The lateral mass slightly overhangs the vertebral artery as it passes from the transverse foramen to the foramen magnum.

The *transverse processes* of the atlas are longer and stronger than those of the other cervical vertebrae, ending slightly anterior, inferior, and medial to the mastoid process. It can be palpated through the lower part of the parotid gland between the mastoid process and ramus of the mandible. The transverse process appears to lack an anterior root and anterior tubercle. Instead, the costotransverse lamella attaches to the lateral mass. The tip of the transverse process is actually the posterior tubercle.

The second cervical vertebra, or *axis*, is also atypical (Fig. 14). It has a body, and fused to its superior surface is the dens, the embryonic body of the atlas (8). It projects upward to intimately relate to the anterior arch of the atlas (Figs. 9 and 10). The superior articular process attaches to the body and pedicle of the axis. It articulates with the inferior surface of the lateral mass of the atlas above. Since the superior and inferior articular processes of the atlas and the superior process of the axis are located relatively anterior, the first and second cervical spinal nerves pass posterior to the corresponding articular processes. The inferior articular process of the axis is a typical inferior articular process, attaching at the junction of the pedicle and lamina. The third cervical nerve, therefore, passes anterior to the inferior articular process of the axis and the superior articular process of C3. All remaining spinal nerves also pass anterior to the articular processes.

The transverse processes of the axis are short and end as a posterior tubercle, there being no anterior tubercle. The transverse foramen is directed upward and laterally to allow the vertebral artery to reach the more laterally placed transverse foramen of the atlas. The spinous process is short and bifed. The vertebral foramen is large.

The seventh cervical vertebra is morphologically transitional between cervical and thoracic vertebrae. It still retains a small transverse foramen, but the vertebral artery does not pass through it. It has a prominent long, horizontal and non-bifed spinous process, which gives the vertebra its name, "vertebra prominens."

LIGAMENTS AND JOINTS BETWEEN VERTEBRAE

Except for the pedicles, all corresponding parts of adjacent vertebrae are joined together by ligamentous tissues: Specific parts of the cervical spine are held together by specific ligamentous tissues—the vertebral bodies by the *intervertebral discs* and by the *anterior* and *posterior longitudinal ligaments*; the articular processes by *joint capsules*; the lamina by *ligamenta flava*; the spinous processes by *interspinous ligaments* and the *supraspinous ligament (ligamentum nuchae)*; the transverse processes by *intertransverse ligaments*; and special ligaments between the atlas, axis, and occipital bone. The latter four of the above can be considered as accessory ligaments to the synovial joints (13).

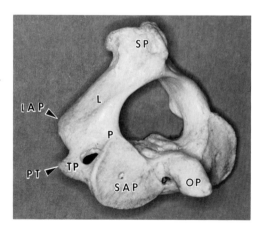

FIG. 14. In this oblique view of axis, note that the second cervical nerve also passes posterior to the articular processes, but all remaining spinal nerves pass anterior to the articular processes. The odontoid process (OP), inferior articular process (IAP), superior articular process (SAP), transverse process (TP) with posterior tubercle (PT) and transverse foramen, short bifed spinal process (SP), lamina (L), and pedicle (P) are shown.

INTERVERTEBRAL DISC

The primary connection between bodies in the cervical region is the *intervertebral disc* (Figs. 10 and 15). Embryologically, the intervertebral disc and adjacent

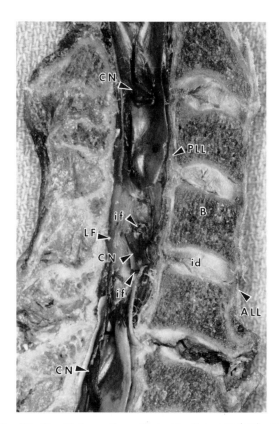

FIG. 15. Sagittal section through the cervical spine showing the concavity of the inferior surface of the vertebral body (B) and low exit of cervical nerves (CN) through the intervertebral foramen (if). The discs show clefts, and the disc between CV5 and CV6 has lost its nucleus pulposus and failed in a repair response. The ligamentum flavum (LF), posterior longitudinal ligament (PLL), anterior longitudinal ligament (ALL), and intervertebral disc (id) are shown.

therefore, the peripheral margins of the disc are not always in the same plane as a centrally placed nucleus pulposus (Fig. 10). The discs contribute to the anterior convexity of the cervical spine by being thicker in front than behind, as the bodies are nearly equal in height, front, and back (Figs. 9 and 15). The discs in the cervical region, as compared to the thoracic region, are larger and contribute more to the length of the cervical spine than do the thoracic discs to the length of the thoracic spine. Functionally, the thicker they are, the more flexible they are.

The vertebral bodies have a layer of hyaline cartilage (*cartilaginous endplate*) resting on a flat subchondral bone plate separating the spongy bone from the disc. This cartilage is the original growth plate of the vertebra and should be considered a key part of the vertebra (9) and not a part of the disc (11). The cartilaginous endplates permit the insertion of the inner one-third fibers of the annulus fibrosis and are essential in the diffusion of nutrients from the subchondral vascular bed into the nucleus pulposus. There is a capillary bed on the cartilaginous endplates that drains into a subchondral venous system. The intervertebral discs display vessels only in the most superficial parts of the annulus. The nucleus pulposus is a completely avascular structure.

From birth to adolescence, the cervical discs increase in height from ~ 0.3 to 0.7 in. Similarly from birth to adulthood, the length of the cervical region increases threefold. At birth, one-third of the length of the spine is due to discs; after age 7, the discs account for only one-fifth of the total length. The disc between the second and third cervical vertebra is the thinnest of all spinal discs (3).

The mature disc consists of two parts, an outer *annulus fibrosis* and an *inner nucleus pulposus*. Structural changes occur during both prenatal and postnatal periods, and developmentally the annulus can be de-

parts of the vertebral bodies above and below are formed from the same somite, and together form a functional unit. The discs are shaped to conform to the surfaces of the bodies to which they are attached, and,

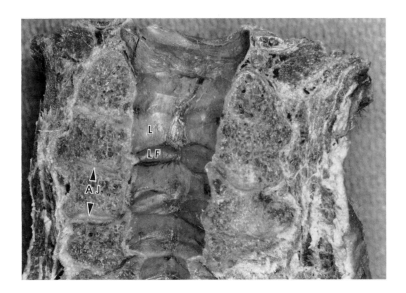

FIG. 16. Coronal section through the articular joints of the cervical spine to show the laminae of the vertebral arch and the ligamenta flava (LF) between them. The lamina (L) and joint spaces (AJ) are shown.

scribed as having four centripetal layers. At full-term, the annulus has an outer collagenous layer and an inner fibrocartilaginous layer, and these are separated from the nucleus pulposus by a transitional layer. During the first two decades, the annulus fibrosis and nucleus pulposus assume adult characteristics as separate structures grossly.

The outer two-thirds of the annulus fibrosis firmly attaches to the bony endplate of the vertebral body above and below. The collagen fibers in the outer portion of the annulus are arranged in lamellae of increasing thickness, with collagen bundles obliquely oriented. In adjacent lamella, the direction of fibers is opposite. The collagen fibers in the posterior portion of the disc run more vertical than oblique, and this may be a cause of the weakness seen clinically in that portion of the disc (15). In addition, the anterior-posterior growth of the vertebral body is mainly the result of the deposition of bone on its anterior surface (12). This may also result in an apparent backward shift (eccentric) of the nucleus pulposus and a relatively weaker posterior portion of the annulus fibrosis.

In infancy abundant mucoid material (mucopolysaccharides within a mucoprotein matrix) is present in the nucleus pulposus, and from age 10 on increasing numbers of collagen fibers and cartilage cells are seen. The nucleus pulposus will rarely ossify in children (2). After 50 years, the nucleus pulposus becomes more difficult to distinguish from the annulus fibrosis, and at age 80 it becomes a firm fibrocartilaginous mass similar in structure to the inner zone of the annulus fibrosis. In fact, it becomes macroscopically (but not microscopically) indistinguishable from the annulus fibrosis (Figs. 10 and 15). The collagen fibers become hyalinized, and, in addition, cleft formation occurs. A horizontal cleft occurs first and may extend nearly throughout the disc. Vertical clefts may also occur with villus-like processes.

Perhaps the most important change with age is the loss of water from the disc. The water content at birth is close to 90%, whereas in late life it may only be 70% (4). The water content is related to the protein-glycosaminoglycan content of the disc, and imbibition pressure appears more important than osmotic pressure. It is generally thought that changes in the protein-glycosaminoglycan content resulting in a loss of water are normal aging changes. Abnormal discs are preceded by earlier than usual changes in this protein-glycosaminoglycan content.

The collagen bundles in the annulus withstand tensile forces very well but when not supported by a firm noncompressible nuclear matrix undergo degenerative changes when subjected to compressive forces (12). Ossification of the outer fibers of the annulus fibrosis heralds the development of cervical spine ankylosis (10).

ANTERIOR AND POSTERIOR LONGITUDINAL LIGAMENTS

The *anterior longitudinal ligament* (Fig. 15) is a strong band that extends from the base of the skull to the sacrum. The cervical portion is broader than that of the thoracic region but narrower than in the lumbar region. It begins above by attaching to the basilar part of the occipital bone, the anterior tubercle of the atlas, and the anterior surface of the body of the axis. It is thickest in its midportion and tapers laterally to fuse with the anterior aspects of the annulus and adjacent parts of the vertebra. It fills the concavity on the front of the bodies of the vertebra. Its most superficial fibers run three to four vertebrae, its intermedial fibers run two to three vertebrae, and its deepest fibers attach to adjacent vertebrae. The individual bundles of collagen fibers making up the ligament are arranged longitudinally.

The *posterior longitudinal ligament* (Fig. 15) is a thick band running from the skull to the sacrum. It begins as the tectorial membrane and attaches to the posterior surface of the axis and continues downward. Its strongest attachments are to the discs and adjacent parts of the vertebrae. It does not extend laterally over the nerve roots. It is only loosely attached to the posterior concavity of the vertebral bodies other than the parts adjacent to the discs, being separated from the bodies by the internal venous plexus and extradural fat. The spinal dura mater has loose attachment by fibrous slips to the posterior longitudinal ligament. In the cervical region, the posterior longitudinal ligament is broad and uniform in width. Its superficial fibers extend three or four vertebrae, whereas its deepest fibers go between adjacent vertebrae, fusing to the annulus fibrosis of the disc. It gives the anterior surface of the vertebral canal a more uniform surface, smoothing the undulating surface of the vertebral bodies and discs.

LIGAMENTS BETWEEN THE ATLAS, AXIS, AND OCCIPITAL BONE

In the occiput, C1 and C1–C2 motion segments provide one-half of total neck flexion and extension; the other half is equally distributed among the joints between the remaining cervical vertebrae. In addition, one-half of total rotation occurs around the odontoid, and the other half is equally distributed among the joints of the other cervical vertebrae. Lateral flexion is equally distributed among all the cervical joints. Ligaments unique to the atlanto-occipital and atlanto-axial motion segments provide stability yet preserve motion (Fig. 9).

The atlas is attached to the occipital bone by the

capsules of the synovial joints between the occipital condyles and the lateral mass of the atlas, and the *anterior and posterior atlanto-occipital membranes.*

The *anterior atlanto-occipital membrane* extends from the anterior arch of the atlas to the anterior margin of the foramen magnum and is continuous laterally with the capsules of the synovial joints. It is strengthened by an upward continuation of the anterior longitudinal ligament, which attaches to the anterior tubercle of the atlas and the basilar position of the occipital bone. The *posterior atlanto-occipital membrane* joins the posterior arch of the atlas to the posterior margin of the foramen magnum. Laterally, there is an opening through the membrane for passage of the vertebral artery into the foramen magnum and for exit of the first cervical nerve.

The integrity of the atlas-axis dynamic relationship is preserved by a number of strong ligaments, including the *transverse ligament of the atlas*, the *cruciform ligament*, the *alar ligaments*, the *apical ligament*, and the *tectorial membrane.*

The *transverse ligament of the atlas* is a strong band that attaches to tubercles on the medial surface of the lateral masses and passes posterior to the dens (Fig. 9). It has articular cartilage on its anterior surface where it is in contact with the dens. The neck of the dens is narrow at this level. In the midline, extensions of this ligament attach superiorly to the occipital bone and inferior to the body of the axis causing the complex to be termed the "cruciform ligament."

The *alar ligaments* are strong bands connecting the upper part of the dens to the rough medial sides of the occipital condyles. The *apical ligament* extends from the dens to the foramen magnum, and is sandwiched between the anterior atlanto-occipital ligament and the upper longitudinal portion of the cruciform ligament of the atlas (Fig. 9).

The *tectorial membrane* is an upward extension of the posterior longitudinal ligament, which broadens as it ascends. It attaches to the body of the axis below and the dura mater of the clivus above. It may extend laterally as far as the capsules of the atlanto-occipital joints.

SYNOVIAL JOINTS BETWEEN ARTICULAR PROCESSES

The articular facets on the adjoining inferior and superior articular processes oppose each other, and the synovial joint thus formed is surrounded by a capsular ligament lined by a synovial membrane. The capsular ligament is attached to the periphery of the articular facets, and is loose and thin. Accessory ligaments of the synovial joints include the *ligamenta flava*, the *interspinous ligaments*, the *ligamentum nuchae*, and the

intertransverse ligaments. The joint capsules and accessory ligaments are richly innervated with prioprioceptive and pain receptors, exceeding that seen in the thoracic and lumbar regions.

Ligamenta Flava

The *ligamenta flava* of the cervical region are thin, broad and long (Fig. 16). They attach to the inner surface of the lamina above and to the superior margin of the lamina below. The left and right ligaments tend to join at the midline, but gaps are present for the exit of veins from the vertebral canal. They extend laterally to the articular processes, where they enter into the fibrous composition of the facet capsule and contribute to the boundary of the intervertebral foramen. The ligaments are composed predominantly of elastic fibers (80%) arranged longitudinally. In the neutral position, the ligamenta flava have a high resting tension. The ligaments are stretched during flexion of the neck and are shortened during extension. Physiologically, the ligament flav do not compress the dura or spinal cord during extension; however, as elasticity is lost, the ligaments can buckle inward posteriorly indenting the spinal canal. However, the ligamenta flava can calcify in the cervical region, causing symptoms of spinal cord compression (5, 6).

Ligamentum Nuchae and Interspinous and Intertransverse Ligaments

In the cervical region, the upward continuation of the supraspinous ligament is the *ligamentum nuchae*, a fibroelastic membrane (Fig. 9). Superficially, it extends from the external occipital protuberance to the spine of the seventh cervical vertebra. Its deep attachments are to the external occipital crest, the posterior tubercle of the atlas, and spinous processes of the remaining cervical vertebrae. It forms an intermuscular septum for attachment of the adjacent muscles on each side. These muscles function to extend and laterally flex the head and neck.

The *interspinous ligaments* are thin and extend the entire length of the spinous processes from ligamenta flava to supraspinous ligaments (Fig. 9). They are less well developed than in the lumbar region. The *intertransverse ligaments* are weak, being represented by a few scattered bundles of collagen. The intertransverse cervical muscles appear to replace these ligaments.

In the cervical spine, total flexion is 45°, total extension is 75° (total flexion/extension is 120°), total rotation is 145°, and total lateral flexion is 65°. Movements of the neck produce dynamic changes in the bony and ligamentous components of the cervical spine as well as adaptive changes in the cervical spinal cord and roots. This adaptation is due to the inherent plasticity of the neural-meningeal tissues. The actual bony relationships change very little regardless of the movement. The effects of neck extension (flexion) are that the anterior longitudinal ligament and anterior annulus tighten (slacken) with widening (narrowing) of the anterior interspace, the posterior longitudinal ligament and posterior annulus slacken (tighten) with bulging of the intervertebral disc into the spinal canal increased (reduced), the inferior facets slide backward (forward) over the superior facets narrowing (widening) the caliber of the intervertebral foramina by 30%, retrolisthesis is increased (reduced), the pedicles are drawn closer together (farther apart) reducing (increasing) the height and size of the intervertebral foramina, the lamina are drawn closer together (farther apart) with bulging inward (tightening) of the ligamenta flava (interspinous ligaments and ligamentum nuchae), the spinal cord anchored by the denticulate ligaments and surrounding dura becomes lax (tightened) and moves slightly in a downward (upward) direction, and the cervical nerve roots become lax (tightened) and decrease (increase) their angulation at the foraminal entrance.

VERTEBRAL CANAL AND ITS CONTENTS

The vertebral foramina of the articulated cervical vertebra form the vertebral canal (Figs. 6 and 12). In life, the canal is completed by the disc, posterior longitudinal ligament, ligamenta flava, and articular capsule of the synovial joints.

The vertebral canal is open above and in alignment with the foramen magnum. The intervertebral foramina form a series of openings in the lateral aspect of the vertebral canal for exit of the spinal nerves, the spinal radicular arteries, and the vertebral veins and plexus. The cervical vertebral canal is large since the cervical spinal cord is the largest part of the spinal cord. The canal becomes more triangular and smaller as one descends.

Within the vertebral canal are the spinal cord, its meninges (and contained cerebrospinal fluid) and extradural fat containing the *internal vertebral plexus* of veins. This venous plexus consists of plexiform sinuses that at each level are most prominent at the narrowest portion of the posterior longitudinal ligament just medial to the pedicles at the mid-portion of the vertebral bodies. The venous plexus is thinnest at the level of the intervertebral disc.

The pia mater intimately invests the spinal cord and has a lateral extension from the lateral side to the spinal cord known as the *denticulate (dentate) ligaments*. Its attachment along the spinal cord is continuous, but laterally it is attached to the arachnoid and dura only at points midway between exiting spinal nerves. The denticulate ligaments act to limit the rostro-caudal and side-to-side movements of the spinal cord during neck motion.

The *arachnoid mater* lies immediately subjacent to the dura and has delicate trabeculae traversing the subarachnoid space. The cranial dura mater has two layers, an inner meningeal and an outer periosteal, but only the meningeal layer of the spinal dura is continuous with the cranial dura, whereas the spinal periosteal layer containing the dura arteries and veins continues on the external surface of the occipital bone as its periosteum.

The anterior and posterior elements of the cervical vertebrae are supplied through each foramen by a branch of the *vertebral artery*. At each level, the vertebral arteries give off branches that supply the longus colli muscles, the anterior aspects of the vertebral column, and the anterior longitudinal ligament. In addition, the vertebral arteries give off branches that enter the intervertebral foramina and pass rostrally and caudally to supply the posterior portion of each vertebra and the posterior longitudinal ligament. Additional branches pass dorsally to supply the posterior elements of the spinal canal. Still other branches pass from the vertebral artery dorsally at each level to supply the external surface of the lamina and the posterior paraspinous muscles.

The cervical spinal cord gives rise to eight cervical nerves; the *dorsal and ventral rootlets* exit the spinal cord and pia mater, traveling laterally as well as ventrally and caudally to lie in the lateral subarachnoid space bathed in cerebrospinal fluid. The dorsal and ventral rootlets join to form the *dorsal and ventral roots*, which together enter a narrow sleeve of arachnoid and dura with distinct separate compartments. This arachnoid sheath that is opacified on myelography. Frequent intradural connections can be seen between adjacent cervical nerve roots. In addition, multiplicity anomalies of the cervical roots with the dorsal and ventral root, each having a separate dural sleeve, are much more frequent than in the lower spinal segments.

The nerve roots enter the *intervertebral foramina* by passing adjacent to the corresponding disc and over the top of the corresponding pedicle (Fig. 11). The anterior root lies anteroinferior to the posterior root. The anterior root is adjacent to the uncovertebral joint, whereas the posterior root is close to the zygoapophyseal joint, especially its superior articular process. Normally, the roots occupy one-third to one-fourth of the foraminal space.

Radicular vessels from the vertebral artery and venous plexus are also prominent components of the intervertebral foramen. The radicular arteries supply ascending and/or descending branches to the anterior and posterior spinal arteries. The most constant of these is a large feeder entering on one or both sides at the C6 or C7 level. In addition, radicular veins drain the epidural venous plexus into the vertebral plexus through the intervertebral foramina.

At the lateral margin or just outside the intervertebral foramina, the dural covering of the nerve root enlarges to accommodate the *spinal ganglion*. The dorsal root ganglion is located in close proximity to the vertebral artery. Just distal to the ganglion and nearly always outside the intervertebral foramina, the anterior and posterior roots join to form the spinal nerve proper.

Distal to the intervertebral foramina, the spinal nerve proper divides into dorsal (*posterior primary rami*) and ventral (*anterior primary rami*) branches. Gray rami communicanti from the sympathetic cervical ganglia are located along the sympathetic chain and the connective tissue between the longus colli and longus capitis muscles posteriorly and the carotid sheath anteriorly. There are no white rami communicanti as the cervical spinal cord has no sympathetic input.

CERVICAL SPINAL NERVES

The first cervical nerve (*suboccipital nerve*) may not have a dorsal root. The nerve exits the vertebral canal through an osteofibrous orifice above the posterior arch of the atlas and posteromedial to the lateral mass (Fig. 11). It lies between the vertebral artery and posterior arch. The first cervical nerve divides into anterior and posterior primary rami as all subsequent spinal nerves do. The anterior primary ramus forms a loop with the second anterior primary ramus and sends fibers to be distributed by the hypoglossal nerve. Together, the anterior primary rami of C1–C4 form the cervical plexus. The posterior primary ramus enters the suboccipital triangle and innervates the muscles forming it. The posterior primary rami are motor only to deep back muscles; the majority of these branches are sensory to cutaneous areas on the back. The first cervical nerve, however, has no cutaneous branches.

The second cervical nerve lies on the lamina of the axis posterior to the lateral mass, in a position that endangers it during surgical approaches in this area (Fig. 11). The posterior boundary of the intervertebral foramina between the axis and third cervical vertebra is the ligamentum flavum, since the articular processes are anterior to the nerve.

The cervical nerves 3 through 7 exit the vertebral canal passing through the intervertebral foramina anterior to the articular processes (Figs. 11 and 12). The foramina are bounded above and below by pedicles, and the nerve is draped over the pedicle below. Thus, the nerve and the pedicle below to which it is most

closely related have the same number. Cervical nerve 8 lies between the seventh cervical vertebra and the first thoracic vertebra. Cervical nerves C3–C7 emerge with a slight oblique slant downward and forward, whereas C8 runs horizontally.

A constant relationship exists between the cervical spinal cord segments, their exiting nerve roots, and the underlying cervical vertebra and disc spaces. Two distinct patterns can be recognized: (a) If the dura ends at S1–S2 then roots C1–C7 emerge 1–2 mm below the inferior edge of the corresponding discs, and the C8 root emerges at the level of the C7–T1 disc. (b) If the dura terminates at S2–S3 then roots C1–C3 emerge below the corresponding disc, roots C4–C6 emerge at the level of the corresponding disc, and roots C7 and C8 emerge above the corresponding disc near the center of the adjacent vertebral body.

The *posterior primary rami* of cervical nerves C3–C8 enter the compartment of deep back muscles as they branch from the spinal nerve lateral to the intervertebral foramina. The sinuvertebral nerve originates from the posterior primary rami and passes into the intervertebral foramina before splitting into ascending and descending branches. These branches supply the corresponding and rostral discs in addition to the surrounding anterior and posterior longitudinal ligaments with pain fibers. Histological studies of discs have demonstrated the presence of fibers as deep as the outer third of the annulus fibrosis. The posterior primary rami reach the posterior compartment muscles by traveling lateral to the articular processes, a position that endangers them to injury when deep lateral exposure of the facet joints is attempted. In addition, deep lateral retraction of the posterior paraspinous muscles can injure the peripheral branches of the posterior primary rami with resultant denervation of these muscles (7). All the posterior primary rami are motor, and the second through fifth are also cutaneous; the cutaneous branches of C6–C8 are variable.

The *anterior primary rami* of the cervical nerves form the cervical plexus (C1–C4) and most of the brachial plexus (C5–T1). The spinal nerves as they exit the intervertebral foramina are coursing anteriorly and laterally, since the groove for the nerve on the upper surface of the transverse process is 40° from a coronal plane. The cervical plexus is characterized by a series of loops that give rise to peripheral nerves. All of the anterior primary rami of the upper four cervical nerves supply muscles and all but the first have cutaneous branches, so there is no dermatome for the first cervical nerve. A branch from the loop between nerves C1 and C2 joins the hypoglossal nerve. These nerve fibers form the nerve to the genioglossus, the nerve to the thyrohyoid and the descendens hypoglossi, a part of the ansa cervicalis. The loop between C2 and C3 gives off the descendens cervicalis, which completes the ansa cervicalis. The ansa cervicalis supplies all of the strap or infrahyoid muscles except the thyrohyoid. The ansa cervicalis leaves the prevertebral fascia, passes through the carotid sheath in relation to the internal jugular vein, and enters the middle cervical fascia to supply these muscles. The loop between C2 and C3 also gives rise to the lesser occipital (C2), great auricular (C2, C3), and transverse cervical (C2, C3) cutaneous nerves. The sternocleidomastoid muscle receives a branch from this loop, which is probably proprioceptive. The supraclavicular nerves arise from the loop between C3 and C4, as do proprioceptive branches to the trapezius muscle. The cutaneous branches pierce the prevertebral and outer investing layers of deep fascia to reach the skin. Nerves C3, C4, and C5 form the phrenic nerve, which descends on the anterior surface of the scalenus anterior muscle before entering the thorax. The three scalene muscles and the levator scapulae muscle are supplied from the rami forming the cervical and brachial plexi, as are the longus colli and longus capitis muscles.

As the rami forming the brachial plexus leave the intervertebral foramina between the origins of the anterior and middle scalene muscles, they form trunks, divisions, and cords within an extension of the prevertebral fascia called the "axillary sheath." Since the subclavian artery passes between the anterior and middle scalene muscles on its way from the thorax to the upper limb, it also passes into the axillary sheath with the plexus.

PREVERTEBRAL MUSCLES

The prevertebral fascia also contains the muscles that extend, rotate, and flex anteriorly and laterally the head and neck (Fig. 12). The scalene muscles are important landmark muscles. These muscles take origin from the transverse processes of the cervical vertebra and insert on the first and second ribs. The scalenus anterior inserts on the scalene tubercle of the first rib. The subclavian vein lies in a groove on the first rib immediately anterior to the scalene tubercle. It joins the internal jugular vein to form the branchiocephalic vein behind the medial end of the clavicle or the sternoclavicular joint. Passing between the scalenus an-

terior and the sternocleidomastoid muscle are the omohyoid and the suprascapular and transverse cervical vessels. Lying directly on the anterior surface of the scalenus anterior are the phrenic nerve and the ascending cervical artery.

The subclavian artery lies in a groove on the upper surface of the first rib immediately posterior to the scalene tubercle. Thus, the subclavian artery and vein are separated by the scalenus anterior muscle. The vagus and phrenic nerve also pass between the artery and vein. Posterior to the artery and anterior to the scalenus medius muscle are the roots and trunks of the brachial plexus.

REFERENCES

1. Engel R, Bogkuk N. The menisci of the lumbar zygapophysial joints. *J Anat* 135:795–809, 1982.
2. Hahn YS, McLone DG, Uden D. Cervical intervertebral disc calcification in children. *The Child's Nervous System* 3:274–277, 1987.
3. Harris HA. The anatomical and physiological basis of physical training. *Br Med J* II 2:939–943, 1939.
4. Hendray NGC. The hydration of the nucleus pulposus and its relation to intervertebral disc derangement. *J Bone Joint Surg [Br]* 40B:132–144, 1958.
5. Inoue N, Motomura S, Murai Y, et al. Computed tomography in calcification of ligamenta flava of the cervical spine. *J Comput Assist Tomogr* 7:704–706, 1983.
6. Iwasaki Y, Akino M, Abe H, et al. Calcification of the ligamentum flavum of the cervical spine. *J Neurosurg* 59:531–534, 1983.
7. Macnab I, Cuthbert H, Godfrey CM. The incidence of denervation of the sacrospinales muscles following spinal surgery. *Spine* 2:294–298, 1977.
8. Ogden JA. *Skeletal injury in the child.* Philadelphia: Lea and Fibiger, 385–390, 1982.
9. Peacock A. Observations on the postnatal structure of the intervertebral disc in man. *J Anat* 86:162–179, 1952.
10. Resnick D. Hyperostosis and ossification in the cervical spine. *Arthritis Rheum* 27:564–569, 1984.
11. Saunders JB, Inman VT. The intervertebral disc. (A critical and collective review.) *Int Abs Surg* [supplementary to *Surg Gyn Obstet*] 69:14–29, 1939.
12. Walmsley R. Development and growth of intervertebral disc. *Edinburgh Med J* 60:341–364, 1953.
13. Williams PW, Warwick R. *Gray's anatomy.* 36th ed. Philadelphia: WB Saunders Company,
14. Yeager VL, Lertprapai N. Heart and aortic arch anomalies. *J Med Assoc Thailand* 53:279– 288, 1970.
15. Zaki W. Aspect morphologique et fonctionnel de l'annulus fibrosus du disque intervertebral de la colonne dorsale. *Arch Anat Pathol* 21:401–403, 1973.

CHAPTER 2

Operative Anatomy and Basic Microsurgical Approaches to the Cervical Spine

Paul H. Young

From a surgical perspective, the cervical spine can be approached from both an anterior and posterior direction (4–8). A review of published reports fails to clearly demonstrate a significant statistical difference in results between anterior and posterior approaches for the management of cervical radiculopathy or myelopathy due to either hard or soft cervical disc compression.

There are a number of advantages and disadvantages of each approach.

Advantages of the anterior approach are that it (a) can be used to approach any level of the cervical spine from C1 to T1 through a natural bloodless tissue plane; (b) is the most direct route to midline anterior soft disc herniations or spondylotic bars; (c) permits adequate decompression of a wide range of pathological lesions projecting into the anterior aspects of the spinal canal (prolapsed and sequestered discs, osteophytic bars, OPLL, displaced bone fragments, tumors, etc.); (d) permits both a decompressive removal and fusion for anteriorly located compressions (such as vertebral body fractures and/or subluxations, degenerative spondylolistheses, tumors, infectious processes, etc.); (e) results in less postoperative recovery than posterior directed approaches (reduced postoperative pain, length of hospitalization, time off work, etc.); (f) when performed for anteriorly located pathology, compared with the posterior approach, has a dramatically reduced incidence of catastrophic postoperative morbidity (such as quadriplegia); (g) may result in the long-term resolution of osteophytes following fusion with restoration of normal disc height and motion segment stabilization; and (h) permits a secondary posterior ap-

proach without concern of instability once a satisfactory anterior fusion has been accomplished.

Disadvantages of the anterior approach are that it (a) provides no reasonable access to the posterior aspects of the spinal canal; (b) provides much less exposure of the spinal cord and nerve roots for pathological processes involving the intradural structures; (c) demands a more extensive procedure than the posterior approach (loss of multiple motion segments) for multilevel spondylosis or canal stenosis; (d) may lead to the development of degenerative changes in bordering motion segments (due to increased stress following the loss of mobility in the operative segment due to the necessity for disc removal); (e) requires additional external stabilization if the posterior elements have been previously disrupted; and (f) cannot be used in the presence of a large neck mass (such as thyromegaly) or open neck wound (such as a tracheostomy).

Advantages of the posterior approach are that it (a) provides the most direct approach to pathological processes occurring within or posterior to the spinal cord or in the posterior aspects of the spinal canal; (b) permits a wide multilevel exposure of the spinal cord and nerve roots (necessary for such conditions as multilevel canal stenosis, tumors, vascular anomalies, etc.) without loss of multiple motion segments; (c) provides easy access to foraminal pathology (soft disc herniation and spondylotic spurs) without the need for an extensive discectomy; (d) does not always necessitate or result in a fusion with motion segment loss as with anterior approaches; and (e) permits immediate access to the facets for unlocking in traumatic dislocations.

Disadvantages of the posterior approach are that it (a) permits no (or only very dangerous) exposure to the pathological processes located anterior to the spinal cord and nerve roots; (b) is incapable of adequately decompressing even single level severe anteriorly directly spondylotic bars, retropulsed bone or disc fragments, etc.; (c) requires a longer postoperative recovery than the anterior approach (with greater muscle discomfort, delayed mobilization, etc.); (d) if directed at decompressing anteriorly located pathology, has an increased risk of catastrophic neurological complications including quadriplegia when compared to the anterior approach; (e) involves more difficult (and dangerous) operative positioning than the anterior approach (particularly in patients with instability); (f) can result in instability or increased spinal mobility leading to subsequent disc deterioration and/or facet spondylosis; and (g) may result in the long-term development of severe neck deformities (such as swan neck deformity) due to disruption or compromise of ligamentum nuchae, paraspinous muscles and/or apophyseal joints.

In general, the final decision as to the direction of approach should be based on a careful analysis of the individual clinical pattern such that the spinal cord and roots are approached from the direction of predominant neural compression. In those situations in which adequate decompression can be achieved with an acceptable risk from either direction, the procedure of choice should be that with which the microsurgeon is most experienced.

ANTERIOR APPROACH (C2–T1)

In this section, the anterior (9–23) and posterior (24–34) cervical exposures *down to* the bony margins of the spinal column are described. Approaches *into* the spinal column for particular pathological processes are described in Chapters 6–14.

Anatomical Landmarks

The following superficial anatomical landmarks can be used to locate levels in the cervical spine (Fig. 1): hard palate (arch of the atlas), angle of the mandible (C2–C3), hyoid bone (C3), thyroid cartilage (C4–C5),

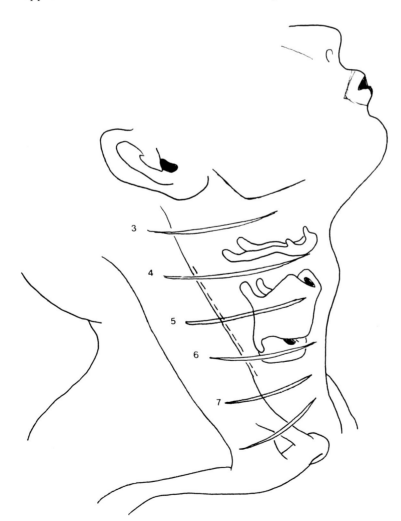

FIG. 1. Superficial anatomical landmarks used for planning anterior incisions.

carotid tubercle (C6), cricoid cartilage (C6–C7), and supraclavicular groove (C7–T1).

Preparation and Anesthesia

Prior to surgery, the patient should be carefully examined for thyromegaly or submandibular gland enlargement that may deny anterior access to the vertebral column. All nonsteroidal antiinflammatory medications and aspirin-containing compounds are stopped 7–10 days prior to surgery. A single dose of a broad-spectrum antibiotic is administered intravenously just prior to the induction of anesthesia (1). Part of the routine for operative preparation should include an accurate assessment of the patient's neck range of motion, especially noting the degrees of painless flexion and extension. This information is vital in determining allowable movement during intubation.

The use of long-acting muscle paralyzing agents with general anesthesia is avoided. Intubation with a flexible endotracheal tube is performed. During intubation in patients with significant cord or radicular compression, a neutral position of the head and neck is maintained to avoid compressing the already compromised spinal cord and nerve roots (i.e., little or no neck hyperextension should be permitted). If significant instability exists or a difficult intubation is anticipated, fiber-optic assisted intubation is performed. A soft flexible esophageal stethoscope is placed for continuous cardiac and respiratory monitoring and to permit intraoperative esophageal localization. Thigh-high ace wraps or antiembolism stockings are applied to the lower extremities to prevent intraoperative peripheral venous stasis.

Positioning

A rolled-towel, rolled-blanket, sand bag, foam roll, or wedge-shaped support is placed under the shoulders for head and neck extension. A smaller rolled-towel is placed under the neck for support (Fig. 2). The head is rotated slightly (10°) to the side opposite the incision (left), and a hollow ring or donut pillow is placed beneath the occiput for further stabilization. Excessive rotation should be avoided as it tenses the sternocleidomastoid muscle producing more difficult retraction. A head traction device (Holter or pin type) may be used in instances that require perfect intraoperative vertebral alignment (anterior plating, multilevel corpectomies with struts, etc.). Shoulder counter traction (using arm or wrist slings) may also be necessary particularly in patients with short-broad necks. Preoperative traction applied to maintain cervical alignment in patients with fractures and/or subluxations should be carefully maintained by the surgeon during the transfer and positioning.

Right- or Left-Sided Approach

Regardless of symptom localization, a right-sided approach is utilized in all cases by a right-handed surgeon. Similarly, a left-sided approach should be used by a left-handed surgeon. The ease of operation afforded a right-handed surgeon from the right side (avoiding the obstruction by the mandible) overcomes the disadvantages of occasionally encountering an aberrant or nonrecurrent laryngeal nerve (~1 out of 200 cases). This important nerve anomaly may pose a surgical hazard as it passes from the carotid sheath to the larynx at the C5–C7 levels. It is noteworthy that similar difficulty can be encountered by the left-handed surgeon approaching from the left side as regards an anomalous thoracic duct emptying into the jugular vein at a higher level than the subclavian vein. In addition in patients with atherosclerotic carotid artery disease, the dangers of intraoperative embolization or occlusion are greater on the more frequently dominant left side.

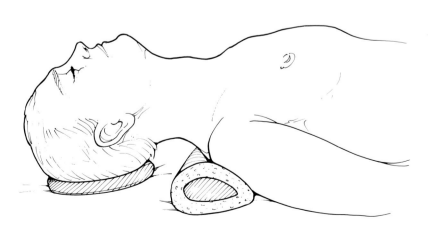

FIG. 2. Positioning for anterior approaches.

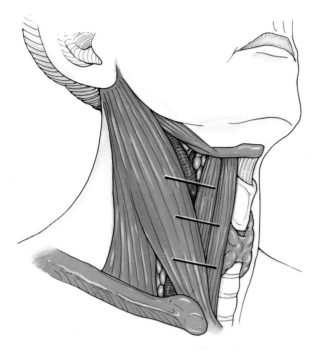

FIG. 3. A transverse incision is made in a skin crease on the right side of the neck centering on the sternocleidomastoid.

Incision

A 3–6-cm transverse skin incision centered on the medial border of the sternocleidomastoid muscle is made preferably along a prominent skin crease or fold (Fig. 3). The superficial anatomical landmarks and a lateral cervical spine roentgenogram are used to identify the disc space(s) of interest. The incision is placed in a slightly oblique fashion along Langer's lines in an attempt to obtain a more cosmetic result. The incision is placed just inferior to the disc space of interest to facilitate a somewhat upward line of vision necessary to align into the plane of the interspace.

If two or three disc spaces are to be explored the incision is placed along the plane just midway between them. For more than three spaces, separate transverse or a cosmetically poor longitudinal incision may be necessary.

Superficial Exposure

The superficial fascia overlying the platysmal muscle is dissected from the superficial surface of the muscle using a fine scissors with care to avoid any interruption of the external jugular vein (or its tributaries) or the superficial transverse cutaneous nerves. The layer of areolar tisue between the platysma and superficial fascia varies tremendously in thickness, clearly related to the patient's general amount of subcutaneous fat.

Using dissecting scissors and a vacular forceps, the platysma muscle layer and its encircling fascia are dissected free of superficial and deep attachments and divided cleanly in a transverse direction along the line of the skin incision (Fig. 4). The edges of the platysma muscle are undercut slightly to produce small flaps of muscle along both upper and lower edges. These musculo-cutaneous flaps provide for a relaxed skin incision that does not interfere with the retractors. Care is taken to avoid injury to the external jugular vein lying beneath the platysma muscle on the external surface of the sternocleidomastoid muscle or the anterior jugular vein lying anteromedially along the lateral aspect of the strap muscles.

The anteromedial border of the sternocleidomastoid muscle is used as a superficial landmark and the carotid artery pulse as a palpable deep landmark to the carotid sheath. The sternocleidomastoid is retracted slightly lateral to expose the middle layer of cervical fascia bridging the sternocleidomastoid muscle to the more medially placed strap muscles. Although sharp dissec-

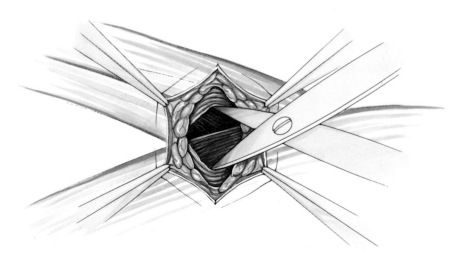

FIG. 4. The skin and subcutaneous tissues are incised in a transverse manner. The platysma is dissected free, revealing the underlying sternocleidomastoid and strap muscles.

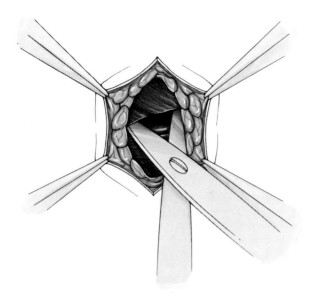

FIG. 5. The fascial plane just medial to the carotid sheath is sharply incised and bluntly dissected to the level of the prevertebral space.

tion is necessary to open the more superficial aspects of this fascia, blunt finger dissection can be used as the separation of the sternocleidomastoid from the infrahyoid (strap) muscles continues down to the level of the carotid sheath (Fig. 5). The omohyoid muscle can be seen crossing perpendicular to the plane of this dissection at the C5–C6 level. This muscle should either be mobilized and retracted inferiorly or superiorly, or transected at its mid-tendonous segment.

It is essential at this stage of the procedure to locate the carotid sheath by palpation of the carotid artery pulse (Fig. 6). The medial fascial attachments of the carotid sheath to the infrahyoid muscles are identified

and opened with sharp dissection under direct visualization. The opening of this fine fascial plane leads directly into the prevertebral space. The full extent of this opening can be easily and safely completed using blunt finger dissection spreading vertically and horizontally. The extent of this dissection will determine the amount of exposure into the prevertebral space. Excessive dissection of this plane providing unnecessary exposure of the prevertebral space should be avoided to prevent inadvertent injury to crossing neurovascular structures.

Prevertebral Neurovascular Structures

The following neurovascular structures frequently cross the interfascial plane between the carotid sheath and the tracheoesophageal groove: the superior middle and inferior thyroid artery and vein, the superior laryngeal nerve, and the nonrecurrent (aberrant) laryngeal nerve.

The *superior, middle*, and *inferior thyroid arteries* and *veins* are retracted superiorly or inferiorly from the field of view or if necessary ligated and transected. The *superior laryngeal nerve* arises from the inferior ganglion of the vagus, passes from behind the carotid artery to generally join the superior thyroid artery, and then crosses the interfascial plane at the C3–C4 level to reach the superior border of the thyroid gland. The *nonrecurrent* or *aberrant laryngeal* nerve generally leaves the vagus nerve at the C5–C7 level and crosses the interfascial plane in conjunction with the middle or inferior thyroid artery or vein to reach the tracheoesophageal groove or larynx. It is essential to recognize the presence of a nonrecurrent laryngeal nerve to avoid inadvertent injury.

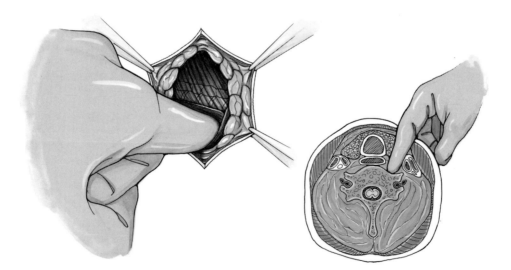

FIG. 6. This fascial plane can be easily developed using finger dissection while palpating the laterally retracted carotid artery.

As a general principle, all neurovascular structures passing behind the carotid sheath fascia, crossing the interfascial plane, and entering the visceral fascia in the neighborhood of the tracheoesophagus or larynx should be preserved. Apparently unrelated thyroid vessels should not be quickly coagulated and/or transected as the superior or aberrant laryngeal nerves may be hidden between them. Most often, even these vascular structures can be carefully dissected free of surrounding fascia and gently retracted rostrally or caudally to preserve their anatomic integrity. Avoiding compression or stretch, both the superior and recurrent laryngeal nerves can be placed behind the blades of self-retaining retractors without resultant injury. Significant compression, tearing, coagulation, or transection of these neural elements, however, will result in permanent neurological impairment.

Deeper Fascial Dissection

Further blunt dissection is used to widen the interfascial plane between the prevertebral fascia overlying the spinal column and attached musculature and the anteriorly located visceral fascia containing the esophagus, trachea, larynx, etc. An assistant-held retractor positioned beneath the visceral fascia is helpful in obtaining initial visualization of the contralateral longus colli muscles easily identified through the prevertebral fascia. In addition, the retractor serves to protect the contents of the visceral fascia from injury during this dissection. The final opening into this interfascial plane is completed by blunt dissection of areolar tissue adhesions until both the right and left anterior tubercles of the vertebra(e) of interest are identified by finger palpation.

Identification of the Midline

At this point, it is essential to clearly identify the midline of the prevertebral space. Using a combination of direct vision (which is facilitated by the use of both an assistant-held retractor gently lifting the contents of the visceral fascia away from the midline and the surgeon's finger retracting the carotid sheath laterally) and finger palpation the following structures are identified to precisely locate the midline: (a) the bilateral tendonous attachments of the longus colli muscles along the anterolateral aspects of the vertebral bodies and disc spaces (the midline of the anterior vertebral bodies and disc spaces is generally free of longus colli attachments, and this can be used as an accurate marker of the true midline); (b) The presence of osteoarthritic spurs projecting from the anterior lips of the vertebral bodies (they are frequently most prom-

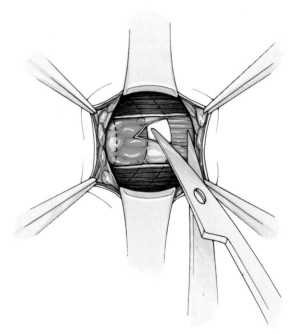

FIG. 7. The fascia overlying the prevertebral space, including the longus colli muscles, is identified and sharply incised, revealing the underlying anterior aspects of the vertebral bodies and disc space.

inent in the midline); and (c) the costal roots and anterior tubercles of both right and left transverse processes (they can be palpated and the midline estimated as a halfway point between; care, however, should be

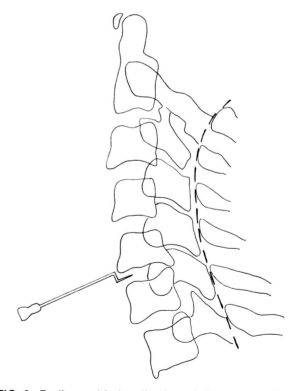

FIG. 8. Radiographic localization of disc space, using a needle with two 90° bends to prevent inadvertent penetration of canal.

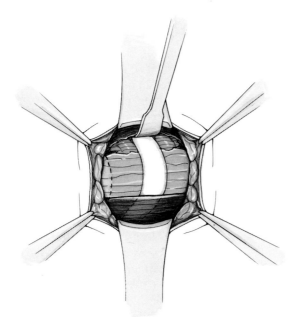

FIG. 9. Using sharp dissection beginning along its medial margins, the periosteal attachments of the longus colli muscles are dissected free, revealing the disc space(s) of interest.

taken to avoid the mistaken identification of the anterior tubercle of C6 as a midline vertebral body spur).

Once the midline has been correctly identified, the three or four thin layers of prevertebral fascia are incised with a combination of sharp and blunt dissection to reveal the underlying vertebral bodies, disc spaces, and longus colli attachments (Fig. 7).

A 20-gauge spinal needle with two short 90° bends (to prevent accidental penetration of the spinal canal) is inserted superficially into the annulus of interest for radiographic confirmation of level (Fig. 8). On occasion, it may be possible to precisely identify the level of interest based on the presence of large anterior spurs as seen on preoperative lateral cervical spine radiographs.

Dissection of the Prevertebral Space

The medial margin of the tendonous attachments of the longus colli muscles are incised over the disc space(s) and vertebral bodies of interest. This dissection should extend halfway up and down the vertebral bodies bordering the disc space(s) of interest. Using a combination of electrocautery dissection and periosteal elevation, the tendonous attachments of the longus colli are removed (Fig. 9) until the most medial part of the transverse process is identified. The costal root of the transverse process is distinguishable as a flat, horizontal bony surface just lateral to the convex surface of the anterior vertebral body. It is located along the horizontal plane of the midline superior surface of the caudal vertebral body or laterally at the base of the uncinate process. Care should be exercised in the use of electrocautery during this dissection to avoid inadvertent injury to surrounding neurovascular and visceral structures. The safety of this maneuver is enhanced using the cutting bipolar coagulator. This dissection should not proceed further lateral than the midportion of the costal element of the transverse process to avoid injury to a tortuous or anomalous vertebral artery, or the sympathetic plexus located on the anterolateral surface of the longus colli muscles.

Numerous small vessels penetrate the anterolateral aspects of the vertebral bodies under cover of the longus colli muscles. These vessels are frequently disrupted in this dissection and may lead to oozing during this stage of the dissection. Complete hemostasis is delayed until direct visualization is permitted by placement of the self-retaining retractor blades beneath the free margins of the longus colli muscles.

Serrated retractor blades of the same length are placed under the freed margins of the longus colli muscles bilaterally under direct vision and distracted laterally using a self-retaining retractor (Cloward- or Caspar-type) (Fig. 10). The serrated blades are helpful as

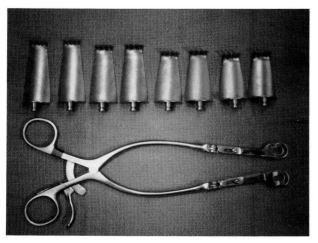

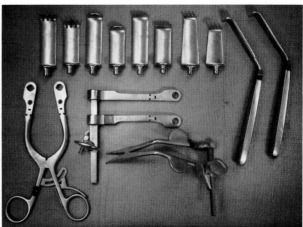

FIG. 10. A: Cloward retractor and blades. **B:** Caspar retractors and blades.

they readily retain their position beneath the longus colli flaps, thereby avoiding pressure or perforation injuries to the cervical viscera and carotid sheath neurovascular structures. Adequate exposure gives a complete view of the anterior portions of the disc space(s) and bordering vertebral bodies. A longitudinal retractor is placed with smooth nonserrated blades to displace overhanging tissues in a rostrocaudal direction.

Wound Closure

Absolute hemostasis of the anterior vertebral bodies (using a combination of mono- and bipolar coagulation) is ascertained. The self-retaining cervical retractors are disarticulated, and the blades carefully removed individually. Particular attention is paid to the serrated blades placed beneath the flaps of longus colli muscles as their rough removal can injure the bordering visceral and neurovascular elements. Upon removal of the blades, the free edges of the longus colli muscle are carefully inspected under the operating microscope for hemostasis as is the remainder of the prevertebral space. Absolute hemostasis is essential to prevent a postoperative prevertebral space hematoma with resultant significant postoperative hoarseness and dysphagia. Extra time spent in this endeavor is of great benefit towards limiting the patient's postoperative morbidity in this regard. In addition, this negates the need for a postoperative drain.

The wound is profusely irrigated with an antibiotic solution. The distracted carotid and visceral sheath structures spontaneously reapproximate themselves towards the midline. If the interfascial plane between the visceral and carotid fascias remains wide open, a few absorbable sutures are placed across this plane to close the dead space. The platysma muscle layer is

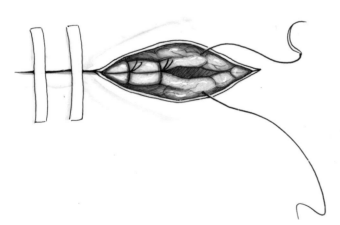

FIG. 11. The wound is closed using a subcutaneous absorbable suture and steri-strips.

reapproximated with several absorbable sutures. Subcutaneous tissue is likewise closed with interrupted absorbable sutures to promote a narrow scar. The skin is held with steri-strips (Fig. 11). A sterile dressing is applied and removed after 24 hr. No additional wound care is necessary other than preserving dryness and cleanliness for the first 7 postoperative days.

POSTERIOR APPROACH (C2–T1)

Anatomical Landmarks

The posterior elements of C2–T1 can be easily palpated in the midline of the posterior spine with the neck bent slightly in flexion. The characteristics of the individual spinous processes are as follows: C2 is longer and bulkier than C3 or C4; C2, C3, and C4 are always bifed; C5 is almost always bifed; C6 is frequently bifed but usually shorter and more slender than C7; C7 is never bifed and more prominent than T1; and T1 is slightly less prominent than C7 but more prominent than T2.

The general position of the facet joints can be palpated approximately two finger-breadths off the midline. The external occipital protuberance is located just above the attachments of the ligamentum nuchae as a contoured protuberant bony ridge that extends several centimeters on each side of the midline.

Preparation and Anesthesia

Careful preoperative evaluation of patients with pulmonary disorders, cardiac abnormalities, or other processes that lead to elevated thoracic venous pressure should be thoroughly evaluated to prevent intraoperative bleeding due to engorged epidural veins. All nonsteroidal antiinflammatory medications and aspirin-containing compounds are stopped 7–10 days prior to surgery. An arterial line, urethral catheter, and central venous line (or triple-lumen catheter) are inserted for intraoperative cardiorespiratory monitoring. Thigh-high ace wraps or antiembolism stockings are also routinely applied.

Part of the routine preoperative preparation should include an accurate assessment of the patient's neck range of motion, especially noting the degrees of painless flexion and extension. This information is vital in determining allowable movements during intubation.

A general anesthetic is administered utilizing a flexible endotracheal tube. During intubation in patients with significant cord or radicular compression, a neutral position of the head and neck is maintained to avoid compressing the already compromised spinal canal or foramen. If significant instability exists or a difficult intubation is anticipated, fiber-optic assisted intubation is performed. The use of long-acting muscle paralyzing agents is avoided. A single dose of a broad-spectrum antibiotic is administered upon the induction of anesthesia. Intravenous steroids (methylprednisolone or dexamethasone) are administered if significant spinal cord or root manipulation is anticipated. Intraoperative somatosensory evoked responses may be a useful adjunct in high-risk posterior cervical procedures (2).

Positioning

Positioning is represented in Fig. 12. Due to the significant risk of air embolism, ischemic complications, and increased instability, the sitting position has been abandoned for routine use in posterior cervical procedures. If the sitting position is deemed absolutely necessary in morbidly obese patients or patients with reduced ventilatory capacity, then Doppler ultrasound is essential for continuous venous air embolism monitoring (3).

The prone position for posterior cervical spine surgery demands firm yet adjustable cervical spine fixation, a degree of cervical flexion for optimal visualization of the interlaminar spaces, the prevention of pressure on eyes or other sensitive facial structures, and the maintenance of adequate ventilation with minimal abdominal compression.

In the absence of significant instability, the patient is turned from the supine to the prone position (following the initiation of general anesthesia) with care to maintain the neck in a neutral position. Particularly in spondylotic myelopathy patients, the surgeon should stabilize the head to be certain that the head,

neck, and shoulders are moved synchronously to avoid stretching a stressed spinal cord against a ventral ridge.

Rolled blankets or padded cushions are applied along the lateral margins of the chest and abdomen to avoid thoracic or abdominal compression (with subsequent elevation of vena caval pressure and secondary engorgement of the epidural venous plexus). A padded horseshoe head rest is utilized with the forehead placed on the toe and the malar eminences on the heels. Special caution is taken to prevent pressure on the orbits and any possibility that intraoperative motion might displace the original position resulting in orbital compromise. Ideally, the neck should be slightly flexed (20°) and angled in a reverse trendelenburg position. Extreme flexion (to enlarge the interlaminar space) should be absolutely avoided as it tenses the spinal cord across the disc spaces and may produce spinal cord ischemia. The chin is positioned slightly backwards in the direction of the occiput. Free access to the endotracheal tube and other monitoring devices must be maintained.

Cervical traction preoperatively in place for patients with instability should be maintained throughout the positioning process. Following placement in the horseshoe head rest, a slightly reduced amount of traction can be reinstituted for stabilization during the operative procedure.

Patients manifesting marked degrees of cervical instability or patients requiring rigid postoperative external stabilization are placed in a halo ring and vest prior to positioning. The stability associated with the halo vest provides a comfortable margin of safety and ease in positioning these patients from supine to prone. Following placement in the prone position, the posterior bars of the halo can be loosened or removed to increase access to the posterior spine region. Additional traction can also be applied to the halo ring if

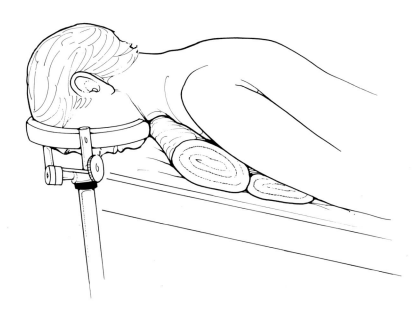

FIG. 12. Positioning in the prone position for posterior spinal procedures.

necessary to add displacement or change alignment during the operative procedure.

Following placement in the prone position, a lateral cervical spine radiograph is obtained to evaluate proper alignment. Adjustments in positioning by changing the position of the horseshoe ring or adding tension to the traction device may be necessary.

Skin folds on the lower cervical and upper thoracic region are stretched free by applying bands of adhesive tape extending from the paracervical region to the shoulders and upper thorax. If intraoperative fluoroscopy or radiography is planned, the patient's arms should be positioned at the sides, with care taken to prevent peripheral nerve compression or thoracic outlet retraction.

Incision

Using spinous process anatomical landmarks, a midline skin incision is made extending across the motion segment(s) of interest. For a single disc or nerve root exposure, a 3-cm incision centered on the disc space of interest may be adequate to expose the appropriate interlaminar space. Larger excisions extending over several or multiple segments may be necessary for multilevel exposures. Cautery hemostasis rather than hemostat retraction should be used along the skin margins to preserve the midline. The spinous process of C7 is used as the primary landmark, permitting the enumeration of the segments above and below in order to precisely identify the level(s) of interest and limit the size of the incision. If doubt exists as to the level, a needle should be inserted into the supraspinous ligament and radiographic confirmation obtained (Fig. 13).

Superficial Exposure

The superficial fascia is incised in the midline to the level of the ligamentum nuchae, which marks the attachments of the trapezius, rhomboid, and levatus scapulae muscles along the spinal axis. For a unilateral single-level interlaminar exposure, the ligamentum nuchae is incised just off the midline ipsilaterally to the side of interest in a curvilinear fashion beginning at the cranial margin of the cephalad and ending at the lower margin of the caudal spinous process. This produces a flap of ligamentum nuchae hinged on the spinous processes encompassing the interlaminar space(s) of interest. This is done in an attempt to spare injury to the bulk of the supra- and interspinous ligamentous complex. For bilateral single-level interlaminar exposures, this same technique is repeated on the contralateral side.

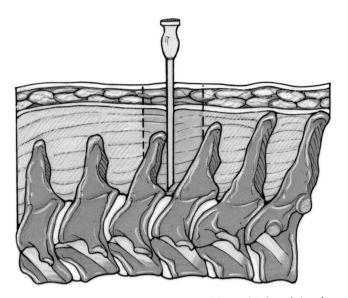

FIG. 13. Needle inserted (too deeply) to obtain a lateral radiograph to identify the level of interest.

For multilevel interlaminar exposures, the ligamentum nuchae incision is extended in a similar paramedian fashion to include the segments of interest (again sparing the midline supra- and interspinous ligamentous complex). For wide posterior decompressions (in which the posterior elements are totally removed), the ligamentum nuchae incision is kept in the midline, as preservation of the suprainterspinous ligamentous complex is impossible. Dissection along the margin (or through the center) of this deep fascia is bloodless, as this avascular plane avoids penetration into the erector spinae muscle mass. The penetration into muscle fibers during this dissection signifies that the fascial incision is progressing too far off the midline. Excessive penetration into or disruption of the erector spinae muscles should be avoided as this can lead to segmental denervation. In the setting of a wide decompression, this can be a factor in the development of permanent kyphosis and other more severe deformities.

Exposure of the Interlaminar Space

The paraspinous muscles attached to the spinous processes, laminae, and apophyseal joints of interest are sharply and carefully dissected in a subperiosteal plane using a soft gauze sponge, and a Cobb or curved periosteal elevator (Fig. 14). Due to the fragile strength of the posterior elements in the cervical spine, this maneuver should be done under direct vision without significant downward force applied to the underlying laminae. This is obviously of even greater importance in those situations where significant posterior element instability exists. If instability is suspected, the pos-

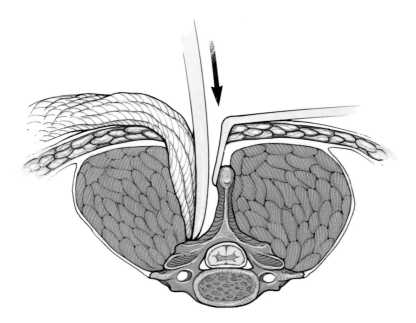

FIG. 14. A subperiosteal dissection of the muscular and ligamentous tissues is accomplished along the laminae of interest. This is carried as far lateral as the facet joint.

terior elements can be somewhat stabilized using toothed clamps placed into the spinous processes and held for external reinforcement. If a wider than normal interlaminar space exists, extreme caution should be exercised in its exposure to avoid penetration through an often thin ligamentum flavum with catastrophic results. Little or no bleeding is encountered if the dissection is kept in the subperiosteal plane along the spinous processes and laminae.

This dissection should continue laterally until the lateral portion of the facet joint capsules are identified. Significant oozing may be encountered at the junction between the interlaminar space and apophyseal joints or in the soft tissue surrounding the apophyseal joint capsules where segmental arteries and their venous plexi supplying adjacent facet joints, transverse pro-

cesses, and posterior elements are located. Care should be taken during exposure and hemostasis not to disrupt the articular capsules of the apophyseal joints.

For multiple-level exposures, the subperiosteal dissection should proceed in a caudal-rostral direction as the muscle attachments to the spinous processes insert obliquely from below. Particularly with multilevel dissections, the integrity of the erector spinae muscles should be protected to avoid denervation and significant postoperative morbidity.

A self-retaining retractor is applied using a narrow serrated blade to reflect the paraspinous muscle mass from the interlaminar space(s) of interest (Fig. 15). Generally, serrated blades can be fixed beneath the muscles in a more stable position than smooth ones.

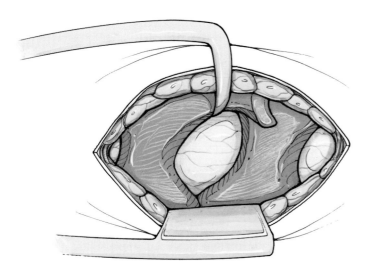

FIG. 15. A self-retaining retractor is inserted, revealing the interlaminar space of interest.

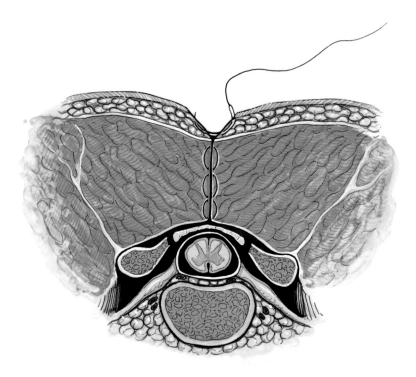

FIG. 16. Closure of the ligamentum nuchae in layers.

For unilateral exposures, a pronged retractor (such as Williams, Caspar, Meyerding, or McCulloch) is inserted with the prong against the supra- and interspinous ligamentous complex. Care should be taken not to lacerate or penetrate this midline ligamentous complex, particularly at its deeper portions, to avoid entering the spinal canal. Total disruption of this important ligamentous complex significantly interferes with dynamic neck stability.

For wider bilateral exposures, retractors with blades on each end are used to reflect the paraspinous muscles. Proper positioning of the blade just superficial to the facet is essential to avoid inadvertent apophyseal capsular injury or inadequate lateral exposure.

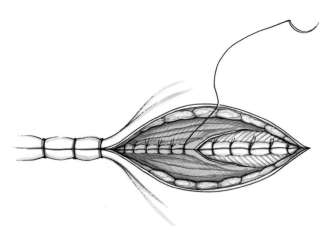

FIG. 17. The last layer of deep fascia, subcutaneous fascia, and skin are also closed in layers.

Closure

The self-retaining retractor is carefully removed avoiding unnecessary abrasion of the surrounding muscle and ligamentous tissue by the serrated blades or pronged hook. The paraspinous muscles are carefully inspected under the operating microscope for hemostasis. In the absence of dural penetration, the paraspinous muscles are injected with 5–10 cc of 0.5% Marcaine, which relieves postoperative pain and muscle spasm in addition to restoring the muscle to its normal paraspinous anatomical location. If penetration of the dura has occurred during the operative procedure, this maneuver should be omitted as the intradural leak of the Marcaine may lead to temporary but frightful spinal cord or root paralysis.

The deepest portion of the ligamentum nuchae is reapproximated using 0 silk (or a similar nonabsorbable suture). Further layers of the ligamentum nuchae are reapproximated utilizing a 0 or 00 Dexon (or similar absorbable suture) (Fig. 16). The subcutaneous tissue is closed in a single layer with a 3-0 or 4-0 absorbable suture. The skin is reapproximated with staples (Fig. 17).

Similar Approaches

Other anterior and posterior approaches designed for specific applications may be considered in the appropriate settings (35–51) (Fig. 18).

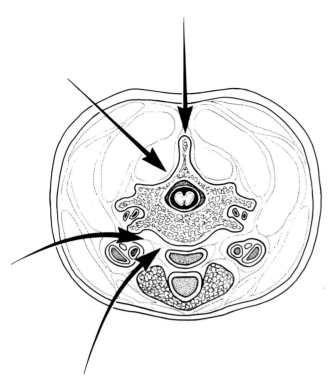

FIG. 18. Common approaches to the cervical spine.

Lateral Approach

The lateral approach is similar to the previously described anterior approach except that it involves passage through the posterior cervical triangle just lateral to the sternocleidomastoid muscle. Instead of retracting the muscle laterally as in the previous approach through the anterior triangle, this approach involves retracting the sternocleidomastoid muscle medially along its lateral border. If retraction of the muscle is not adequate for visualization, division of the muscle either partially or entirely may be necessary. Blunt dissection through the fat pad just lateral to the carotid sheath gains entrance into the prevertebral space.

Advantages of this approach include improved exposure of the antero-lateral structures including the transverse process, nerve root, and vertebral artery; and less retraction of the visceral fascia and its contents.

Disadvantages of this approach include that it exposes to a greater degree (and risks injury to) the sympathetic plexus, phrenic nerve, and brachial plexus; involves severe retraction or division of the sternocleidomastoid muscle; involves severe retraction of the carotid sheath and its contents; and does not permit a true midline view of the vertebral bodies or disc space.

Anterolateral Approach

This is a multisegmental approach that employs a greater degree of sternocleidomastoid muscle and carotid sheath lateral retraction than the previously described anterior approach. Both the longus colli and longus capitis muscles are identified. The lateral attachments of the longus capitis are incised, and the muscle is gently dissected from lateral to medial beginning at the anterior tubercles and extending along the costal roots of the transverse processes. Care is taken to avoid injury to the sympathetic chain or ganglia, which lie anterior to the transverse processes, either embedded in the posterior carotid sheath or in the connective tissue plane between the carotid sheath and the longus colli muscles. If embedded in the muscle layer, the sympathetic chain as well as the cervical ganglion should be retracted together with the muscle. Care is also taken to avoid injury to the laterally placed nerve roots or the unroofed vertebral artery as it runs between adjoining foramen transversaria. The vertebral artery is particularly susceptible as it lies between the bony grooves on adjoining vertebrae surrounded by only a venous plexus. Bleeding encountered in this dissection can be easily controlled with a combination of bipolar coagulation and gel-foam packing.

This exposure affords excellent identification of the vertebral artery over as many segments as necesary and allows exploration of the foramena transversaria, the components of the transverse processes, and the foramena and the lateral aspects of the disc spaces. The nerve roots in their entirety (including branches) can also be clearly identified.

Posterior Paramedian Approach

This approach involves a paramedian exposure with splitting of the trapezius, serratous posterior superior, and splenius capitis muscle bundles parallel to their fibers. The deeper muscle layer including the multifidus and semispinalis is then similarly separated to gain access to the interlaminar space(s).

Advantages of this approach over the previously described posterior approach include no disruption of the ligamentum nuchae.

Disadvantages include direct penetration of muscle tissue with denervation, and increased blood loss and postoperative pain.

REFERENCES

Intraoperative Monitoring and Care

1. Dempsey R, Rapp RP, Young B. Prophylactic parenteral antibiotics in clean neurosurgical procedures. A review. *J Neurosurg* 69:52–57, 1988.

2. Hargadine JR. Intraoperative monitoring of somatosensory evoked potentials. In: Rand RW, ed. *Microsurgery*. 3rd ed. St. Louis: CV Mosby, 92–110, 1985.

3. Michenfelder JD, Miller RH, Groinert GA. Evaluation of an ultrasonic device (Doppler) for the diagnosis of venous air embolism. *Anesthesiology* 36:164–167, 1972.

Anterior/Posterior Approaches

4. Cotler HB, Kaldis MG. In: Spinal fusion. *Anatomy and surgical approaches of the spine*. Springer-Verlag, 1990.

5. Louis R. *Surgery of the spine: surgical anatomy and operative approaches*. Springer-Verlag, 1982.

6. Mayfield FH. Cervical spondylosis: a comparison of the anterior and posterior approaches. *Clin Neurosurg* 13:181–188, 1965.

7. Perry J. Surgical approaches to the spine. In: Pierce D, Nichol V, eds. *The total care of spinal cord injuries*. Boston: Little, Brown, 53–79, 1977.

8. Raynor RB. Anterior or posterior approach to the cervical spine: an anatomical and radiographic evaluation and comparison. *Neurosurgery* 12:7–13, 1983.

Anterior Approach

9. Cloward RB. The anterior approach for the removal of ruptured cervical discs. *J Neurosurg* 15:602–617, 1958

10. Fang HS, Ong GB. Direct anterior approach to the upper cervical spine. *J Bone Joint Surg [Am]* 44(A):1588–1604, 1962.

11. Hodgson AR, Yau ACMA. Anterior surgical approach to the spinal column. In: Apley AG, ed. *Recent advances in othopaedics*. Baltimore: Williams & Wilkins, 289–323, 1964.

12. Hodgson AR. Approach to the cervical spine C3–C7. *Clin Orthop* 39:129–134, 1965.

13. Hoff JT, Wilson CB. Microsurgical approach to the anterior cervical spine and spinal cord. *Clin Neurosurg* 26:523–528, 1979.

14. Hoff JT. Cervical spondylosis. In: Wilson CB, Hoff JT, eds. *Current surgical management of neurologic disease*. Churchill Livingstone, 1980.

15. Hoff J, Waters D. Anterior approaches to the cervical spine. *Clin Neurosurg* 30:606–625, 1982.

16. Hoff JT. Surgical approaches to disease of the anterior cervical spine. *Contemp Neurosurg* 6:1–6, 1984.

17. Kosary IZ, Braham J, Shacked I, Shacked R. Microsurgery in anterior approach to cervical discs. *Surg Neurol* 6:275–277, 1976.

18. Lunsford LD, Bissonette DJ, Janetta PJ, Sheptak PE, Zorub DS. Anterior surgery for cervical disc disease. *J Neurosurg* 53:1–11, 1980.

19. Robinson RA. Approaches to the cervical spine C1–T1. In: Schmidek HH, Sweet WH, eds. *Current techniques in operative neurosurgery*. New York: Grune & Stratton, 205–302, 1978.

20. Robertson JT. Anterior operations for herniated cervical disc and for myelopathy. *Clin Neurosurg* 25:245–250, 1978.

21. Schmidek HH. The anterolateral approach to the cervical spine in the management of cervical spondylosis and its complications. In: Schmidek H, Sweet W, eds. *Current techniques in operative neurosurgery*. New York: Grune & Stratton, 303–322, 1978.

22. Southwick WO, Robinson RA. Surgical approaches to the vertebral bodies in the cervical and lumbar regions. *J Bone Joint Surg [Am]* 39A:631, 1957.

23. Spetzler RF. The microscope in anterior cervical spine surgery. *Clin Orthop* 168:17–23, 1982.

Posterior Approach

24. Epstein JA, Carras R, Lavine LS, Epstein BS. The importance of removing osteophytes as part of the surgical treatment of myeloradiculopathy in cervical spondylosis. *J Neurosurg* 30:219–226, 1969.

25. Fager CA. Rationale and techniques of posterior approaches to cervical disk lesions and spondylosis. *Surg Clin North Am* 56:581–592, 1976.

26. Fager CA. Posterior surgical tactics for the neurological syndromes of cervical disc and spondylotic lesions. *Clin Neurosurg* 25:218–244, 1978.

27. Fager CA. Posterolateral approach to ruptured median and paramedian cervical disk. *Surg Neurol* 20:443–452, 1983.

28. Fager CA. *Atlas of spinal surgery*. Lea & Febiger, 1989.

29. Raynor RB, Pugh J, Shapiro I. Cervical facetectomy and its effect on spine strength. *J Neurosurg* 63:278–282, 1985.

30. Piepgras DC. Posterior decompression for myelopathy due to cervical spondylosis. Laminectomy alone versus laminectomy with dentate ligament section. *Clin Neurosurg* 24:509–515, 1977.

31. Rogers L. The treatment of spondylotic myelopathy by mobilisation of the cervical cord into an enlarged spinal canal. *J Neurosurg* 18:490–492, 1961.

32. Schneider RC. Treatment of cervical spine disease. In: Schneider RC, Kahn EA, Crosby EC, Taren JA, eds. *Correlative neurosurgery*. 3rd ed. Springfield, IL: Charles C Thomas, 1094–1174, 1982.

33. Scoville WB. Cervical spondylosis treated by bilateral facetectomy and laminectomy. *J Neurosurg* 18:423–428, 1961.

34. Watkins RG. *Surgical approaches to the spine*. Springer-Verlag, 1983.

Other Approaches

35. Fager CA. Posterolateral approach to ruptured median and paramedian cervical discs. *Surg Neurol* 20:443–452, 1983.

36. Hacuba A. Trans-unco-discal approach. A combined anterior and lateral approach to cervical discs. *J Neurosurg* 45:284–291, 1976.

37. Hodgson AR. Approach to the cervical spine C3–C7. *Clin Orthop* 39:129–134, 1965.

38. Kehr P. Anterolateral approaches to the cervical spine for management of cervical vascular and cervical radicular syndromes. *Contemp Neurosurg* 6:1–6, 1984.

39. Kehr P. Combined anterolateral and anteromedial approaches of the lower cervical spine. In: *Cervical Spine I*. 297–303, 1987.

40. Louis E, Ruge D. Lateral approach to the cervical spine. In: Wilse LL, Ruge D, eds. *Spinal disorders*. London: Henry Kimpton Publishers, 132–136, 1977.

41. Nanson EM. The anterior approach to upper dorsal sympathectomy. *Surg Gynecol Obstet* 104:118–120, 1957.

42. Riley LH. Cervical disc surgery: its role and indications. In: *Symposium on Disease of the Intervertebral Disc Orthopaedic Clinics of North America*. Philadelphia: WB Saunders, 443–452, 1971.

43. Riley LH. Surgical approaches to the anterior structures of the cervical spine. *Clin Orthop* 91:16–20, 1973.

44. Verbiest H, Paz Y, Geuse HD. Anterolateral surgery for cervical spondylosis in cases of myelopathy and nerve root compression. *J Neurosurg* 25:611–615, 1966.

46. Verbiest H. A lateral approach to the cervical spine: technique and indications. *J Neurosurg* 28:191–203, 1968.

47. Verbiest H. The lateral approach to the cervical spine. *Neurosurgery* 20:295–305, 1973.

48. Verbiest H. Anterolateral operations for fractures and dislocations in the middle and lower parts of the cervical spine. *J Bone Joint Surg [Am]* 51A:1489–1530, 1969.

49. Verbiest H. From anterior to lateral operations on the cervical spine. *Neurosurg Rev* 1:47–67, 1978.

50. Whitesides TE Jr, Kelly RP. Lateral approach to the upper cervical spine for anterior fusion. *South Med J* 59:879–883, 1966.

51. Whitesides TE Jr, McDonald AP. Lateral retropharyngeal approach to the upper cervical spine. *Orthop Clin North Am* 9:1115–1127, 1978.

CHAPTER 3

Cervical Spinal Cord and Roots

Basic Neurological Anatomy and Clinical Syndromes

Paul A. Young and Paul H. Young

CERVICAL SPINAL CORD

The seven cervical vertebrae surround and protect the eight cervical segments of the spinal cord. Rostrally, the cervical cord is continuous with the medulla oblongata of the hindbrain at the foramen magnum. Caudally, it is continuous with the first thoracic segment of the spinal cord, which is located at the level of the intervertebral disc between the seventh cervical and first thoracic vertebrae. Each of the eight cervical spinal cord segments provides attachment for a pair of spinal nerves, which are numbered according to the segment of attachment. Cervical nerves 1–7 emerge from the vertebral canal in the intervertebral foramina above the pedicles of their respective vertebrae whereas spinal nerve C.8 emerges in the intervertebral foramen between pedicles of the seventh cervical and first thoracic vertebrae. Actually, in the cervical region, the intervertebral foramina contain the nerve roots because the spinal ganglia and nerves lie just distal to the foramina. The vertebral relationships of the cervical segments of the spinal cord and the cervical roots are shown in Fig. 1.

INNERVATION OF THE CERVICAL VERTEBRAE

The innervation of the cervical vertebrae (3) is represented in Fig. 2.

The vertebral column is surrounded by *dorsal and ventral nerve plexi*, which are interconnected. The *dorsal plexus* is related to the posterior longitudinal ligament. In the cervical region, this plexus receives bilateral contributions from the *sinu-vertebral* or *meningeal nerves*, and the perivascular plexi on the vertebral arteries. The *ventral plexus* is related to the anterior longitudinal ligament. It receives bilateral contributions from the *sympathetic trunk*, its gray communicating rami, and the perivascular vertebral plexi. The contributing nerves reach the anterior longitudinal plexus both deeply and superficially to the longus colli muscle.

The anterior longitudinal ligament plexus gives off bundles of nerve fibers that penetrate the vertebral bodies along with the radially arranged blood vessels. Further small branches are given off towards the outer zone of the anulus fibrosus.

The posterior longitudinal ligament plexus gives off four types of small branches: those that cross the epidural space to reach the ventral surface of the spinal dura, those radiating along blood vessels into the bodies of the vertebrae, those passing onto epidural blood vessels, and those that pass to the outer layers of the anulus fibrosus.

The *sinu-vertebral nerves* in the cervical region are made up of plexiform branches of the gray communicating rami of the sympathetic ganglia and from the perivascular plexi of the vertebral arteries. At any particular level, there are usually one or two thick and one to four thin sinu-vertebral nerves. The sinu-vertebral nerves give off short and long ascending, short and long descending, dichotomizing, and crossing

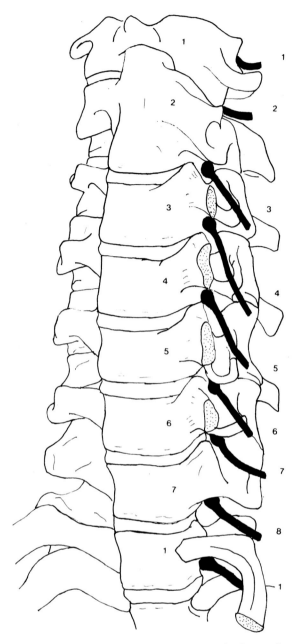

FIG. 1. Relationships between the cervical vertebrae, spinal cord segments, and exiting roots.

GROSS ANATOMY

In general, the spinal cord tapers from rostral to caudal ends (4). However, because of the cervical enlargement, which extends from C4–T1, the lower cervical segments are larger than the upper. Thus, the transverse diameter of C1 is ~12 mm, whereas at C8 it is ~13–14 mm. The sagittal diameter is relatively consistent at ~9 mm.

The external surface of the cervical cord is marked by grooves along its entire length. The most prominent groove is the anterior median fissure, which is ~3 mm deep and contains the anterior spinal vessels and the initial parts of their sulcal branches. The posterior median sulcus is much shallower. Pairs of posterolateral and anterolateral sulci contain the attachments of the dorsal and ventral rootlets of the cervical spinal nerves. The posterior spinal vessels are located at the posterolateral sulci. A shallow posterior intermediate sulcus is located on each side between the posterior median and posterolateral sulci.

Closely investing the cervical spinal cord is the *pia mater*, which is continuous with the pia investing the brain. The *arachnoid* loosely invests the cervical cord and is also continuous with the cranial arachnoid. The arachnoid is attached to the inner surface of the *dura mater*, which is continuous at the foramen magnum with the inner or visceral layer of the cranial dura. The outer or endosteal layer of the cervical dura is represented by the vertebral canal periosteum.

The cervical cord is anchored to the dura by the *denticulate ligaments*. Medially, these form a continuous longitudinal attachment to the spinal pia on each lateral surface midway between the attachments of the dorsal and ventral rootlets. Laterally, the denticulate ligaments form triangular, tooth-like processes that attach to the dura.

Three spaces are related to the cervical cord and its meninges. The epi- or extradural space is between the dura and the periosteum lining the vertebral canal. It contains loose connective tissue, fat, and the *internal vertebral venous plexus*. This plexus forms a valveless communication between the cranial dural sinuses above and the veins of the thoracic, abdominal, and pelvic cavities below. It, therefore, provides a possible route for the spread of infections or neoplasms and the flow of emboli. A potential subdural space exists between the dura and arachnoid. Between the arachnoid and pia is the *subarachnoid space*, which contains the cerebrospinal fluid as well as the spinal blood vessels and nerve rootlets enroute to and from the spinal cord.

The spinal dura mater contains nerves ventrally and dorsally (5). Ventrally there is a dense and longitudinally oriented plexus. It receives contributions from three sources: the sinu-vertebral nerves, the posterior

branches. In addition to supplying the posterior longitudinal ligament plexus, they give branches to the superficial and posterior parts of the anulus and the ventral part of the spinal dura. The functional components of the sinu-vertebral nerves include sympathetic as well as somatic and visceral sensory fibers. In regard to regional distribution, each vertebral segment or disc is usually supplied by the corresponding sinu-vertebral nerve as well as those arising from the segments immediately craniad and caudad.

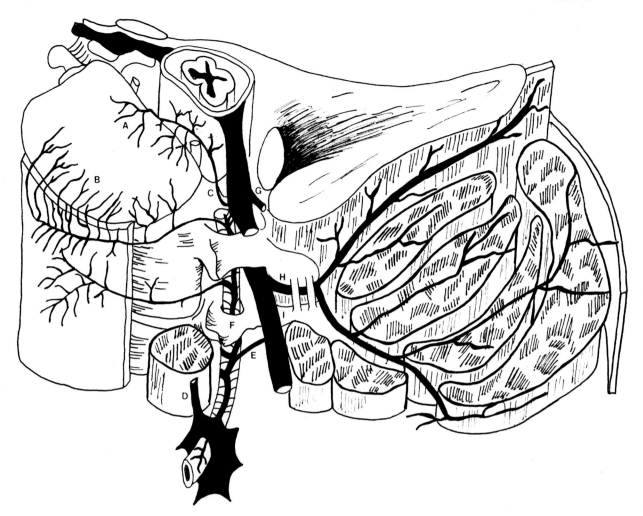

FIG. 2. Innervation of the cervical vertebral column. **A:** Dorsal nerve plexus. **B:** Ventral nerve plexus. **C:** Sinu-vertebral nerve. **D:** Sympathetic trunk. **E:** Gray ramus communicantes. **F:** Vertebral perivascular plexus. **G:** Dorsal root ganglion. **H:** Dorsal ramus. **I:** Ventral ramus.

longitudinal ligament plexus, and the perivascular plexi of the radicular branches of the segmental arteries.

The ventral dural nerves overlap as many as eight segments, the four craniad and four caudad. The dorsal dural nerves are much smaller than the ventral, do not form a distinct plexus, and are limited to the lateral quarters or sides of the dura; hence, they do not reach the median or midline of the dura. These dorsal dural nerves are derived from the ventral dural plexus via the "intersleeval" parts of the dura.

The functional components of the dural nerves are mainly nociceptive, although some vasomotor and viscerosensory fibers may also exist.

INTERNAL FEATURES

Throughout the spinal cord, the gray matter is internal and the white matter external (10). The gray matter consists of nerve cell bodies, dendrites, preterminal and terminal axons, capillaries, and glia. It is divided into three main parts: *dorsal* or *posterior horn, ventral* or *anterior horn*, and *intermediate zone*.

The neurons are arranged in layers or *cytoarchitectonic laminae*. These are used for the precise localization of functionally similar neurons that are used in describing the locations of origins and terminations of functional paths. Ten laminae make up the spinal gray (Fig. 3). The dorsal horn includes laminae I through VI, numbered from dorsal to ventral. The intermediate zone is lamina VII, and the ventral horn contains lamina VIII in its most medial part and clusters of large alpha motoneurons scattered elsewhere that form lamina IX. Lamina X is in the commissural area around the central canal.

The neurons of the cervical cord are also arranged in longitudinal columns of functionally similar cells referred to as *nuclei*. The most clinically important nuclei in the dorsal horn are the marginal (LI), substantia

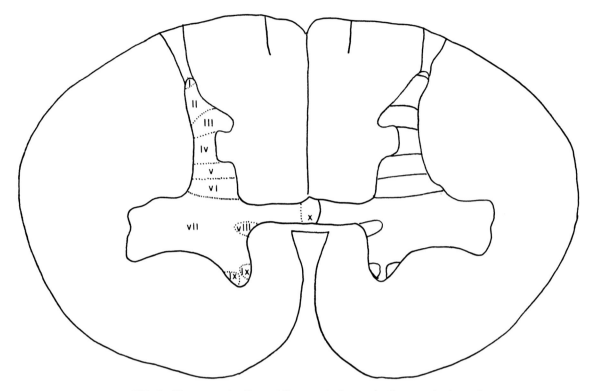

FIG. 3. The organization of the central gray in the cervical cord.

gelatinosa (LII), and proper sensory (LIV, V, VI). The marginal and proper sensory nuclei are intimately associated with the conduction of pain (Fig. 3)—the marginal chiefly with fast pain and the proper sensory chiefly with slow pain. The substantia gelatinosa consists of local circuit neurons that play an important role in the modulation of pain. The *ventral horn* is comprised of large motoneurons somatotopically arranged so that the more medial motoneurons innervate more proximal muscles, whereas the more lateral innervate the distal muscles. The specific muscles innervated by motoneurons in the segments of the spinal cord related to the cervical vertebrae are given in Fig. 4–12.

The white matter is divided into three areas: the posterior, the anterior, and the lateral funiculi.

In the cervical spinal cord, the *posterior funiculus*, also called the "dorsal column," is comprised chiefly of the gracile tract medially and the cuneate tract laterally (Figs. 13 and 14). Both convey the discriminative general sensations (tactile, two-point, vibratory, joint position, stereognosis, graphesthesia) from the spinal nerve dermatomes, the gracile tract from T7 to S5, and the cuneate from T6 to C1. The sacral dermatomes are localized posteromedially, the cervical laterally. Interruption of the dorsal column results in the loss of the above sensations below the level of the lesion on the ipsilateral side (Fig. 13 and 14).

In general, the *lateral funiculus* is related to motor activity posteriorly and to pain and thermal impulses anteriorly. Almost the entire posterior half of the lat-

eral funiculus is comprised of the lateral corticospinal tract, which originates primarily from the contralateral motor cortex. Input to the cervical segments is represented medially, to the sacral laterally. Interruption of the lateral corticospinal tract results in a spastic weakness, exaggerated tendon reflexes, increased resistance to passive stretch, and an extensor plantar response ipsilaterally (Figs. 13 and 14).

Separating the lateral corticospinal tract from the posterolateral surface of the lower cervical segments is the dorsal spinocerebellar tract. This tract arises from the ipsilateral dorsal nucleus of Clarke (Clarke's column) and carries information pertaining to tension of individual muscle spindles from the ipsilateral lower limb to the anterior lobe of the cerebellum. Interruption of the dorsal spinocerebellar tract results in ataxia in the ipsilateral lower limb (Figs. 13 and 14).

The anterior part of the lateral funiculus contains nerve fibers related to the transmission of pain and thermal impulses from contralateral dermatomes. These fibers form the neo- and paleospinothalamic and the spinoreticular tracts. The neospinothalamic tract transmits the fast pain associated with pin-prick, whereas the paleospinothalamic and spinoreticular tracts transmit the slow pain impulses associated with tissue damage. These tracts actually extend into the *anterior funiculus*; hence, they are located in the *anterolateral quadrant* of the spinal cord. Somatotopic localization exists with the contralateral sacral dermatomes being represented near the surface, whereas

C_1

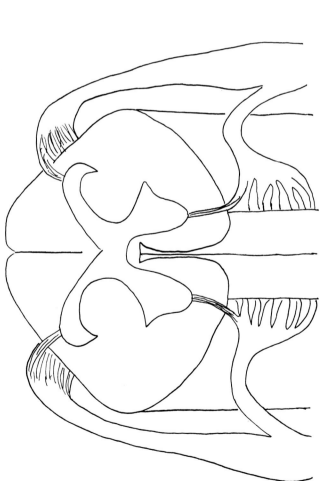

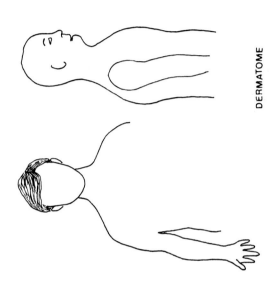

EXAM

MOTOR:
    Head flexion, rotation, lateral flexion and
      extension
    Fixation and steadying the neck
SENSORY:
    None

DERMATOME

MYOTOME

Sternocleidomastoid (C1C4 CNX11)
Longus capitis (C1C4)
Rectus capitis anterior (C1C2)
Rectus capitis lateralis (C1)
Rectus capitis posterior (C1)
Obliquus capitis inferior (C1)
Obliquus capitis superior (C1)
Infrahyoid muscles (C1C3)

FIG. 4. Segmental innervation at C1.

C₂

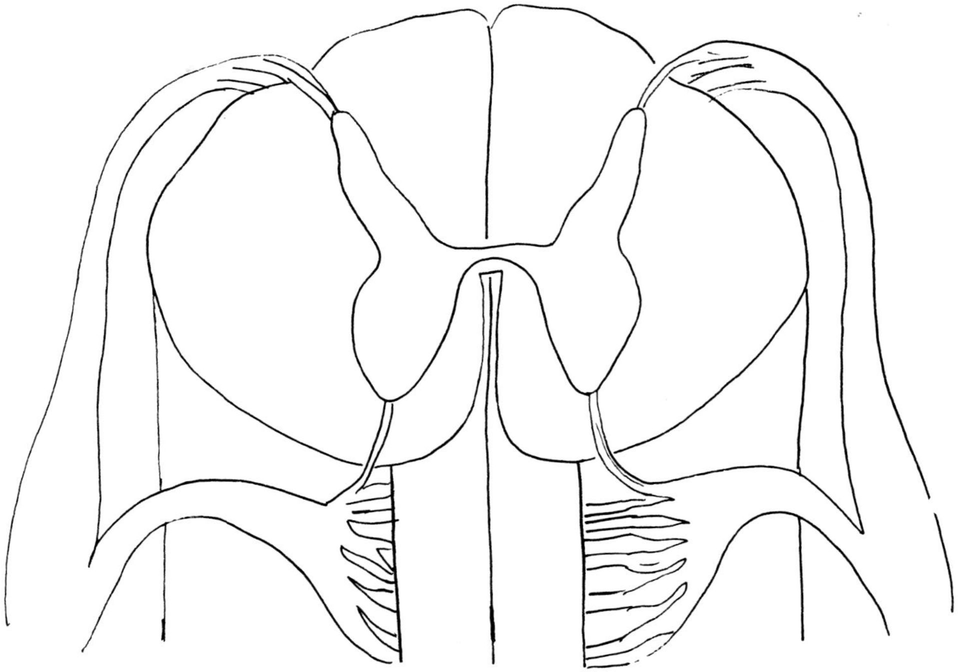

EXAM

MOTOR:
  Head flexion, extension, lateral flexion
    and rotation
  Fixation and steadying neck
REFLEX:
  Sternocleidomastoid reflex
SENSORY:
  Suboccipital pain

DERMATOME

MYOTOME

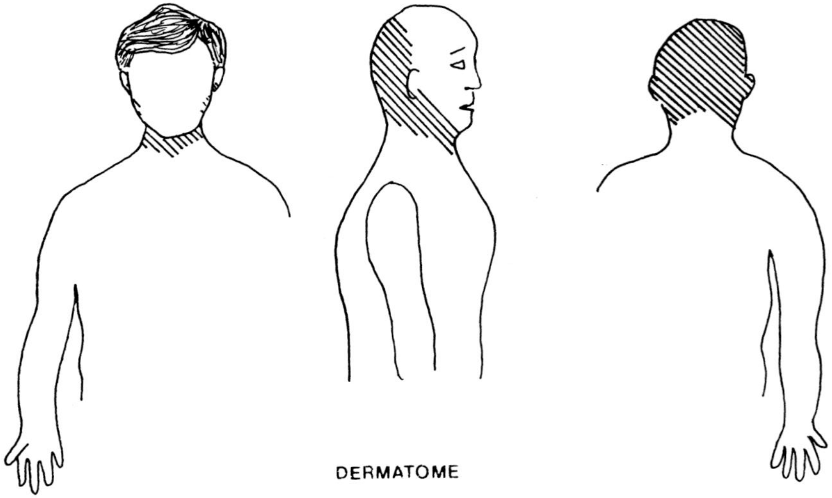

Sternocleidomastoid (C1C4 CNX1)
Trapezius (C2C4 CNX1)
Longus capitis (C1C4)
Longus colli (C2C6)
Rectus capitis anterior (C1C2)
Splenius capitis (C2C4)
Splenius cervicis (C2C4)
Semispinalis capitis (C2C4)
Infrahyoid muscles (C1C3)

FIG. 5. Segmental innervation at C2.

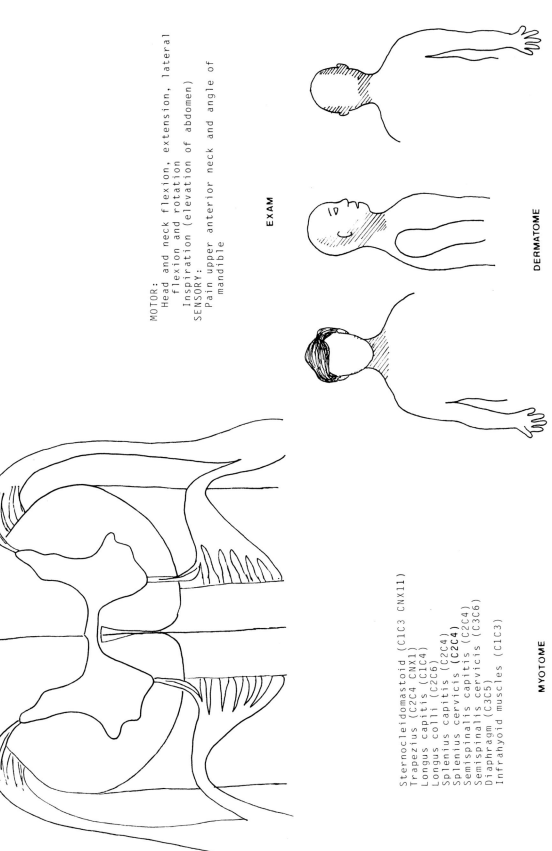

C₃

MOTOR:
    Head and neck flexion, extension, lateral
       flexion and rotation
    Inspiration (elevation of abdomen)
SENSORY:
    Pain upper anterior neck and angle of
       mandible

EXAM

DERMATOME

```
Sternocleidomastoid (C1C3 CNX11)
Trapezius (C2C4 CNX1)
Longus capitis (C1C4)
Longus colli (C2C6)
Splenius capitis (C2C4)
Splenius cervicis (C2C4)
Semispinalis capitis (C2C4)
Semispinalis cervicis (C3C6)
Diaphragm (C3C5)
Infrahyoid muscles (C1C3)
```

MYOTOME

FIG. 6. Segmental innervation at C3.

MOTOR:
  Head and neck flexion, extension, lateral
    flexion and rotation
  Inspiration (elevation of abdomen)
REFLEX: Scapulohumeral reflex
SENSORY:
  Pain upper posterior neck and suprascapular region

EXAM

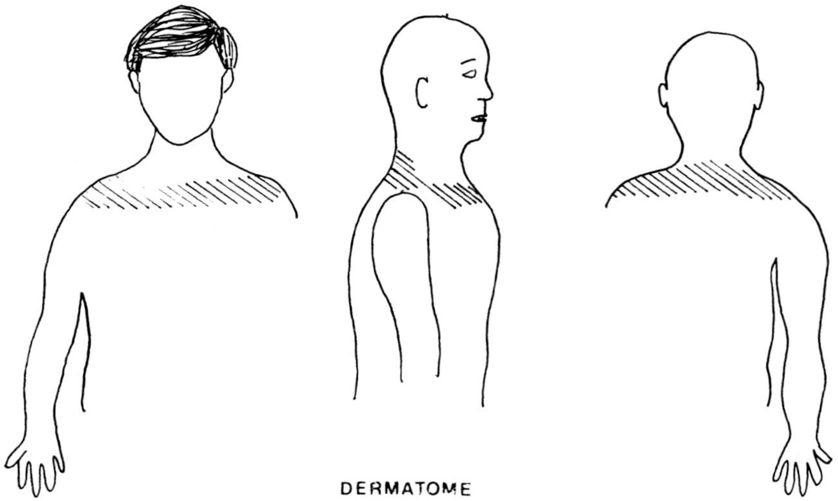

C₄

DERMATOME

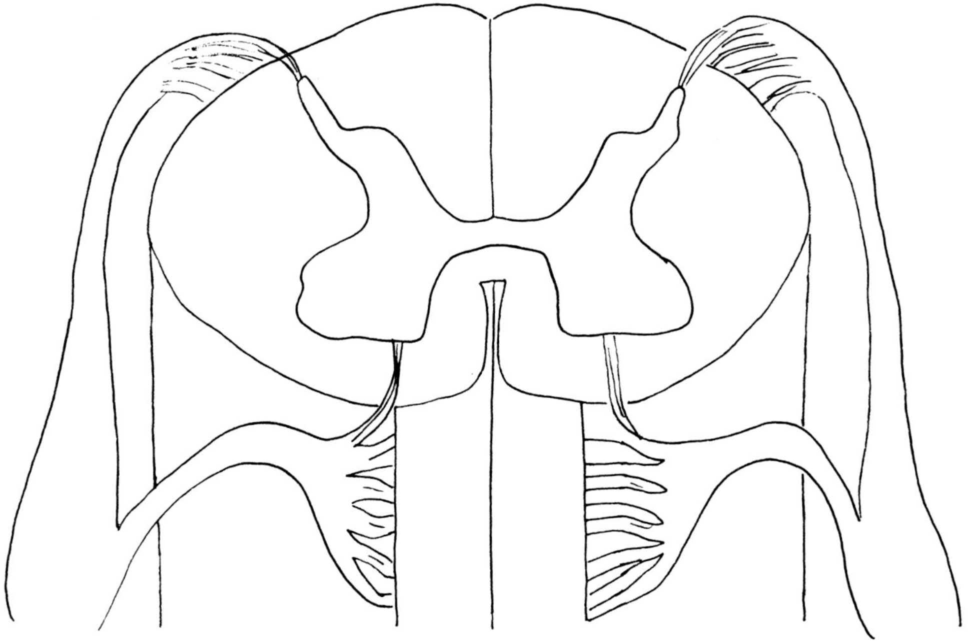

Trapezius (C2C4)
Scalenus anterior (C4C7)
Scalenus posterior (C4C8)
Longus capitis (C1C4)
Longus coli (C2C6)
Splenius capitis (C2C4)
Splenius cervicis (C2C4)
Semispinalis capitis (C2C4)
Semispinalis cervicis (C3C6)
Diaphragm (C3C5)

MYOTOME

FIG. 7. Segmental innervation at C4.

C₅

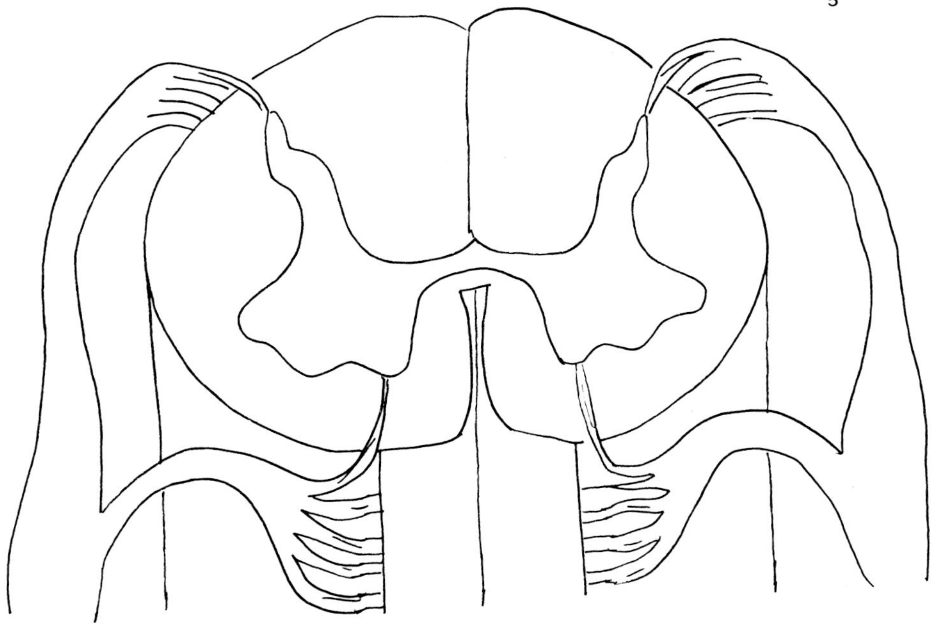

MOTOR:
Adduction arm from behind to front
Forward thrust shoulders
Medial adduction and elevation scapula
Adduction arm
Abduction arm
Lateral rotation arm
Flexion forearm
REFLEXES:
Deltoid reflex
Pectoralis reflex
Biceps reflex
Brachioradialis reflex
SENSORY:
Pain and numbness lateral upper arm
and shoulder

EXAM

DERMATOME

Latissimus dorsi (C5C8)
Scalenes, anterior, posterior and medial (C4C8)
Pectoralis major and minor (C5T1)
Serratus anterior (C5C7)
Levator scapulae (C5)
Rhomboids (C4C5)
Supraspinatus (C5)
Infraspinatus (C5C6)
Teres minor (C5)
Biceps brachii (C5C6)
Brachialis (C5C6)
Brachioradialis (C5C6)
Deltoid (C5C6)

MYOTOME

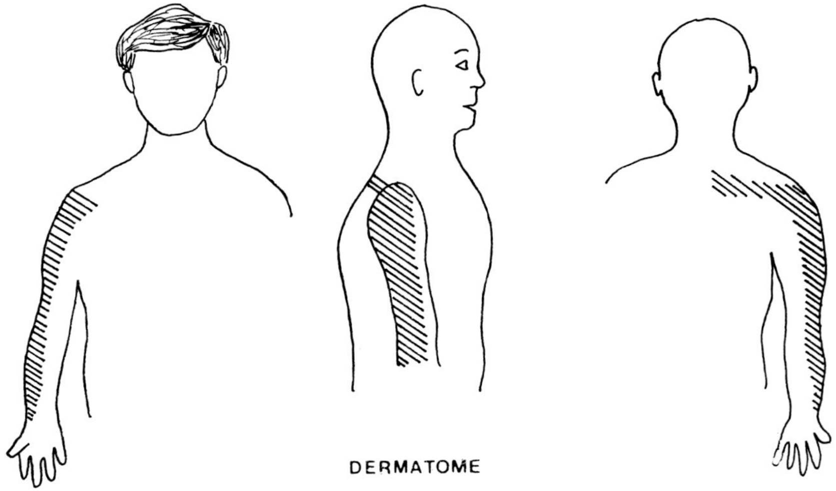

FIG. 8. Segmental innervation at C5.

C₆

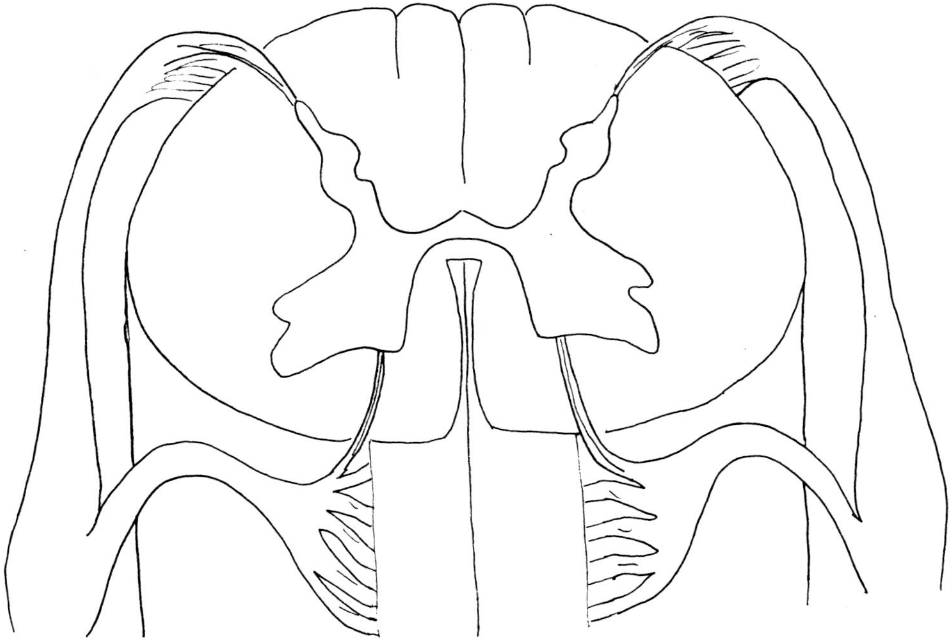

EXAM

MOTOR:
Wrist extension
Medial rotation arm
Adduction arm front to back
Adduction arm
Flexion forearm
Pronation forearm
Radial flexion hand
Flexion terminal phalanx thumb
Abduction metacarpal thumb
Flexion proximal phalanx thumb
REFLEXES:
Biceps reflex
Brachioradialis reflex
Pronator reflex
Wrist extension reflex
Wrist flexion reflex
SENSORY:
Pain medial border scapulae, lateral
arm and dorsal forearm
Numbness thumb and index finger

MYOTOME

Biceps brachii (C5C6)
Brachioradialis (C5C6)
Latissimus dorsi (C5C8)
Coracobrachialis (C6C7)
Pronator teres (C6C7)
Flexor carpi radialis (C6C7)
Flexor pollicis longus (C6C7)
Abductor pollicis brevis (C6C7)
Flexor pollicis brevis (C6C7)
Opponens pollicis (C6C7)
Extensor digitorum communis
Extensor carpi radialis (C6C7)

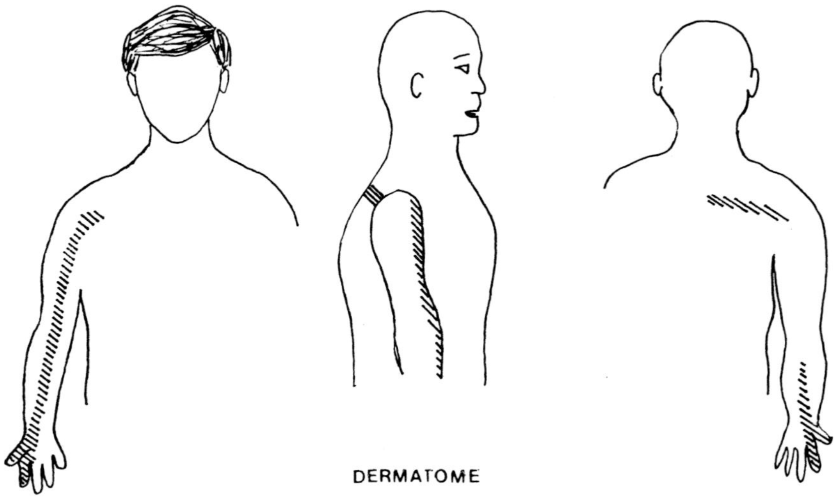

DERMATOME

FIG. 9. Segmental innervation at C6.

MOTOR:
   Adduction arm
   Flexion forearm
   Flexion hand
   Flexion middle phalanx, index and middle fingers
   Flexion terminal phalanx index and middle fingers
   Flexion proximal phalanx and extension two distal
     phalanges index, middle, ring and little fingers
   Ulnar flexion hand
REFLEXES:
   Triceps reflex
   Thumb reflex
   Finger flexion reflex
SENSORY:
   Pain in forearm
   Numbness in middle finger

EXAM

DERMATOME

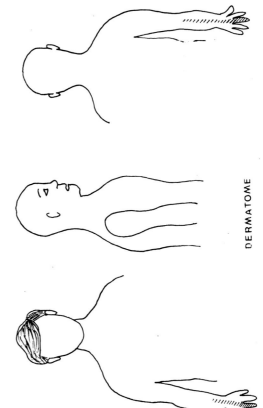

MYOTOME

Triceps brachii (C6C7)
Latissimus dorsi (C5C8)
Coracobrachialis (C6C7)
Palmaris longus (C7T1)
Flexor digitorum sublimis
Flexor digitorum profundus
Lumbricals–two lateral (C6C7)
Flexor carpi ulnaris (C7T1)

C7

FIG. 10. Segmental innervation at C7.

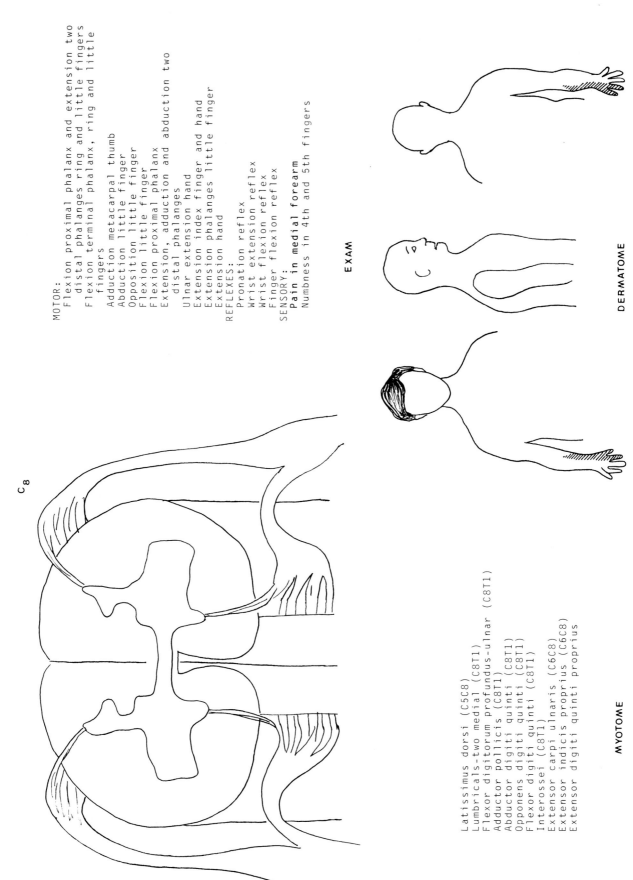

MOTOR:
Flexion proximal phalanx and extension two
  distal phalanges ring and little fingers
Flexion terminal phalanx, ring and little
  fingers
Adduction metacarpal thumb
Abduction little finger
Opposition little finger
Flexion little finger
Flexion proximal phalanx
Extension, adduction and abduction two
  distal phalanges
Ulnar extension hand
Extension index finger and hand
Extension phalanges little finger
Extension hand
REFLEXES:
Pronation reflex
Wrist extension reflex
Wrist flexion reflex
Finger flexion reflex
SENSORY:
Pain in medial forearm
Numbness in 4th and 5th fingers

EXAM

C_8

DERMATOME

Latissimus dorsi (C5C8)
Lumbricals-two medial (C8T1)
Flexor digitorum profundus-ulnar (C8T1)
Adductor pollicis (C8T1)
Abductor digiti quinti (C8T1)
Opponens digiti quinti (C8T1)
Flexor digiti quinti (C8T1)
Interossei (C8T1)
Extensor carpi ulnaris (C6C8)
Extensor indicis proprius (C6C8)
Extensor digiti quinti proprius

MYOTOME

FIG. 11. Segmental innervation at C8.

T₁

MOTOR:
    Flexion terminal phalanges ring and little
        fingers
    Adduction metacarpal of thumb
    Abduction little finger
    Opposition little finger
    Flexion little finger
    Flexion proximal phalanx
    Extension, adduction, and abduction two
        distal phalanges
REFLEXES:
    Wrist extension reflex
    Wrist flexion reflex
    Finger flexion reflex
SENSORY:
    Pain medial elbow
AUTONOMIC:
    Horner,s Syndrome

EXAM

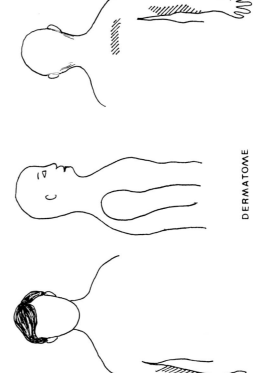

DERMATOME

Flexor digitorum profundus (C8T1)
Adductor pollicis (C8T1)
Abductor digiti quinti (C8T1)
Flexor digiti brevis (C8T1)
Interossei (C8T1)

MYOTOME

FIG. 12. Segmental innervation at T1.

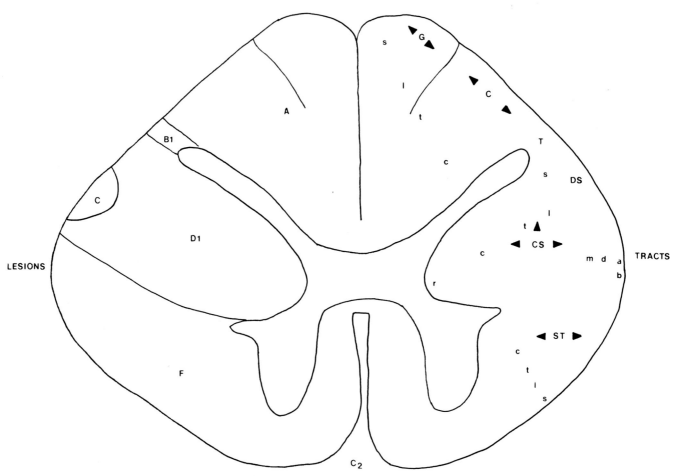

FIG. 13. Clinically important white matter pathways in upper cervical cord (C2). *Lesions*: **A:** Ipsilateral loss of tactile, vibratory, and position senses. **B1:** Ipsilateral loss of pain in V, dermatome. **B2:** Ipsilateral loss of C7–C8 dermatomes. **C:** Ipsilateral gait ataxia. **D1:** Ipsilateral spastic hemiplegia (upper motor neuron syndrome). **D2:** Ipsilateral spastic monoplegia (upper motor neuron syndrome). **F:** Contralateral pain and thermal loss. *Tracts*: C, cervical; T, thoracic; L, lumbar; S, sacral; G, gracile fasciculus; C, cuneate fasciculus; T, spinal trigeminal tract; L, tract of Lissauer; DS, dorsal spinocerebellar tract; CS, lateral corticospinal tract; ST, spinothalamic tract; r, respiratory path; m, micturition path; d, defecation path; a, rectum; b, bladder/urethra.

the contralateral cervical are near the gray matter. Interruption of the anterolateral quadrant results in the loss of pain and thermal sensation in the contralateral dermatomes below the level of the lesion (Figs. 13 and 14).

Also within the lateral and anterior funiculi are the so-called descending supraspinal tracts that influence spinal motor activity. Thus, the rubrospinal and lateral vestibulo- and reticulospinal tracts are chiefly in the lateral funiculus, whereas the medial vestibulo- and reticulospinal tracts as well as the tectospinal tract are in the anterior funiculus. Also within the anterior funiculus is the variable uncrossed component of the pyramidal tract, the anterior corticospinal tract.

Several tracts of clinical importance include the descending paths associated with respiration, micturition, erection, ejaculation, and defecation, and the ascending paths associated with the sensations that accompany these phenomenon (Figs. 13 and 14). All

of these tracts convey impulses bilaterally; hence, unilateral lesions affect neither the sensations nor the actions of these organs associated with the elimination of waste or reproductive products.

In addition to the tracts in the various funiculi, the dorsolateral fasciculus or tract of Lissauer consists of a group of fibers between the dorsal gray horn and the surface of the cord at the posterolateral sulcus and is related to the transmission of pain impulses. In the more rostral cervical segments, these fibers chiefly belong to the spinal trigeminal tract and carry pain and also some thermal impulses from the ipsilateral side of the face, especially the area supplied by the ophthalmic division of the trigeminal nerve. In the more caudal cervical segments, the tract of Lissauer transmits pain and thermal impulses from the dermatome of its respective segment as well as one or two segments below.

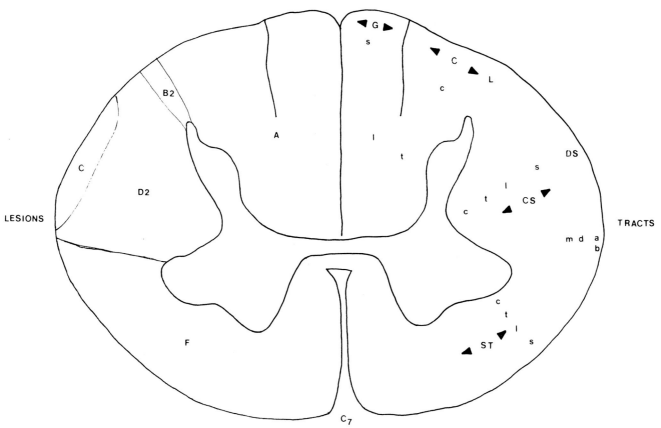

FIG. 14. Clinically important white matter pathways in lower cervical cord (C7). *Lesions:* **A:** Ipsilateral loss of tactile, vibratory, and position senses. **B1:** Ipsilateral loss of pain in V, dermatome. **B2:** Ipsilateral loss of C7–C8 dermatomes. **C:** Ipsilateral gait ataxia. **D1:** Ipsilateral spastic hemiplegia (upper motor neuron syndrome). **D2:** Ipsilateral spastic monoplegia (upper motor neuron syndrome). **F:** Contralateral pain and thermal loss. *Tracts:* C, cervical; T, thoracic; L, lumbar; S, sacral; G, gracile fasciculus; C, cuneate fasciculus; T, spinal trigeminal tract; L, tract of Lissauer; DS, dorsal spinocerebellar tract; CS, lateral corticospinal tract; ST, spinothalamic tract; r, respiratory path; m, micturition path; d, defecation path; a, rectum; b, bladder/urethra.

BLOOD SUPPLY

Extrinsic Arteries

Extrinsic arteries are described here (1,2). The cervical spinal cord receives its blood supply from the single *anterior spinal* and the paired *posterior spinal arteries*, all three of which are reinforced along their lengths by radicular arteries.

The *anterior spinal artery* is located in the anterior median fissure and is formed in the cranial cavity by fusion of the anterior spinal branches of the vertebral arteries immediately before the formation of the basilar artery. The parent anterior spinals usually fuse within 2 cm of their origin, but on occasion they remain separate as far caudally as C5.

The *posterior spinal arteries* arise most often from the posterior inferior cerebellar arteries, sometimes from the vertebral arteries, and on rare occasions from posterior radicular arteries. The artery on each side zig-zags caudally along the posterolateral surface of the cord to midcervical levels. Between C3 and C5, each vessel moves medial to where the posterior root-

lets enter at the posterolateral sulcus. In the lower cervical region, they communicate freely with small arteries running parallel but lateral to the rootlets. The posterior spinal arteries are extremely variable in size, sometimes one being so small that it appears to be absent. Medially directed branches from the posterior spinal arteries on each side connect to form an arterial plexus on the posterior surface of the cord.

The anterior spinal and posterior spinal arteries are reinforced along their lengths by *radicular arteries*. In the upper six cervical segments, radicular arteries may arise from the vertebral artery or the ascending cervical branch of the thyrocervical trunk. A large radicular artery to the lower cervical cord at the C5 or C6 level usually arises from the deep cervical artery, a branch of the costocervical trunk. Sometimes, however, this radicular vessel arises from the ascending cervical artery. Anterior and posterior radicular arteries reach the spinal cord by traveling along the anterior surfaces of the respective roots of the spinal nerves (Fig. 15). In the cervical region, the number of anterior radicular arteries ranges from one to six and

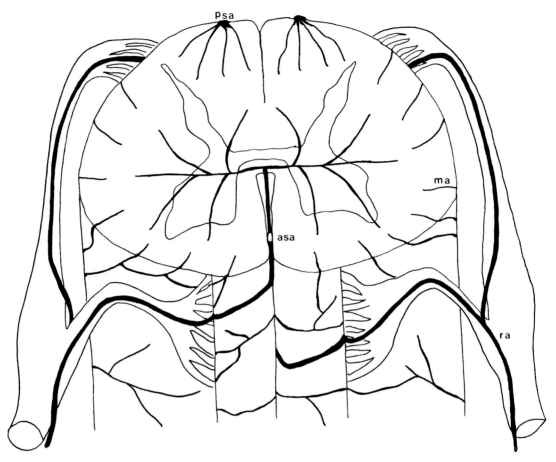

FIG. 15. Extrinsic blood supply of the cervical cord. PSA, posterior spinal artery; ASA, anterior spinal artery; RA, radicular artery; MA, marginal artery.

are as frequent on one side as on the other. The number of posterior radicular arteries varies from zero to eight, but in 75% of the time there are two or three. These usually occur at lower cervical levels, with the level of C6 showing the greatest frequency of occurrence. The levels of the posterior radiculars do not necessarily coincide with the anterior. When they do, the posterior artery is a branch of the anterior. Blood in the anterior spinal artery flows downward from its origin to about the second cervical segment. In the cervical segments below this, the flow is upward from the anterior radicular arteries.

The filling of the anterior spinal artery in the cervical cord depends upon at least one major radicular artery. The input of this artery divides the cervical spinal cord into a rostral cervicocranial and a caudal cervicothoracic arterial territory. Interruption of this major medullary source, regardless of the cause, will result in ischemic degeneration in one arterial dominion or the other.

Blood flow in the posterior spinal arteries is downward in the cranial cavity. Where reinforced by the posterior radicular arteries, the flow is upward and downward.

The pial plexus (vasa corona) on the sides of the spinal cord receives small branches from the anterior and posterior spinal arteries as well as from some of the radicular arteries. The branches supplying this plexus are so small that an effective functional anastomosis between the anterior and posterior spinal systems does not exist.

Intrinsic Arteries

Intrinsic arteries are represented in Fig. 16 and described here (6–8,11).

Central or *sulcal branches* (sulcocommissural) of the anterior spinal artery pass posteriorly in the anterior median fissure and enter the cord at the anterior white commissure. Here, they arch laterally to one side or the other. Arteries to the right alternate with those to the left, but on occasion two consecutive arteries go to the same side. In the upper cervical cord, the anterior spinal artery gives rise to five to seven sulcal branches per centimeter; in middle and lower cervical levels, the density is five to eight per centimeter. These sulcal branches are end-arteries since no anastomoses occur except at capillary levels.

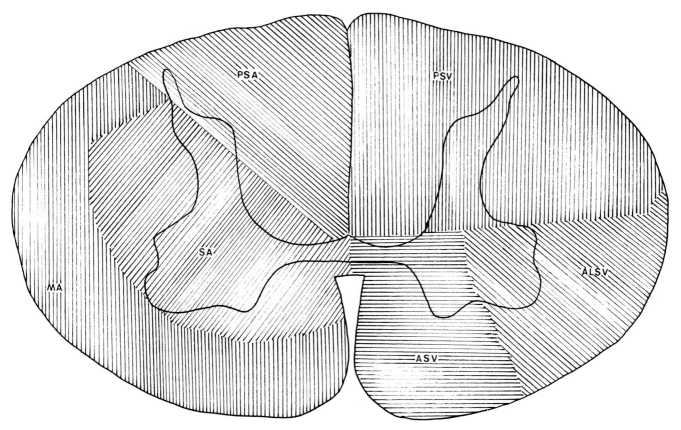

FIG. 16. Intrinsic blood supply of the cervical cord. PSA, posterior spinal artery; PSV, posterior spinal vein; SA, sulcal artery; MA, marginal artery; ASV, anterior spinal vein; ALSV, anterolateral spinal vein.

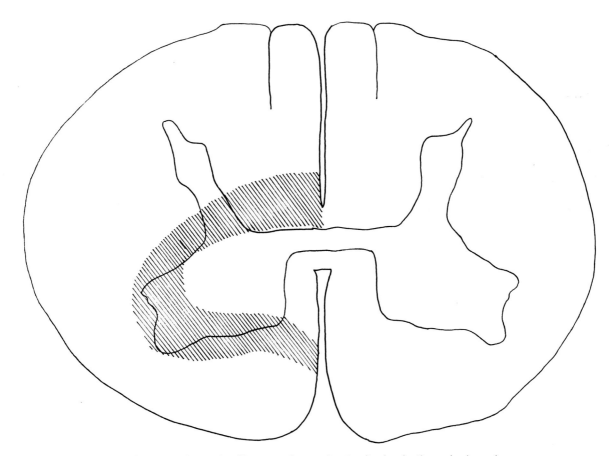

FIG. 17. "Water-shed" zone of vascular territories in the spinal cord.

The pial anterior plexus gives off branches that penetrate the white matter along the entire circumference of the cord except along the borders of the anterior median fissure. A heavier concentration of these penetrating branches occurs at the posterolateral sulcus. All enter the spinal cord perpendicular to the surface and pass directly inwards.

The anterior spinal artery, via its sulcal and pial branches, supplies the anterior two-thirds of the spinal cord (Fig. 16). This includes the lateral and anterior funiculi, the anterior third of the posterior funiculi, and all of the gray matter anterior to the substantia gelatinosa. The posterior spinal arteries supply, via the posterior pial plexus, the posterior third of the cord. This includes the posterior two-thirds of the posterior funiculi, the dorsolateral fasciculus of Lissauer, and the marginal (LI) and substantia gelatinosa (LII) parts of the dorsal horn of the gray matter.

The pial arterial plexus supplies the peripheral parts of the cord, whereas the sulcal arteries supply the central gray matter. Overlap between the two systems occurs in the inner third to quarter of the white matter, and outer edge of the gray matter except the posterior half of the posterior horn (Fig. 17).

VENOUS DRAINAGE

The cervical spinal cord veins run parallel to the arteries within the cord, and on the cord and roots of the spinal nerves. However, they are far more variable than the arteries.

Blood from the capillaries of the gray matter passes to the surface by veins running radially, parallel to the penetrating arteries, and by veins located along the sulcal arteries. The latter drain into a single anterior spinal vein located deep to the artery in the anterior median fissure. This vein also receives tributaries from the pial veins on the anterior surface of the cord. The anterior spinal vein empties into anterior radicular veins, which are located on almost every other anterior root.

Veins in the white matter drain into the radially arranged veins coming from the gray matter. At the surface, these intrinsic veins join the pial venous plexus. Posteriorly, there may be a pial plexus, but usually there are one or two posterior spinal veins that are larger than the anterior spinal. The posterior spinal veins drain into posterior radicular veins located on every second or third posterior root.

The anterior and posterior radicular veins anastomose with the epidural and vertebral body veins. Occasionally, a conspicuous vein passes from the posterior surface of the cord at approximately C3 to the dura near the midline.

REFERENCES

1. Chakravorty BG. Arterial supply of the cervical spinal cord (with special reference to the radicular arteries). *Anat Rec* 170:311–330, 1972.
2. Crock HV, Yoshizawa H. *The blood supply of the vertebral column and spinal cord in man.* New York: Springer-Verlag, 1977.
3. Gerbrand JG, Baljet B, Drukker J. Nerves and nerve plexuses of the human vertebral column. *Am J Anat* 188:282–296, 1990.
4. Williams and Warwick, eds. *Gray's anatomy.* 36th British ed. Edinburgh, London, Melbourne, and New York: Churchill Livingstone, 1980.
5. Groen GJ, Baljet B, Drukker J. The innervation of the spinal dura mater: anatomy and clinical implications. *Acta Neurochirurg* 92:39–46, 1988.
6. Hassler O. Blood supply to the human spinal cord. A microangiographic study. *Arch Neurol* 15:302–307, 1966.
7. Herren RY, Alexander L. Sulcal and intrinsic blood vessels of human spinal cord. *Arch Neural Psych* 41:686–687, 1939.
8. Lazorthes B, Gouaze A, Zadek JO, Santini JJ, Lazorthes Y, Burdin P. Arterial vascularization of the spinal cord: recent studies of the anastomotic substitution pathways. *J Neurosurg* 35:253–262, 1971.
9. Murphy F, Simmons JCH, Brunson B. Ruptured cervical discs, 1939 to 1972. *Clinical Neurosurgery* 20:9–17, 1973.
10. Truex–functional neuroanatomy of the spinal cord. *Clin Neurosurg* 20:29–55, 1973.
11. Turnball IM, Brieg A, Hassler O. Blood supply of cervical spinal cord in man. A microangiographic cadaver study. *J Neurosci* 24:951–965, 1966.

CHAPTER 4

Degenerative Cervical Disc Disorders

Pathophysiology and Clinical Syndromes

Paul H. Young

A rapidly evolving understanding of the complex pathophysiology surrounding cervical disc disease has occurred over the past six decades. Mixter and Barr (101) introduced the basic relationship between radicular pain syndromes and associated nerve root compression by demonstrating that the relief of radicular compression resulted in relief of the pain syndrome. The subsequent introduction of Pantopaque (157) pioneered an ability to diagnose cervical disc difficulties particularly spondylosis with midline bars and lateral spurs. For the first time, it was possible to differentiate between these surgically treatable conditions and other nonsurgical entities such as spinal syphilis, multiple sclerosis, combined system disease, amyotrophic lateral sclerosis, and other degenerative conditions. As a consequence of this diagnostic ability, an increasing number of patients were subjected to posterior decompressive procedures, which provided not only treatment for a reversible cause of neurologic disability but also impetus for a better understanding of the pathophysiology of degenerative cervical spine disease.

PATHOPHYSIOLOGY OF CERVICAL DEGENERATIVE DISC DISEASE IN SPONDYLOSIS

The pathophysiology of cervical degenerative disc disease in spondylosis is described here (1–20). The pathological substrate of cervical spondylosis is a circumferential degeneration of structures surrounding the cervical spinal canal (Fig. 1), including interver-

tebral disc (nucleus pulposus and annulus fibrosis), vertebral body cartilaginous endplates, anterior and posterior longitudinal ligaments, uncovertebral joints, zygoapophyseal (facet) joints, laminae, and ligamenta flava.

The advancing sequence of pathological changes in each of these anatomical structures bordering the

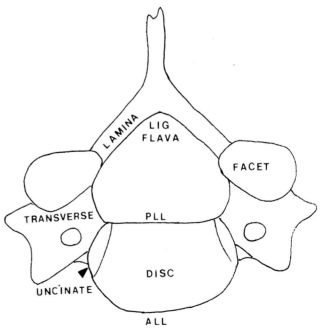

FIG. 1. The structures surrounding the spinal canal that are directly affected by spondylosis.

spinal canal (and spinal cord) can be summarized as follows:

Nucleus pulposus (normally a noncompressible gel):
—diminished water content and increased fibrous tissue

↓

—degeneration and fragmentation

↓

—disc resorption with decreased intradiscal pressure, shrinkage, and decreased vertical height

↓

—reduced ability to distribute axial forces evenly

↓

—decreased elasticity and increased (over normal) mobility

↓

—progressive internal disruption of disc

↓

—progressive resorption of disc with replacement by degenerative fibrous tissue

Annulus fibrosis (normally elastic with high tensile strength):
—increased axial weight load due to shrinkage of the nucleus

↓

—collapse of fibers—center lamellae buckle inward, peripheral lamellae bulge outward

↓

—circumferential tears, fissuring, and cracking

↓

—coalescence of radial and annulus tears

↓

—mechanical breakdown with instability

↓

—bulging of annulus

↓

—abnormal movements of motion segment

↓

—extrusion of nuclear material (rare)

Vertebral body cartilaginous endplates (normally vascularized cartilage providing nutrition of the nucleus pulposus):
—motion segment abnormalities with abnormal stresses

↓

—increased deposition of cartilaginous tissue (sclerosis)

↓

—loss of blood vessels in the cartilage with increased numbers of blood vessels in the subcartilaginous vertebral body

↓

—reactive hyperostosis and osteophytic bridging

↓

—increase subchondral vertebral body diameter (increased weight bearing surface)

↓

—circumferential hypertrophic osteophytic ridge

↓

—bony ankylosis

Posterior longitudinal ligament (also anterior longitudinal ligament) (normally a strong motion segment stabilizer):
—increased stress with reactive fibrosis

↓

—supported by hypertrophic osteophytic ridge for restabilization of degenerative interspace

↓

—stretching of the dura with epidural fibrosis

↓

—penetration by extrusion of nucleus (rare but more frequent laterally than medially)

Uncovertebral joints (joints of Luschka) (normally a lateral cleft in disc with colloid deposited):
—uncinate process progressively overrides the opposing indented surface

↓

—joint space destroyed

↓

—reactive hypertrophy

↓

—spur formation posterolaterally into foramen and posteromedially into canal

Zygoapophyseal (facet) joints (normally a gliding type synovial joint):
—abnormal joint mobility with joint strain

↓

—synovial reaction and degeneration of the articular cartilage

↓

—tears in capsule and ligaments

↓

—thinning of capsule with capsular laxity

↓

—articular subluxation (minor degree)

↓

—periarticular and capsular fibrosis

↓

—erosion of articular surface

↓

—capsular hypertrophy

Posterior arch (laminae and ligamenta flava) (normally a segmented, flexible, and elastic canal roof):
—segmental instability and strain

↓

—compensatory hypertrophy with decreased elasticity

↓

—inward folding upon neck extension thereby reducing spinal canal height

These spondylotic changes involving spinal column supporting structures cumulatively result in a circumferential narrowing of the spinal canal (Fig. 1). Thus, the spondylotic changes can be considered to be primarily affecting the spinal column and its ligamentous supporting tissues and secondarily affecting neurovascular elements by narrowing the spinal canal, intervertebral foramina, and foramina transversalis.

This narrowing produces neurological symptomatology by compressing the enclosed spinal cord, spinal roots, and vertebral artery and its radicular branches.

Although the spondylotic spine itself generally is asymptomatic (except for perhaps axial pain syndromes), secondary compression of the above structures frequently results in significant symptomatology and often leads the patient to seek medical attention.

PATHOPHYSIOLOGY OF CERVICAL MYELOPATHY

Four key factors are particularly important in the development of cervical myelopathy in the setting of cervical spondylosis (21–44): (a) the development of canal compression by spondylotic ridges, bars, or spurs; (b) the presence of a congenitally narrow spinal canal; (c) the adequacy of spinal cord radicular and medullary circulation; and (d) the effects of repetitive biomechanical motion on the cervical spinal cord and its vascular supply.

Development of Spondylotic Compressive Ridges, Bars, or Spurs

The development of spondylotic compressive ridges, bars, or spurs leads to direct compression of the spinal cord matter (Fig. 2). Within the cervical spinal cord, there is a differential vulnerability to direct compression of descending and ascending white fiber tracts. The corticospinal tract is most sensitive followed by the anterior horn cells, anterior funiculus, and posterior funiculus. The pathological sequence of events within the compressed cervical cords are: distortion of spinal cord tissue and blockage of axoplasmic flow, then increased cord tension by the dentate ligaments restraining the spinal cord anteriorly in the canal, then demyelination of compressed axons, then gliosis (scarring), and, finally, cystic degeneration and central gray cavitation.

Congenitally Small Spinal Canal

The actual production of cord compression depends not only on the presence of a protruding spondylotic bar or spur but also on the overall premorbid size of

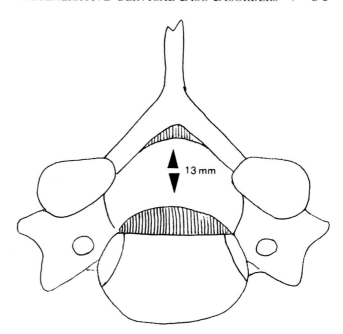

FIG. 2. Midline spondylotic bar decreasing the size of the spinal canal.

the spinal canal (45–62). Larger than average spinal canals can accommodate large spondylotic intrusions without neural compression. The sagittal diameter of the midcervical spinal canal ranges in the normal population from 14 to 23 mm (Fig. 3). Generally only those patients with spinal canals of ≤14 mm will develop a

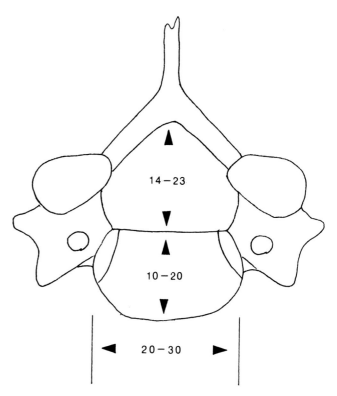

FIG. 3. Normal range of diameters for the cervical spinal canal.

spondylotic myelopathy. It has been shown that athletes possessing a narrow cervical canal have a high incidence of transient quadriplegia secondary to hyperflexion, hyperextension and compressive forces (58). As a consequence, it is certainly possible, based on simple radiographic measurements of cervical canal diameter, to predict those patients at greatest risk for the eventual development of a spondylotic myelopathy.

Adequacy of Spinal Cord Radicular and Medullary Circulation

Cervical cord blood flow is dependent on the integrity of both the anterior and posterior spinal arteries in addition to the radicular supply from the vertebral arteries (63–79) (Fig. 4). Both intrinsic and extrinsic spinal cord ischemia can develop following spondylotic compression. Factors related to *intrinsic spinal cord ischemia* include direct intermittent compressive occlusion of the anterior spinal artery against anterior spurs with transient ischemia of the anterior two-thirds of the spinal cord, compression of the sulcal and terminal branches of the anterior spinal artery due to direct anterior spinal cord compression, spinal cord vascular stasis due to tethering of the cord against an anterior spondylotic compressive force by the dentate ligaments, obliteration of venous channels due to flattening of the anterior spinal cord, spinal cord capillary-venous stasis and local edema with absent spinal cord pulsation, and cumulative local spinal cord ischemia progressing to microscopic infarction.

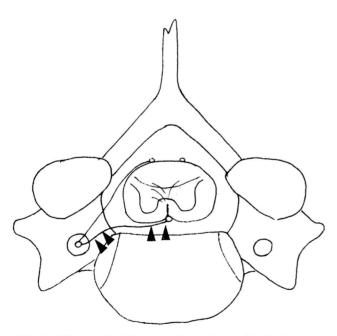

FIG. 4. Effects of midline and lateral spondylotic bars on spinal cord medullary and radicular arteries.

Extrinsic spinal cord ischemic factors predominate in the lower cervical spine as follows: The largest (and most important) radicular arteries arise in the C5, C6, or C7 segments; the proximal vertebral artery and its most proximal radicular branches (C5, C6, C7) have a greater incidence of atherosclerotic occlusion; and there is an increased frequency of osteoarthritic foraminal encroachment in the lower cervical region (C5, C6, C7) resulting in radicular artery compression.

Effects of Repetitive Biomechanical Motion on the Spinal Cord

Dynamic motion within the compromised cervical spinal canal has both direct compressive as well as secondary ischemic effects upon the spinal cord (80–95).

Compressive Effects

The functional diameter of the spinal canal is significantly reduced by full flexion and hyperextension of the neck. The increased tension in the spinal cord with flexion diminishes the anteroposterior diameter of the spinal cord with direct pressure on the anterior columns and indirect intramedullary pressure on the lateral columns. Full flexion results in a stretched and flattened spinal cord anteriorly where osteophytic protrusion into the spinal canal exists. This flattening and widening of the cord produces intermittent narrowing and elongation of the anterior spinal and transverse arteries with cumulative ischemic affects. In addition, these compressive forces result in a stress pattern which is maximal in the central gray area. These sheer forces may also compress the small venulae present in this area leading to increasingly inadequate gray matter perfusions.

With hyperextension, the ventral compression is reduced and the anteroposterior spinal cord diameter is increased. In addition, however, buckling inward of the ligamenta flava occurs with direct posterior cord compression. Repeated full flexion-hyperextension motions produce cumulative compressive and vascular affects upon the spinal cord. In addition, further compression affects may be seen if motion segment instability exists secondary to spondylotic changes.

PATHOPHYSIOLOGY OF SPONDYLOTIC RADICULOPATHY

Osteophytic compression of the intervertebral foramina can occur from either the uncovertebral or apophyseal joint borders (96–102) (Fig. 5). Compression alone of the exiting nerve root initially affects the

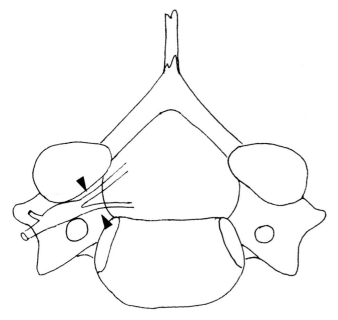

FIG. 5. Radicular compression by both uncovertebral and apophyseal joint spondylotic process producing foraminal narrowing.

larger *A*-fibers resulting in the characteristic radiculopathic syndrome of weakness, numbness and reflex loss. In addition to foraminal compression, however, uncovertebral and facet spondylosis leads to the development of epidural adhesions and perineural inflammation. The combination of nerve root compression and inflammation produces the radicular pain so characteristic of a spondylotic radiculopathy.

Finally, the biomechanical affects of repetitive hyperextension and lateral flexion towards the side of foraminal encroachment further diminish the caliber of the foramen leading to the additional cumulative affects of repeated nerve root compression.

VERTEBRAL ARTERY AND TRANSVERSE FORAMEN COMPRESSION

Osteophytic protrusions into the foramina transversalis can result in compression of the vertebral artery (123,132). This occurs most commonly in the lower cervical spine (C5–C6–C7), corresponding to the area most frequently afflicted by joint spondylosis. The compression of the vertebral artery by posteriorly projecting uncovertebral spurs is increased by head rotation and neck hyperextension. In most situations, the natural flexibility of the arterial wall particularly in accommodating slowly developing compressions makes this condition only rarely symptomatic. Violent neck movements, however, can produce acute vertebral artery injuries as the vessel is suddenly stretched across tight osteophytic spurs.

Klippel-Feil Syndrome

The *Klippel-Feil syndrome* constitutes a group of congenital anomalies affecting the cervical vertebra (103). This generally includes the congenital fusion of vertebral bodies and posterior elements and may involve the partial loss of vertebral segments (hemivertebra). The abnormal mobility generally associated with this condition frequently leads to the development of motion segment instability and/or degenerative spondylosis at adjacent vertebral segments.

OSSIFICATION OF THE POSTERIOR LONGITUDINAL LIGAMENT

Ossification of the posterior longitudinal ligament, a nonspondylotic-related condition, occurs when the posterior longitudinal ligament progressively is replaced by bone (104–107). This process represents true ossification as Haverson canals are present in the ossified tissue. The etiology of this condition is unknown but it has a particularly high incidence in the Japanese population. It usually occurs beyond the age of 40 and tends to affect males more than females. It may involve the entire spine or be limited to two or three segments. The ossified posterior longitudinal ligament is frequently tightly adherent to the dura resulting in intraoperative dural compromise. It tends to affect the mid and upper cervical spine more frequently than the lower cervical spine, which is in contradistinction to spondylosis which more commonly affects the lower cervical spine. This condition much more frequently leads to a myelopathy than a radiculopathy.

INCIDENCE AND PREVALENCE OF CERVICAL SPONDYLOSIS

Cervical spondylosis is a common occurrence in the general population (108–116). Radiographic evidence of significant spondylosis can be found in 25–50% of people by age 50 and in 75–90% of people by age 65. Fortunately, little correlation exists between the presence of radiographic evidence of spondylosis and the presence or absence of symptomatology. There is an association between cervical and lumbar spondylosis such that those affected in the neck which have a two and a half times more likely chance of being affected in the lumbar region. There appears to be no sex predilection, but there is an increased incidence in those who use cigarettes, dive, engage in occupations that involve a great deal of driving, work with vibrating equipment, or do heavy manual labor.

Intervertebral disc spondylotic changes occur in order of decreasing frequency at the C5–6, C6–7, C4–5, C3–4, and C7–T1 interspaces, with 94% of spondylotic changes found at the lower three cervical segments (C4–5, C5–6, C6–7). This is thought to reflect the motion segments subjected to the most stress and strain. The apophyseal joints on the other hand are more commonly affected at the C2–3 and C3–4 levels.

Spondylotic myelopathy is the most common cause of spinal cord dysfunction over the age of 55. Unlike cervical spondylosis which shows no sex predilection, spondylotic myelopathy affects males 4:1. The direct cause-effect relationship between the spondylotic process and the development of a spondylotic myelopathy is so significant that compressive myelopathies not related to trauma or rheumatoid subluxation are quite rare above the C4 segment.

CLINICAL SYNDROMES

Presentation and Natural History

The clinical presentation of cervical spondylosis includes both radicular (95%) and myelopathic (5%) symptomatology (117–122).

Radiculopathy

The radiculopathy usually presents insidiously although an acute traumatic event may trigger the onset of difficulty even though this is not a primary factor. Fortunately, patients that initially present with a radiculopathy only rarely go on to develop a myelopathy. Unfortunately, two-thirds of patients with a radiculopathy will continue to remain symptomatic and only one-third will develop a spontaneous long term remission.

Myelopathy

A spondylotic myelopathy may present as a series of episodes each marking the appearance of new symptoms (75%), as insidiously progressing without remissions (20%), or as rapidly regressing followed by lengthy periods of remission (5%).

A myelopathy may initially appear alone, as a minor symptom in conjunction with a severe radiculopathy, or, most commonly, as a significant component of a mild or moderate myeloradiculopathy. Once the symptoms of a myelopathy have occurred, a complete remission almost never occurs; in fact, even a significant improvement of neurologic deficits (particularly the motor abnormalities) is quite uncommon. Following presentation and initial conservative treatment, most patients with a spondylotic myelopathy suffer through long periods of nonprogressive disability with a minority suffering continued progressive deterioration.

Those patients, however, presenting with the most marked myelopathic findings in association with drastically reduced spinal canal dimensions over several levels may expect a steadily progressive course of deterioration.

CLINICAL PRESENTATION

Spondylotic Radiculopathy

The majority (95%) of patients with cervical spondylosis present with and experience only nonmyelopathic symptomatology (123–137). The natural history of radicular symptomatology is as follows:

Initial Symptoms (age 20–30)

Initial symptoms, age 20–30, are acute episodic unilateral neck pain with muscle spasm aggravated by movement with resolution in 4–7 days.

Progressing Symptoms (age 30–40)

Progressing symptoms, age 30–40, are poorly localized but radicular type pain that is too diffuse for radiculopathic localization; deep aching, primarily proximal pain (scapular) associated with distal tingling; and pain lasting for weeks at a time.

Advanced Symptoms (Age 40–50)

Advanced symptoms, age 40–50, are chronic, deep, poorly localized, aching pain (proximal greater than distal) with paravertebral muscle spasm; radicular numbness and tingling (distal greater than proximal); and episodes of motor-reflex loss which accurately define the affected root(s).

Chronic Symptoms (age 60–70)

Chronic symptoms, age 60–70, are steady, severe, suboccipital, interscapular, or shoulder pain; and severe radiculopathic symptomatology, but, as the root loses function, the radicular pain resolves spontaneously.

Spondylotic Myelopathy

Initial Symptoms

Initial symptoms are stiffness, heaviness, and weakness in legs associated with cramping, muscle spasms, and easy fatigue ability.

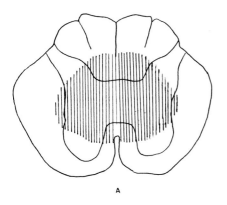
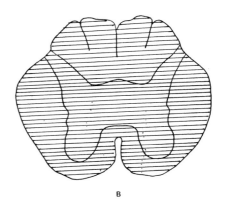
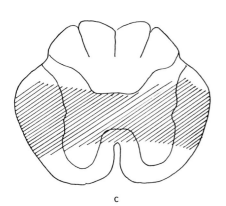
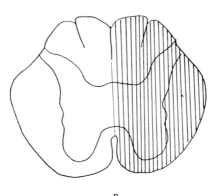
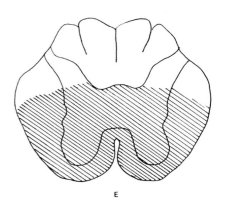

FIG. 6. Myelopathic syndromes associated with cervical spondylosis. **A:** Central cord syndrome. **B:** Transverse lesion. **C:** Motor system involvement. **D:** Brown-Sequard syndrome. **E:** Anterior cord syndrome.

Progressive Symptoms

Progressive symptoms are upper motor neuron dysfunction; and spastic paraparesis with increased reflexes, clonus, and extensor plantar response.

Advanced Symptoms

Advanced symptoms are a combination of upper and lower motor neuron findings.

Chronic Symptoms

Chronic symptoms are marked weakness, atrophy, spasticity, or diminished reflexes.

Several different spinal cord syndromes can be recognized in spondylotic myelopathy (Fig. 6): central cord syndrome (lower motor neuron lesion in upper extremities out of proportion to upper motor neuron lesion in lower extremities), transverse lesion (combined corticospinal, spinothalamic, and dorsal column involvement), motor system involvement (combined corticospinal and anterior horn cell involvement), Brown-Sequard's syndrome (hemicord symptomatology), and anterior cord syndrome (preservation of the posterior columns).

ASSOCIATED SPONDYLOTIC SYMPTOMATOLOGY

Axial symptoms are headache, neck pain, occipital neuralgia, lump in throat, or dysphasia.

Neural symptoms may include autonomic symptoms—sweating, flushing, dizziness, lacrimation, nausea, and vomiting, etc.

Vascular symptoms (vertebral artery symptoms) are vertigo, dizziness, diplopia, homonymous hemianopsia, hemisensorimotor syndromes, ataxia, and drop attacks.

PHYSICAL SIGNS OF SPONDYLOSIS

Neck Range of Motion

The cervical spine range of motion should be examined actively, passively, and against resistance. Asymptomatic or pain-producing limitations of motion are evidence of motion segment(s) spondylosis.

Radicular and Cord Compression Signs

Neck Compression Test

Radicular symptoms are produced by laterally flexing, slightly rotating, and compressing the patient's head.

Spurling Sign

The production of radicular symptoms occurs with hyperextension and contralateral rotation of the neck.

Lhermitte's Sign

An axial shock-like discomfort or extremity tingling is produced by head and neck full flexion or extension.

Babinski's and Hoffmann's Signs

Babinski's and Hoffmann's signs are the combination of lower motor neuron involvement at the level of the lesion (atrophy of muscle with absent or diminished reflex) and upper motor neuron findings below the level of the lesion (hyperreflexia and gait disturbance); flaccidity and atrophy of upper extremity muscles, especially intrinsic hand muscles; and upper motor neuron involvement with lower extremity spasticity and increased reflexes.

Inverted Radial Reflex

Diminished brachial radialis reflex (lower motor neuron, C6) is associated with flexion of the fingers (upper motor neuron involvement below the lesion).

Valsalva's Test

Radicular symptomatology is produced by maneuvers that increase intraabdominal pressure.

Axial Manual Traction Test

Radicular symptoms are improved by 10–15 lb of axial traction.

Shoulder Abduction Tests

Radicular symptoms are improved by elevating the hand over the patient's head in a sitting position.

Sensory, Motor, and Reflex Abnormalities

Radiculopathy

Sensory abnormalities are radicular loss of sensory function (dorsal column and/or spinothalamic) and dissociated sensory loss (dorsal column on one side and spinothalamic on the other).

Motor and reflex abnormalities are loss of dexterity in the arms or hands (difficulty writing or buttoning clothes); and muscle atrophy, weakness, or diminished reflex in appropriate radicular distribution.

Myelopathy

Abnormalities are difficulty walking, unsteadiness, and diminished balance; a broad-based, unsteady gait; clonus; and jaw reflexes that remain normal with diminished abdominal reflexes.

Myelopathic gait abnormalities are classified as follows (137): grade 0, root signs and symptoms only—no evidence of cord involvement; grade I, signs of cord involvement but normal gait; grade II, mild gait involvement but able to be employed; grade III, gait abnormality prevents employment; grade IV, able to ambulate only with assistance; and grade V, chair bound or bedridden.

DIFFERENTIAL DIAGNOSIS

A number of common disorders affecting the cervical spine may resemble the symptoms of cervical spondylosis. These disorders include cervical spine musculo-ligamentous strain with hyperflexion or hyperextension injury; cervical spine fracture; rheumatoid arthritis; ankylosing spondylitis; vertebral osteomyelitis; compressive neuropathy (such as thoracic outlet syndrome, carpal tunnel syndrome, ulnar neuropathy, etc.); bursitis, arthritis, neuritis, myositis, etc.; acromioclavicular joint pain; temporomandibular joint pain (TMJ); tumor invading the apex of the lung (Pancoast's tumor); brachial plexus tumor; pain related to intraabdominal organs (diaphragm, gall bladder, pancreas, etc.); metastatic disease; carotid and vertebral artery atherosclerosis; aneurysm of the aortic arch; spasmodic torticollis; psychiatric illness; and malingering.

In addition, the symptoms of other conditions may resemble the initial symptoms of myelopathy. These include multiple sclerosis, amyotrophic lateral sclerosis (ALS), low-pressure (communicating) hydrocephalus, cerebrovascular disease (stroke, TIA, etc.), and spinal cord tumor.

DIAGNOSTIC TESTS

Plain Radiographs

A thorough cervical spine radiographic evaluation for spondylosis includes anterior-posterior, lateral, open mouth, and oblique films, as well as flexion and extension views (138–140). The normal sagittal diameter of the lower cervical canal (C3–C7) is 17 ± 1 mm. A sagittal diameter of ≤12 mm is critical to the production of a cervical myelopathy. In fact, in a patient with myelopathy, if the minimal sagittal diameter at every level in the cervical spine is >13 mm on plain lateral views, then it is unlikely that a spondylotic process is responsible.

A helpful formula to estimate the cervical sagittal canal diameter on any lateral cervical spine film (regardless of magnification factors) is Pavlov's ratio (140): AP canal diameter = AP body diameter, and

$$\frac{\text{AP diameter spinal canal}}{\text{AP diameter body}} = 1$$

so, at 0.8 or less there is a small canal.

Radionucleid Bone Scan

Cervical spine radionucleid scanning has little application in the evaluation of pathology in the spondylotic spine. This test is helpful, however, in evaluating the presence and extent of metastatic disease as a possible cause of neck pain.

Computed Tomography

Cervical computed axial tomography (CAT) provides a better definition of normal bone structures and bony abnormalities than any other diagnostic modality (141–153). It provides accurate information regarding the size and shape of the spinal canal. In addition, it is very helpful in the patient with associated traumatic laminar or posterior element fractures. Axial, sagittal, coronal, oblique, and three-dimensional images are presently available (Fig. 7).

Myelography

Since the introduction of the nonionic contrast agents (iopamidol and iohexol), myelography has be-

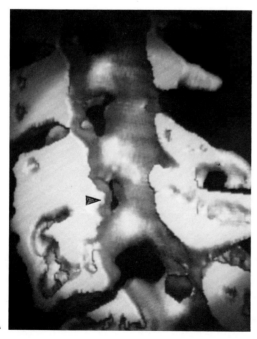
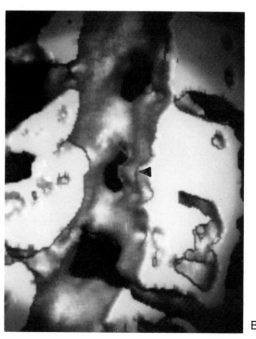

A

B

FIG. 7. Three-dimensional CT images of a severely spondylotic intervertebral foramina. **A:** Left. **B:** Right. Compare the affected foramen *(arrows)* to normal foramen below.

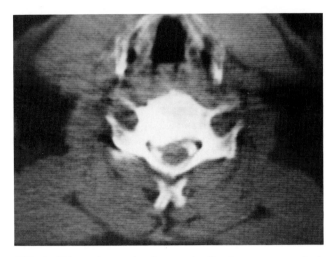

FIG. 8. CT-myelography demonstrating large paracentral and foraminal spur distorting the spinal cord.

come the diagnostic modality of choice for patients with radiculopathic or myelopathic symptomatology (154–157). The addition of computed tomography to myelography makes this the single most formative method in this condition (Fig. 8). This test provides the following major advantages over other diagnostic tests: demonstrates excellent bony detail, permits precise visualization of the spinal cord in the axial plane, and relates the size and shape of the spinal cord to the size and shape of the spinal canal.

Magnetic Resonance Imaging

Magnetic resonance imaging (MRI) is rapidly becoming the primary diagnostic modality of choice for patients with cervical spondylotic radiculopathy and myelopathy (158–173) (Fig. 9). The T1-images are most sensitive in providing anatomical detail, whereas the T2-images are most sensitive to pathological changes within the spinal cord. Intrinsic spinal cord pathology such as intramedullary syringomyelia, hematoma, edema, infarction, or tumor can be precisely defined only by this test.

In the myelopathic patient, an MRI may show spinal cord changes at the level of compression consistent with myelomalacia or lesions consistent with cystic necrosis and syrinx formation. These changes may be confined to the level of compression or extend longitudinally up and down the spinal canal. Dynamic MRI can also be used to identify motion changes affecting the spinal cord; sagittal flexion and extension views are able to show the mechanisms of neural compression. Finally, MRI is as good as radionucleid bone scanning or gadolinium scanning in detecting osteomyelitis and discitis.

The current preoperative evaluation of radiculopathy and myelopathy should demand a precise anatomical demonstration of both the compressive spondylotic agents as well as the compressed neural or vascular structures. Plain film radiography, MRI, and/ or computed tomography (CT) myelography are presently the commonly available diagnostic modalities of choice. At present, nearly all soft disc herniations can be precisely localized by MRI, forming the basis for surgical strategies. Spondylotic compressions on the other hand are generally not fully defined by MRI, requiring the addition of CT myelography prior to surgical intervention.

Physiological Testing

Physiological testing includes electromyogram (EMG) and somatosensory evoked potentials (SSEP) (175–181). EMG can be helpful to confirm the presence of injured axons indicative of a nerve root injury secondary to a compressive radiculopathy. With EMG, the presence of fibrillation implies dead axons and an

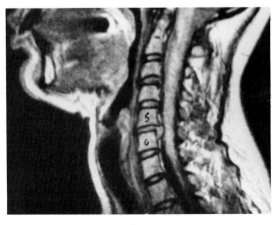
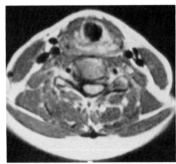
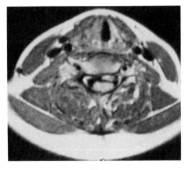

A   B   C

FIG. 9. MRI demonstrating large soft disc extrusion. **A:** Sagittal image. **B and C:** Coronal images.

associated nerve root injury, whereas the presence of the H-reflex suggests a compromise of interneurons acting on spinal cord motor neurons indicative of spondylotic compression of the gray matter.

Recent refinements including SSEP can be used to differentiate a radiculopathy and myelopathy or decide upon the level of involvement. Motor evoked potentials (MEP) are also recently available. The combination of these tests may help differentiate root, plexus, peripheral nerve, and muscle disorders which may at times mimic a radiculopathy. They also may uncover associated co-existing problems.

TREATMENT

Conservative

The following nonoperative modalities are helpful in the treatment of cervical spondylotic disease with or without associated radiculopathy and myelopathy (see Chapter 15.): nonsteroidal antiinflammatory medications, analgesics, muscle relaxants, immobilization with a soft collar, heat treatment, ultrasound, massage, TENS unit, axial traction, and exercise.

A majority of patients with spondylotic radiculopathy or myelopathy will improve symptomatically at least initially with conservative treatment. The improvement in myelopathic patients can only be anticipated if the symptoms have been present for ≤2 years.

The decision to proceed with operative treatment must be firmly based on a clear concept of the origin of pain whether it be root, cord, disc, facet, foramen, spur, ridge, etc. The indications for a surgical procedure in patients with cervical spondylosis are disabling persistent and progressive or recurrent neck pain in the absence of neurologic signs in patients who have failed conservative treatment over an extended period (plateau pain without neurologic deficit is not an indication for surgery); neck pain and radiculopathic pain with or without neurological signs unresponsive to conservative measures; acute monoradiculopathy due to root compression with appropriate sensory, motor, and reflex changes; symptomatology occurring as a result of cervical myelopathy; dysphasia (very rare); and symptoms of vertebral artery ischemia due to foramen transversalis stenosis.

REFERENCES

Etiology of Spondylosis

1. Brain R. Cervical spondylosis. *Ann Intern Med* 41:439–441, 1954.
2. Brain L, Wilkinson M. *Cervical spondylosis and other disorders of the cervical spine.* 1st ed. Philadelphia: W.B. Saunders, 226, 1967.
3. Adams P, Eyre DR, Muir H. Biochemical aspects of development and aging of human intervertebral discs. *Rheumatol Rehabil* 16:22–29, 1977.
4. Coventry MB, Ghormley RK, Kernohan JW. The intervertebral disc: Its microscopic anatomy and pathology: III. Changes in the intervertebral disc concomitant with age. *J Bone Joint Surg [AM]* 27, 1945.
5. Ehni G. *Cervical arthrosis. Diseases of the cervical motion segments (spondylosis, disk rupture, radiculopathy, and myelopathy).* Chicago: Year Book Medical Publishers, 1984.
6. Ehni B, Ehni G, Patterson RH. Extradural spinal cord and nerve root compression from benign lesions of the cervical area. In: Youmans JR., ed. Philadelphia: W.B. Saunders, 2878–2917, 1990.
7. Hendry N. The hydration of the nucleus pulposus. *J Bone Joint Surg [Br]* 40B:132–144, 1968.
8. Hickey SD, Huckins DW. Relation between the structure of the annulus fibrosis and the function and failure of the intervertebral disc. *Spine* 5:106, 1980.
9. Lipson SJ, Muir H. Experimental intervertebral disc degeneration: morphological and proteoglycan changes over time. *Arthritis Rheum* 24:12–21, 1981.
10. Lipson SJ, Muir H. Proteoglycans in experimental intervertebral disc degeneration. *Spine* 6:194–210, 1984.
11. Murphey R, Semmes J. Ruptured cervical discs. *Am Surg* 32:83, 1966.
12. Oda J, Tanaka H, Tsuzuki N. Intervertebral disc changes with aging of human cervical vertebra from the neonate to the 80s. *Spine* 13:1205–1211, 1988.
13. Payne EE, Spillane JD. The cervical spine: an anatomical pathological study of 70 specimens using a special technique with particular reference to the problems of cervical spondylosis. *Brain* 80:471–596, 1957.
14. Pemberton R. *Arthritis and rheumatoid conditions: their nature and treatment.* Philadelphia: Lea and Febiger, 156, 1929.
15. Penning L. *Functional pathology of the cervical spine.* Baltimore: Williams and Wilkins, 1968.
16. Rothman, Simeone: *The spine. Volumes I and II.* Philadelphia: WB Saunders, 1975.
17. Sokoloff L. Remodeling of articular cartilage. In: Schattesskirchner M, ed. *Rheumatology. Volume 7.* Basel: S Karger, 11, 1982.
18. Spurling RG. *Lesions of the cervical intervertebral disc.* Springfield IL: Charles C. Thomas, 1956.
19. Symonds CP. The interrelation of trauma and cervical spondylosis in compression of the cervical cord. *Lancet* 1:451–454, 1953.
20. Wilkinson M. *Cervical spondylosis.* 2nd ed. Philadelphia: WB Saunders, 1–9, 1971.

Pathophysiology of Myelopathy

21. Bohlman HH. Cervical spondylosis with moderate to severe myelopathy: a report of seventeen cases treated by Robinson anterior cervical discectomy and fusion. *Spine* 2:151–161, 1977.
22. Bohlman HH, Emery SE. The pathophysiology of cervical spondylosis and myelopathy. *Spine* 13:843–846, 1988.
23. Clark E, Robinson PK. Cervical myelopathy. A complication of cervical spondylosis. *Brain* 79:483, 1956.
24. Crandall PH, Batzdorf U. Cervical spondylotic myelopathy. *J Neurosurg* 25:57–66, 1966.
25. Epstein JA, Davidoff LM. Chronic hypertrophic spondylosis of the cervical spine with compression of the spinal cord and its nerve roots. *Surg Gynecol Obstet* 93:27–39, 1951.
26. Epstein JA, Carras LA, Epstein BS, et al. Myelopathy in cervical spondylosis hyperlordosis. *J Neurosurg* 32:421–426, 1970.
27. Epstein JA, Carras R, Hyman RA, Costa S. Cervical myelopathy caused by developmental stenosis of the spinal canal. *J Neurosurg* 51:362–367, 1979.
28. Ferguson RT, Caplan LR. Cervical spondylitic myelopathy. *Neurol Clin* 3:373–382, 1985.

29. Gooding MR. Pathogenesis of myelopathy in cervical spondylosis. *Lancet* 2:1180–1181, 1974.
30. Guidetti B, Fortuna A, et al. Cervical spondylosis myelopathy. In: Grote W, et al., eds. *Advances in neurosurgery 8.* New York: Springer-Verlag, 104–111, 1980.
31. Hoff JT, Wilson CB. The pathophysiology of cervical spondylotic radiculopathy and myelopathy. *Clin Neurosurg* 24:474–487, 1977.
32. Hukuda S, Ogata M, Katsuura A. Experimental study on acute aggravating factors of cervical spondylotic myelopathy. *Spine* 13:15–20, 1988.
33. Lindblom K. Intervertebral disc degeneration considered as a pressure atrophy. *J Bone Joint Surg [AM]* 39A:933–945, 1957.
34. Liversedge LA, Hutchinson EC, Lyons JB. Cervical spondylosis simulating motor neurone disease. *Lancet* 2:652–659, 1953.
35. Mair WGP, Druckman R. The pathology of spinal cord lesions and their relation to the clinical features in protrusion of cervical intervertebral disks. *Brain* 76:70–91, 1953.
36. Nurick S. Pathogenesis of the cervical spinal cord disorder associated with cervical spondylosis. *Brain* 95:87–100, 1972.
37. O'Connell JEA. Involvement of the spinal cord by intervertebral disc protrusions. *Br J Surg* 43:225–247, 1955.
38. Ono K, Ota H, Tada K, Yamamoto T. Cervical myelopathy secondary to multiple spondylotic protrusions, a clinicopathologic study. *Spine* 2:109, 1977.
39. Phillips DG. Surgical treatment of myelopathy with cervical spondylosis. *J Neurol Neurosurg Psychiatry* 36:879–884, 1973.
40. Robinson RA, Afeiche N, Dunn EJ, Northrup BE. Cervical spondylotic myelopathy: etiology and treatment concepts. *Spine* 2:89–99, 1977.
41. Scoville WB. Cervical spondylosis treated by bilateral fascectomy and laminectomy. *Neurosurgery* 18:423–428, 1961.
42. Schneider RC, Cherry G, Pantek H. Syndrome of acute central cervical spinal cord injury with special reference to the mechanisms involved in hyperextension injuries of the cervical spine. *J Neurosurg* 11:546–577, 1954.
43. Schneider RC. Treatment of cervical spine disease. In: *Correlative neurosurgery.* 3rd ed. Springfield, IL: Charles C. Thomas, 1094–1174, 1982.
44. Taylor AR. Mechanism and treatment of spinal cord disorders associated with cervical spondylosis. *Lancet* 1:717–720, 1953.

Pathophysiology

Canal Size

45. Arnold JG Jr. The clinical manifestations of spondylochrondrosis (spondylosis) of the cervical spine. *Ann Surg* 141:872–889, 1955.
46. Burrows EH. The sagittal diameter of the spinal canal in cervical spondylosis. *Clin Radiol* 14:77–85, 1963.
47. Chrispin AR, Lees F. The spinal canal in cervical spondylosis. *J Neurol Neurosurg Psychiatry* 26:166–170, 1963.
48. Edwards WC, LaRocca H. The development segmented sagittal diameter of the cervical spinal canal in patients with cervical spondylosis. *Spine* 8:20–27, 1983.
49. Ehni G. Developmental variations, including shallowness, of the cervical spinal canal. In: Post JD, ed. *Radiographic evaluation of the spine.* New York: Masson, 469–474, 1980.
50. Epstein JA, Carras R, Hyman RA, Costa S. Cervical myelopathy caused by developmental stenosis of the spinal canal. *J Neurosurg* 51:362–367, 1979.
51. Estrin T, Crandall PH. Cervical spondylitic radiculopathy and myelopathy. A long-term follow-up study. *Arch Neurol* 33:618–625, 1976.
52. Mair WGP, Druckman R. The pathology of spinal cord lesions and their relation to the clinical features in protrusions of cervical intervertebral discs. *Brain* 76:70, 1953.
53. Moiel RH, Raso E, Waltz TA. Central cord syndrome resulting from congenital narrowness of the cervical spinal canal. *J Trauma* 10:502–510, 1970.
54. Nordquist L. The sagittal diameter of the spinal cord and subarachnoid space in different age groups. *Acta Radiol [Suppl]* 227:1–96, 1964.
55. Ogino H, Tada K, Okada K, Yonenobu K, Yamamoto T, Ono K, Namiki H. Canal diameter, anteroposterior compression ratio, and spondylotic myelopathy of the cervical spine. *Spine* 8:1–15, 1983.
56. Ono K, Ota H, Tada K, Yamamoto T. Cervical myelopathy secondary to multiple spondylotic protrusions: a clinico-pathologic study. *Spine* 2:109–125, 1977.
57. Penning L. *Functional pathology of the cervical spine.* Baltimore: Williams and Wilkins, 1968.
58. Torg JS, Pavlov H, Genuario SE, Sennett B, Wisneski RJ, Robie BH, Jahre C. Neuropraxia of the cervical spinal cord with transient quadriplegia. *J Bone Joint Surg [Am]* 68A:1354–1370, 1986.
59. Wilkinson HA, LeMay ML, Ferris EJ. Roentgenographic correlations in cervical spondylosis. *Am J Roentgenol* 105:370–374, 1969.
60. Wilkinson M. *Cervical spondylosis: its early diagnosis and treatment.* 2nd ed. Philadelphia: W.B. Saunders, 1971.
61. Wolf BS, Khilnani M, Malis L. Sagittal diameter of the bony cervical spinal canal and its significance in cervical spondylosis. *Mt Sinai J Med (NY)* 23:283–292, 1956.
62. Verbiest H. Further experiences on the pathological influence of a developmental narrowness of the bony lumbar vertebral canal. *J Bone Joint Surg [Br]* 37B:576–583, 1955.

Vascular Factor

63. Brieg A, Turnbull IM, Hassler O. Effects of mechanical stresses on the spinal cord in cervical spondylosis: a study of fresh cadaver material. *J Neurosurg* 25:45, 1966.
64. Brieg A. *Adverse mechanical tension in the central nervous system.* 2nd ed. New York: John Wiley & Sons, 264, 1978.
65. Doppman JL. The mechanism of ischemia in anteroposterior compression of the spinal cord. *Invest Radiol* 10:543, 1975.
66. Gooding MR. Pathogenesis of myelopathy in cervical spondylosis. *Lancet* 2:1180–1181, 1974.
67. Gooding MR, Wilson CB, Hoff JT. Experimental cervical myelopathy: Effects of ischemia and compression of the canine cervical spinal cord. *J Neurosurg* 43:9–17, 1975.
68. Hoff J, Nishimura M, Pitts L, Vilnis V, Tuerk K, Lagger R. The role of ischemia in the pathogenesis of cervical spondylotic myelopathy: a review and new microangiographic evidence. *Spine* 2:100–108, 1977.
69. Hutchinson EC, Yates PO. The cervical portion of the vertebral artery. A clinicopathological study. *Brain* 79:319–330, 1956.
70. Hukuda S, Wilson C. Experimental cervical myelopathy: Effects of compression and ischemia on the canine cervical cord. *J Neurosurg* 37:631–652, 1972.
71. Jellinger K. Spinal cord arterioscleroses and progressive vascular myelopathy. *J Neurol Neurosurg Psychiatry* 30:195–206, 1967.
72. Mannen T. Vascular lesions in the spinal cord of the aged. *Geriatrics* 21:151–160, 1966.
73. Schneider RC. The syndrome of acute anterior spinal cord injury. *J Neurosurg* 12:95–122, 1955.
74. Schneider RC, Thompson JM, Bebin J. The syndrome of acute central cervical cord injury. *J Neurol Neurosurg Psychiatry* 21:216–227, 1958.
75. Shimomura Y, Hukuda S, Mizuno S. Experimental study of ischemic damage to the cervical spinal cord. *J Neurosurg* 28:565–581, 1968.
76. Suh TH, Alexander L. Vascular system of the human spinal cord. *Arch Neurol Psychiatry* 41:659–677, 1939.
77. Taylor AR. Vascular factors in the myelopathy associated with cervical spondylosis. *Neurology* 14:62–68, 1964.
78. Turnbull IM, Breig A, Hassler O. Blood supply of cervical spinal cord in man: a microangiographic cadaver study. *J Neurosurg* 24:951–955, 1966.
79. Turnbull IM. Microvasculature of the human spinal cord. *J Neurosurg* 35:141–147, 1971.

Biomechanics

80. Adams CBT, Logue V. Studies in cervical spondylotic myelopathy: I. Movement of the cervical roots, dura and cord, and their relation to the course of the extrathecal roots. *Brain* 94:557–568, 1971.
81. Adams CBT, Logue V. Studies in cervical spondylotic myelopathy: II. The movement and contour of the spine in relation to the neural complications of cervical spondylosis. *Brain* 94:569, 1971.
82. Brief A. *Biomechanics of the central nervous system.* Stockholm: Almquist & Wicksell, 1960.
83. Brief A. *Adverse mechanical tension in the central nervous system.* Stockholm: Almquist & Wicksell, 1978.
84. Kirkaldy-Willes WH, Dupries PR, Yong-Hing K. Biomechanics and aging of the spine. In: Youman JR, ed. *Neurological surgery. Volume 3.* Philadelphia: WB Saunders, 2605–2628, 1990.
85. Murone I. The importance of the sagittal diameters of the cervical spinal canal in relation to spondylosis and myelopathy. *J Bone Joint Surg [Br]* 56B:30–36, 1974.
86. Nugent GR. Clinico-pathologic correlations in cervical spondylosis. *Neurology* 9:273, 1959.
87. Panjabi MM, Pelker RR, White AA. Biomechamics of the spine. In: *Neurosurgery.* Wilkins & Rengachary McGraw-Hill, 2219–2228, 1985.
88. Panjabi M, White A. Biomechanics of nonacute cervical spinal cord trauma. *Spine* 13:838–842, 1988.
89. Penning L, van der Zwaag P. Biomechanical aspects of spondylotic myelopathy. *Acta Radiol* 5:1090–1103, 1966.
90. Raynor RB, Koplik B. Cervical cord trauma: the relationship between clinical syndromes and force of injury. *Spine* 10:193–197, 1985.
91. Schneider RC. The syndrome of acute anterior spinal cord injury. *J Neurosurg* 12:95, 1955.
92. Taylor AR. The mechanism of injury to the spinal cord in the neck without damage to the vertebral column. *J Bone Joint Surg [Br]* 33B:543, 1951.
93. White AA, Johnson, RM, Panjabi MM, Southwick, WO. Biomechanical analysis of clinical stabilization in the cervical spine. *Clin Orthop Rel Res* 109:85–96, 1975.
94. White AA, Panjabi MM. *Clinical biomechanics of the spine.* JB Lippincott, 1978.
95. White AA, Panjabi MM. Biomechanical considerations in the surgical management of cervical spondylotic myelopathy. *Spine* 13:856–860, 1981.

Radiculopathy

96. Dillin W, Booth R, Cuckler J, Balderston R, Simeone F, Rothman R. Cervical radiculopathy: a review. *Spine* 11:988–991, 1986.
97. Epstein JA, Epstein BS, Lavine LS, et al. Clinical monoradiculopathy caused by arthrotic hypertrophy. *J Neurosurg* 49:387, 1978.
98. Gregorius FK, Estrin T, Crandall PH. Cervical spondylotic radiculopathy and myelopathy. *Arch Neurol* 33:618–625, 1976.
99. Hoff JT, Wilson CB. The pathophysiology of cervical spondylotic radiculopathy and myelopathy. *Clin Neurosurg* 24:474–487, 1977.
100. Mitchell PEG, Hendry NGC, Billewicz WZ. The chemical background of intervertebral disk prolapse. *J Bone Joint Surg [Br]* 43B:141–151, 1961.
101. Mixter WJ, Barr JS. Rupture of the intervertebral disk with involvement of the spinal canal. *N Engl J Med* 211:210–215, 1934.
102. Spurling RG, Scoville WB. Lateral rupture of cervical intervertebral discs: common cause of shoulder and arm pain. *Surg Gynecol Obstet* 78:350–358, 1944.

OpII and Klippel-Feil Syndrome

103. Avery LW, Rentfro CC. The Klippel-Feil syndrome: a pathological report. *Arch Neurol Psychol* 36:1068, 1936.
104. Bakay L. Ossification of the posterior longitudinal ligament. *Neurosurgery* 288:2243–2244, 1985.
105. Hirabayashi K, Miyakawa J, Satomi K, et al. Operative results and postoperative progression of ossification among patients with ossification of cervical posterior longitudinal ligament. *Spine* 6:354–364, 1981.
106. Miyazaki K, Kirita Y. Extensive simultaneous multisegment laminectomy for myelopathy due to the ossification of the posterior longitudinal ligament in the cervical region. *Spine* 11:531–542, 1986.
107. Nagashima C. Cervical myelopathy due to ossification of the posterior longitudinal ligament. *J Neurosurg* 37:653–660, 1972.

Incidence

108. Anehnig. *Cervical arthrosis diseases of the cervical motion segments.* Chicago: Yearbook Medical Publisher, 1984.
109. Friedenberg Z, Miller W. Degenerative disc disease of the cervical spine. *J Bone Joint Surg [Am]* 45A:1171–1175, 1963.
110. Gore DR, Sepic SB, Gardner GM. Radiographic findings of the cervical spine in asymptomatic people. *Spine* 11:521–524, 1986.
111. Holt S, Yates PO. Cervical spondylosis and nerve root lesions: Incidence and routine necropsy. *J Bone Joint Surg [Br]* 48B:407, 1966.
112. Kelsey J, Githens P, Walter SD, et al. An epidemiological study of acute prolapse cervical intervertebral disc. *J Bone Joint Surg [Am]* 66A:907–914, 1984.
113. Lunsford L, Bissonette B, et al. Anterior surgery for cervical disc disease. *J Neurosurg* 53:1–111, 1980.
114. Murphey F, Simmons JCH, Brunson B. Ruptured cervical discs, 1939–1972. *Clin Neurosurg* 20:9–17, 1973.
115. Nakano N, Nakano T. Relationship between osteophytes and symptoms in cervical spondylosis in the cervical spine. *Spine* 1:148–152, 1987.
116. Pallis C, Jones AM, Spillane JD. Cervical spondylosis, incidence and implications. *Brain* 77:274–289, 1954.

Natural History

117. Gregorius FK, Estrin T, Crandall PH. Cervical spondylotic radiculopathy and myelopathy: a long-term followup study. *Arch Neurol* 33:618–625, 1976.
118. LaRocca H. Cervical spondylotic myelopathy: natural history. *Spine* 13:854–855, 1988.
119. Lees F, Turner JWA. Natural history and prognosis of cervical spondylosis. *Br Med J* 2:1607–1610, 1963.
120. Murphey F, Simmons JCH. Ruptured cervical discs: experience with 250 cases. *Am J Surg* 32:83–88, 1966.
121. Symon L, Lavender P. The surgical treatment of cervical spondylotic myelopathy. *Neurology* 17:117–127, 1967.
122. Nurick S. The natural history and the results of surgical treatment of the spinal cord disorder associated with cervical spondylosis. *Brain* 95:101–108, 1972.

Symptomatology

123. Bakey L, Leslie EV. Surgical treatment of vertebral artery insufficiency caused by cervical spondylosis. *J Neurosurg* 23:596–602, 1965.
124. Brain WR, Northfield D, Wilkinson M. The neurological manifestations of cervical spondylosis. *Brain* 75:187–225, 1952.
125. Clark CR. Cervical spondylotic myelopathy: history and physical findings. *Spine* 13:847–849, 1988.
126. Cusick JF. Monitoring of cervical spondylotic myelopathy. *Spine* 13:877–880, 1988.

127. Edwards WC, La Rocca SH. The developmental segmental sagittal diameter in combined cervical and lumbar spondylosis. *Spine* 10:42–49, 1985.
128. Facer JA. Osteophytes of the cervical spine causing dysphagia. *Arch Otolaryngol* 86:341–345, 1967.
129. Fantis A. Spinal symptoms accompanying cervical root compression syndromes. In: Grote W, et al., eds. *Advances in Neurosurgery. Volume 8*. New York: Springer-Verlag, 47–49, 1980.
130. Ferguson RJC, Caplan LR. Cervical spondylitic myelopathy. *Neur Clin North Am* 3:373–382, 1985.
131. Grain WR, Moorefield D, Wilkinson M. The neurological manifestations of cervical spondylosis. *Brain* 75:187–225, 1952.
132. Hardin CA, Williamson WP, Steegmann AT. Vertebral artery insufficiency produced by cervical osteoarthritic spurs. *Neurology* 10:855–858, 1960.
133. Hilding DA, Tachdjian MO. Dysphagia and hypertrophic spurring of the cervical spine. *N Engl J Med* 263:11, 1960.
134. McNab I. Symptoms in cervical disc degeneration. In: *Spine*. Philadelphia: JB Lippincott, 388–394, 1983.
135. Maran A, Jacobson I. Dysphagia associated with cervical spondylosis: cervical osteophytes presenting with pharyngeal symptoms. *Laryngoscope* 81:412, 1971.
136. Meeks LW, Renshaw TS. Ankylosing vertebral hyperostosis and dysphagia. In: Bailey RW, ed. *The cervical spine*. Philadelphia: Lea and Febiger, 242–249, 1974.
137. Nurick S. Classification of disability in spondylitic myelopathy: the natural history and the results of surgical treatment of the spinal cord disorder associated with cervical spondylosis. *Brain* 95:101, 1972.

Plain Films

138. McRae DL. The significance of abnormalities of the cervical spine. *Am J Roentgenol* 84:3–25, 1960.
139. Penning L. Some aspects of plain radiography of the cervical spine and chronic myelopathy. *Neurology* 12:513–519, 1962.
140. Torg JS, Pavlov H, Robie B, Jahre C. Pavlov's radio: a simplified, accurate and specific method for determining stenosis of the cervical spinal canal. Presented at the 15th annual meeting of the Cervical Spine Research Society, Washington DC, December 5, 1987.

CT/CT Myelography

141. Alker G. Neuroradiology of cervical spondylotic myelopathy. *Spine* 13:850–853, 1988.
142. Capesius P, Smaltino F, Kaiser M, Meoli S, Gambardella A. Computed tomography of the cervical spinal canal. *J Neurosurg Sci* 25:265–270, 1981.
143. Coin CG, Coin JT. Computed tomography of cervical disc disease: technical considerations with representative cases reports. *J Comput Assist Tomogr* 5:275–280, 1981.
144. Daniels DL, Grogan JP, Johansen JG, et al. Cervical radiculopathy: computed tomography and myelography compared. *Radiology* 151:109–113, 1984.
145. Fujiwara K, Yonenobu K, Hiroshima K, Ebara S, Yamashita K, Ono K. The morphometry of the cervical spinal cord and its relation to pathology in cases with compressive myelopathy. *Spine* 13:1212–1216, 1988.
146. Iwasaki Y, Abe H, Isu T, Miyasaka K. CT myelography with intramedullary enhancement in cervical spondylosis. *J Neurosurg* 63:363–366, 1985.
147. Kaiser MC, Capesius P. CT diagnosis of cervical hernias. In: *Cervical spine I*. Springer-Verlag, 93–96, 1987.
148. Miyasaka K, Isu T, Iwasaki Y, Abe S, Takei H, Tsuru M. High resolution computed tomography in the diagnosis of cervical disc disease. *Neurorad* 24:253–257, 1983.
149. Modic MT, Masaryk TJ, Mulopulous GP, et al. Cervical radiculopathy: prospective evaluation with surface coil MR imaging, CT with metrizamide and metrizamide myelography. *Radiology* 161:753–759, 1986.
150. Osborne DR, Heinz ER, et al. Role of computed tomography in the radiological evaluation of painful radiculopathy after negative myelography: foraminal neural entrapment. *Neurosurgery* 14:147–153, 1984.
151. Penning L, Wilmink JT, van Woerden HH, Knol E. CT myelographic findings in degenerative disorders of the cervical spine: clinical significance. *AJNR* 140:793–801, 1986.
152. Russell EJ, D'Angelo CM et al. Cervical disk herniation: CT demonstration after contrast enhancement. *Radiology* 152:703–712, 1984.
153. Thijssen HOM, Keyser A, Horstink MWM, et al. Morphology of the cervical spinal cord on computed myelography. *Neurorad* 18:57–62, 1979.

Myelography

154. Gebarski SS, Gabrielsen TO, Knake JE et al. Iohexol versus metrizamide for cervical myelography: double blind trial. *AJNR* 6:923–926, 1985.
155. Kaplan JO, Quencer RM, Stokes NA, Post JD. Improved technique for cervical metrizamide myelography. *Radiology* 135:519–520, 1980.
156. Marinacci AA. Correlation between the operative findings in cervical herniated discs with the electromyelograms and opaque myelograms with particular reference to simulators of root compression. *Bulletin LA Neurol Soc* 30:118–130, 1965.
157. Steinhausen, TD, Dungan CE, Furst JB, et al. Iodinated organic compounds as contrast media for radiographic diagnosis: III. Experimental and clinical myelography and iodophenylundecylate (Pantopaque). *Radiology* 43:230–235, 1944.

MRI

158. Al-Mefty O, Harkey LH, Middleton TH, Smith RR, Fox JL. Myelopathic cervical spondylotic lesions demonstrated by magnetic resonance imaging. *J Neurosurg* 68:217–222, 1968.
159. Clark CR, Igram CM, El-Khoury GY, Ehara S. Radiographic evaluation of cervical spine injuries. *Spine* 13:742–747, 1988.
160. Daniels D1, Hyde JS, Kneelon KN, et al. The cervical nerves and foramina: Local coil MR imaging. *AJNR* 7:129–133, 1980.
161. Dernbach PD, Weinstein MA, Little JR. Magnetic resonance imaging of spinal disorders. *Clin Neurosurg* 34:261–281, 1988.
162. Epstein NE, Hyman RA, Epstein JA, Rosenthal AD. Technical note: dynamic MRI scanning of the cervical spine. *Spine* 13:937–938, 1988.
163. Flanagan BD, Lufkin RB, McGlade C, et al. MR imaging of the cervical spine: neural vascular anatomy. *AJNR* 8:27–32, 1987.
164. Han JS, Kaufman B, El Youse SJ. NMR imaging of the spine. *AJNR* 141:1137–1145, 1983.
165. Heindel W, Friedmann G, Bonke J, et al. Artifacts in MR imaging after surgical intervention. *J Comput Assist Tomogr* 10:596–599, 1986.
166. Hyman RA, Edwards JE, Merten CW, Naidich JB, Vacirca ST, Stein HL. Evaluation of degenerative disease of the spine with MR imaging. *Radiology* 153:204, 1984.
167. Lyons CJ, Betz RR, Mesgarzadeh M, Revasz G, Bonakdarpour A, Clancy M. The effect of magnetic resonance imaging on metal spine implants. *Spine* 14:670–672, 1989.
168. McAfee PC, Bohlman HH, Han JS, Salvagno RT. Comparison of nuclear magnetic resonance imaging and computer tomography in the diagnosis of upper cervical spinal cord compression. *Spine* 11:295–304, 1986.
169. Modic MT, Weinstein MA, Pavlicek W, et al. Nuclear magnetic resonance imaging of the spine. *Radiology* 148:757–762, 1983.
170. Modic MT, Masaryk TJ, Ross JS, et al. Cervical radiography: value of oblique MR imaging. *Radiology* 163:227–231, 1987.

171. Norman D, Mills CM, Brant-Zawadzki M, Yeates A, Crooks LE, Kaufman L. Magnetic resonance imaging of the spinal cord and canal: potentials and limitations. *AJNR* 6:1147–1152, 1984.

172. Ross JS, Masaryk TJ, Modic MT. Postoperative cervical spine: MR assessment. *J Comput Assist Tomogr* 11:955–962, 1987.

173. Ullrich CG. Magnetic resonance imaging of the cervical spine and spinal cord. In: *Cervical Spine I*. Springer-Verlag, 97–101, 1987.

Angiography

174. DiChiro G, Fisher RL. Contrast radiography of the spinal cord. *Arch Neurol* 11:125–143, 1964.

EMG/SEP

175. Borromeo U, Cherubino P, Cosi V. Pre- and postoperative evaluation in patients affected by spondylotic myelopathy. In: *Cervical Spine II*. Springer-Verlag, 192–198, 1989.

176. Kotani H, Saiki K. Yamasaki H, Hattori S, Kawai S, Omote K. Evaluation of cervical cord function in cervical spondylitic myelopathy and/or radiculopathy using both segmental conductive spinal evoked potentials (SEP). *Spine* 11:185–190, 1986.

177. Matsukado Y, Yoshida M, Goya T, Shimosi K. Classification of cervical spondylosis or disc protrusion by preoperative evoked spinal electrogram. *J Neurosurg* 44:435–441, 1976.

178. Ryan TP, Britt RH. Spinal and cortical somatosensory evoked potential monitoring during corrective spinal surgery with 108 patients. *Spine* 11:352–361, 1986.

179. Satomi K, Okuma T, Kenmotsu K, Nakamura Y, Harabayashi K. Level diagnosis of cervical myelopathy using evoked spinal cord potentials. *Spine* 13:1217–1224, 1988.

180. Siivola J, Sulg I, Heiskari M. Somatosensory evoked potentials in diagnosis of cervical spondylosis and herniated disc. *Electroencephalogr Clin Neurophysiol* 52:276–282, 1981.

181. Yannikas C, Shahani BT, Young RR. Short latency somatosensory evoked potentials from radial, median, ulnar and peroneal nerve stimulation in the assessment of cervical spondylosis. *Arch Neurol* 43:1264–1271.

CHAPTER 5

Instrumentation and Use of the Operating Microscope as Applied to the Cervical Spine

Paul H. Young

It is clear that the skillful use of the operating microscope increases the precision of surgical procedures. The advantages of the operating microscope, including magnification (variable), stereoscopic vision (even through a small opening), improved lighting, and image duplication (real-time and recorded video, assistant arms, 35 mm photography), greatly enhance the ability of the surgeon to preserve the integrity of normal tissue. It is often suggested that operating loops can achieve these same results due to their ability to magnify tissue, but fixed magnification, the loss of stereoscopic vision (particularly in small openings), inadequate lighting, and the inability to use video attachments suggest the opposite. In this section, the principles and benefits of using the operating microscope for cervical spine procedures will be emphasized (1–3).

OPTICAL PRINCIPLES

The surgeon's ability to visualize normal and pathological anatomical structures is significantly enhanced by four properties of the operating microscope: *variable magnification, stereoscopic vision, coaxial illumination*, and *video/photographic duplication*.

Magnification

The overall magnification of objects viewed through the operating microscope depends on the eye piece magnification, the focal length of the microscope tube, the focal length of the objective, and the magnification

setting being used.

$$\text{actual magnification} = \frac{\text{tube length}}{\text{objective length}}$$
$$\times \text{ eyepiece magnification} \times \text{magnification setting}$$

Most cervical spine procedures are performed at a magnification of between four and twelve.

Stereoscopic Vision

Many procedures on the cervical spine take place in a limited field through a narrow opening and as a consequence it is essential that the surgeon maintain binocular, stereoscopic vision in the far depths of the operative field. Of the many advantages of the operating microscope, this is the most important for the cervical spine surgeon. The average interpupillary distance is ~60 mm so that the unaided eyes (even when using magnification loops) require a surgical opening of 60 mm in order to maintain stereoscopic vision. The distance between the anterior lens of the binocular tube, however, is only 16–24 mm so that the operating microscope may require only a 16 mm opening to permit stereoscopic vision. Thus, the operating microscope is able to preserve stereoscopic vision through very small openings by reducing the critical interpupillary distance necessary for binocular vision (Fig. 1).

Coaxial Illumination

Objects viewed through microscopes with coaxial illumination have light directed onto them along the

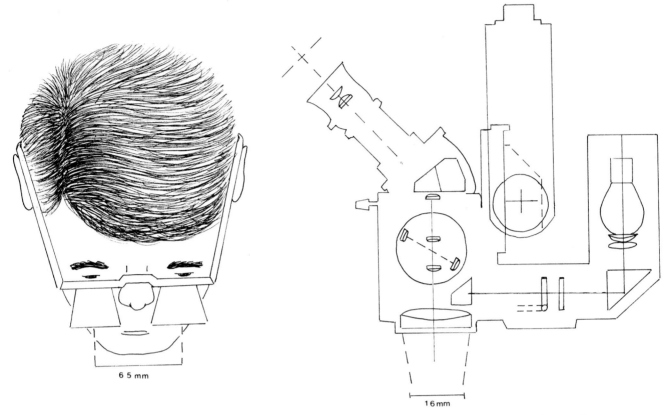

FIG. 1. Stereoscopic vision in a deep hole is possible only if the superficial opening is equal to the surgeon's interpupillary distance. The operating microscope decreases this distance (and the size of the opening) dramatically.

visual axis of the microscope. This type of lighting provides a sharply defined beam of light that is confined to the field of vision only, without the light scatter observed with the use of headlights (frequently used with loops).

Video/Photographic Duplication

Video and photographic attachments permit real-time and recorded reproductions of the surgical image. Real-time video (and assistant arms) enhance the ability of operating room nurses and assistant surgeons to participate in delicate procedures. The surgeon's ability to maintain precision through a long and tedious operative procedure is increased as a result of co-workers who can visualize every step and thus better assist with the procedure.

OPERATING MICROSCOPE COMPONENTS

Operating microscope components are shown in Fig. 2.

Eye Piece

Eye piece magnifications are 10, 12.5, 16, and 20. The 12.5 and 16 magnification eye pieces are most commonly used for cervical spine.

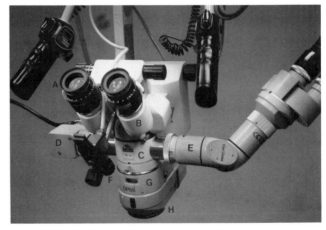

FIG. 2. Operating microscope components. **A:** Eye piece. **B:** Ocular. **C:** Beam splitter. **D:** Video camera. **E:** Assistant tube. **F:** Body. **G:** Magnification chamber. **H:** Objective.

Ocular

Prior to surgery, the surgeon should calibrate the eye pieces to his or her own visual correction and tape them in that position to prevent dislodgement by microscope movement and draping. If the surgeon does not use the ocular diapter adjustment, those attempting to view the procedure will not see a focused image and attempts at documentation through video recording or 35 mm photography will fail. In addition to the diapter adjustment, the ocular permits the surgeon to adjust to her or his own interpupillary distance.

Binocular tubes in straight, angled, and variable-angled types are available. The use of loops over long periods of time in the cervical spine force the surgeon to work with his or her neck in a somewhat flexed position, which is tedious and certainly uncomfortable. By adjusting the angle of the binocular tube from 90° to 190°, the surgeon can obtain comfortable neck positions for procedures on the cervical spine in the supine, prone, and even sitting positions.

Microscope Body

The microscope body contains the optical pathway and magnification chamber. The size and shape of the microscope body varies depending on the manufacturer. Each has a distinctive tube focal length, which is important in determining final magnification.

Magnification Chamber

The magnification chamber is either manually controlled by a control knob or automatically adjusted by a foot petal. Because the final image magnification is dependent upon other factors (including the tube focal length, objective distance, and eye piece magnification), the numbers inscribed on the magnification chamber seldom denote true magnification.

It is important to remember that the higher the magnification, the smaller the surgeon's field of vision.

Coaxial Illumination

Several types of illumination systems are available, including tungston, hallogen, and metal halide.

Tungston

The tungston incandescent light source utilizes either a 6 V–30 W or 6 V–50 W bulb.

Hallogen

The most commonly used light source today is the 12 V–100 W hallogen bulb. The hallogen source is mounted either directly on the microscope body or at some distance from it, with the light being transmitted through a fiber-optic cable.

Metal Halide

The most intense light available today is the 250 W metal halide lamp (Superlux 40) (Fig. 3). Light of this intensity has proven important in procedures using magnification through a small opening.

Objective Lens

The objective lens determines the focal length of the operating microscope, i.e., the distance between the lens and the operating field. This corresponds to the operating space available. Objectives are commonly available in focal lengths from 150 to 400. The 300 and 350 mm objectives are most applicable for a majority of cervical spine procedures. With a 300 mm objective, the focal length is 30 cm so that structures lying 10 cm below the surface of the skin can be reached while still maintaining a 20 cm gap between the surface of the skin and the operating microscope. In addition, the larger the objective focal length, the larger the diameter of illumination from coaxial light sources.

Beam Splitter

A beam splitter is frequently placed between the body of the microscope and the binocular tube. It consists of a set of mirrors that split the optical path into two beams without diminishing the quality of the

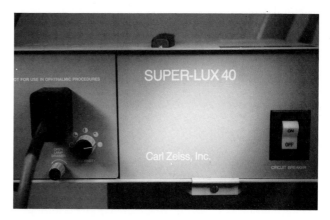

FIG. 3. Superlux-40 metal halide light source is the most intense currently available.

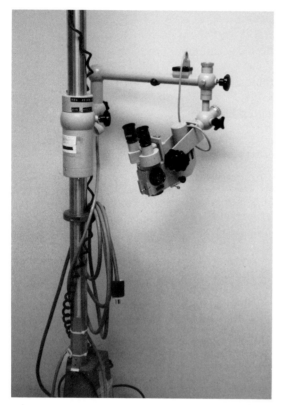

FIG. 4. Zeiss-Opmi II floor stand commonly available in most operating rooms.

down. The first automatic scope, the Zeiss-Opmi II, was introduced in the late 1960s and is on a motorized stand that permits automatic changes in the height of the microscope by foot pedals (Fig. 4). In addition, focusing and magnification changes can be controlled automatically by foot pedals.

More recently developed Zeiss-Universal S2 and S3 stands possess a canter-levered arm, which permits easier positioning and movement of the microscope. Wilde and Storz have developed similar canter-levered floor stands with a counter-balancing action that permits the microscope to be effortlessly moved by the surgeon (Fig. 5). The contraves microscope stand employs electromagnets that, when released, permit the microscope to be placed in any desired position. By utilizing either hand controls or a special mouth switch, the surgeon will certainly find this the most mobile and easily maneuverable microscope stand available today (Fig. 6).

The optics of the Wilde and Storz microscopes employ a wider optical path than the traditional Zeiss, but these superior optics have now been duplicated by the Zeiss-Opmi MD series. In addition, the Zeiss MD model employs a double optical system for a true stereoscopic view by an assistant working 180° from the surgeon.

image. It does, however, reduce the brightness of the light. Most beam splitters are 50/50, providing each visual path with 50% of the light.

Video/Photography

The beam splitter permits the use of various accessories such as the binocular assistant tube, video camera, and 35 mm camera. Video and camera adapters are available that permit the use of most 35 mm cameras and video cameras on the operating microscope. Recently, a three-dimensional video system has been developed that permits a true stereoscopic duplication of the surgeon's view for observation and documentation.

Microscope Stand

Zeiss, Wilde, Storz, Aus Jena, and Siemens are the major microscope manufacturers. The Zeiss-Opmi I microscope was developed in the early 1950s and can still be found in many operating rooms. This is a completely manual microscope that can be moved into any position and firmly held by adjusting control knobs. It is focused by manually moving the microscope up and

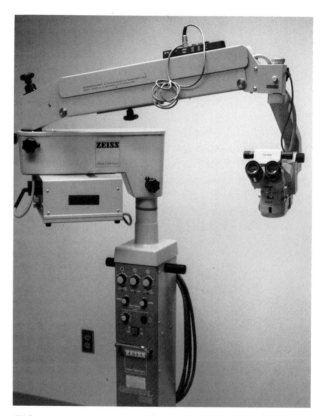

FIG. 5. Zeiss-Universal S3 stand with balancing arm.

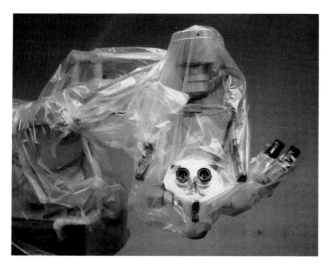

FIG. 6. Contraves operating microscope stand draped and ready for surgery.

SETTING UP THE OPERATING MICROSCOPE FOR CERVICAL SPINE PROCEDURES

Be certain that an angled or variably angled binocular tube is in place. A straight binocular tube is nearly impossible to use in the supine or prone position.

Check the eye pieces (oculars) to be certain they are inserted as far as possible into the binocular tube. Adjust the oculars for interpupillary distance and optical corrections. Secure the diapter adjustment with tape. Be certain that the eye pieces are free of dust. If necessary, clean with a soft cloth dampened with water.

Check the objective to be certain that a 300 or 350 mm objective is in place. Again, clean with a soft dampened cloth to remove fingerprints or dust.

Test the light source to be certain that it functions properly.

With the light source on, look through the microscope and focus on the end of your thumb. Check various magnifications to be certain that the optic pathway is functioning properly.

Check video and photographic attachments. Add film or batteries if necessary. Be certain that the video, photographic, and assistant images are properly oriented to the surgeon's image. This can be adjusted by rotating the video or 35 mm camera. The assistant's view can be adjusted at the base of the assistant's binocular tube.

Adjust the microscope stand so that it is stable and balanced yet freely movable.

Once a sterile plastic drape has been applied, remove the plastic strips covering the eye pieces and a small plastic lens covering the objective to clear the optic pathway of any distortions (Fig. 6).

ADVANTAGES/DISADVANTAGES OF THE OPERATING MICROSCOPE IN THE CERVICAL SPINE

Advantages

Advantages of the operating microscope are (a) better visualization, (b) ability to work through small incisions with less tissue disruption and reduced postoperative morbidity, (c) more precise tissue dissection, (d) more precise identification of pathology, (e) less chance of inadvertent spinal cord, root, or dural injury, (f) better visualization of epidural blood vessels with more meticulous hemostasis and less blood loss, and (g) reduced operative time.

Disadvantage

The disadvantage of the operating microscope is the potential greater risk of infection.

OTHER INSTRUMENTATION

High-Speed Drill

The precise removal of bone is greatly facilitated by the use of a high-speed burr. The Midas Rex system using the M-8 dissecting tool permits the precise removal of bone under direct visualization (Fig. 7). Other drill systems may be employed when a slower revolutions per minute (rpm) speed or angled hand piece is desired.

Cutting burrs are used to quickly remove dense cortical bone, but diamond burrs should always be used as the dural, epineural, or vascular surfaces are approached. Constant irrigation is crucial to prevent the

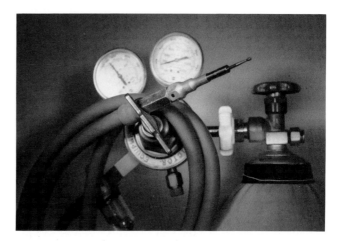

FIG. 7. Midas Rex high speed drill with M-8 dissecting tool.

thermocoagulation of bone that may damage existing bone forming cells, crucial for satisfactory bone healing and fusion. Dissecting tools or burrs that appear dull should be immediately replaced. This may occur after only a few seconds of thermal breakdown, again emphasizing the need for constant irrigation. Irrigation can be accomplished either through a suction-irrigation system or the bulb-syringe method. Irrigation fluids in contact with root or cord structures should be kept at body temperature to prevent the danger of thermal injury to sensitive neural structures.

Sponges of any kind should be absolutely prohibited from the operative field during the use of drills. Even the most clever surgeon will at some time inadvertently catch the edge of a small sponge in the wound, resulting in a rotary "weed-eater," tearing apart everything in its path.

Before applying a power tool to a bony surface, the instrument should be thoroughly checked by the surgeon. Particular attention should be paid to the structural integrity of the instrument. Inadequately attached tools have the potential of becoming flying missles with resultant injury to surrounding tissues.

Foot pedals for motor instruments should be controlled by the surgeon or an assistant who has visual access to the operative field so that the power can be adjusted very quickly without the need for repeated instructions from the surgeon. Surgeons unfamiliar with the use of power equipment or inexperienced in the use of power equipment in the cervical spine should gain practice with its use in the laboratory setting. The potential for danger in using power equipment in a small operative field surrounded by vital tissues and organs need not be emphasized.

The precise removal of bone enclosing neural and vascular elements involves repetitive side-to-side or back and forth motions. Absolutely no pressure is applied to the blind end of the dissecting tool or burr. All bone cutting or removal is done using the sides of the tool under direct visualization. This prevents injury to adjacent structures and inadvertent plunging of the instrument once a bony plane has been completely removed.

Advantages

Advantages of the high-speed burr are that it (a) is able to quickly and precisely remove bone under constant direct visualization, (b) avoids compression of sensitive tissues adjacent to bone, (c) prevents tension on bone surrounding points of removal, (d) avoids leaving sharp spicules or edges of bone, (e) promotes hemostasis by its thermal action, and (f) permits the removal of bone at angles impossible with other instrumentation.

Disadvantages

Disadvantages of the high-speed burr are that it (a) is dangerous if used improperly and can result in sudden and severe injury to surrounding tissue, (b) may produce thermal injury to bone forming cells, and (c) may introduce infection into the operative field by flying bone debris.

Suction

Continuous suction can be applied throughout microsurgical procedures by positioning a suction tip in the operator's nondominant hand. At various times, this can be utilized as a sucker, dissector, retractor, pointer, or coagulator. Suction diameters commonly range from 6 to 18 gauge (1–3 mm in caliber) and 16–20 cm in length. The largest gauge suction that permits good visualization should be used to remove debris during bone drilling. In addition, a large bore suction can be used to "vacuum sweep" soft tissue or bony debris excised with a rongeur. This avoids the necessity of repetitively removing instruments from the surgical field and from direct vision, thereby improving the precision of its use and diminishing the length of the procedure and the risk of inadvertent surrounding tissue injury.

A Frazier- or Ferguson-type suction tip has been adapted to permit continuous regulation of suction during its use. Suction control can also be managed by applying a suction regulator along the suction tubing. Suction tubes with additional holes near the end of the shaft have been developed to limit the amount of suction along dural and neural elements. These are most helpful during intradural exposures of neural elements.

It is helpful to have several suction tubes of the same size available so that they can be rapidly exchanged during the cleaning process. The use of suction over a small cotton pledget is a helpful adjunct to the control of epidural venous bleeding. The tamponading affect of pressure beneath the suction tube is frequently all that is necessary to completely control the bleeding while the suction action through the shaft of the suction tube clears the field of blood.

Bipolar Coagulation

Bipolar coagulation should be available to obtain both superficial and epidural hemostasis.

In using bipolar coagulation, it is important to remember that there is no significant current flow or coagulation from either tip alone as the current flows only *between* the tips. In addition, when the tips directly touch each other, the current is short-circuited, so no coagulation occurs. It is essential that tissue to be coagulated be held between the tips. Insulated tips prevent inadvertent coagulation of tissue touching both shafts away from the tips.

A variety of insulated bipolar forceps are available in a variety of tip sizes, lengths, and angulations. The bipolar tips must be kept meticulously clean to prevent burning and sticking. In addition, it is helpful to keep the tips of the forceps and the surrounding tissues moist during coagulation by applying a few drops of irrigating solution or using a self-irrigating bipolar coagulator.

The bipolar forceps should be used at low voltage (3–4 V) to coagulate bleeding epidural venous structures. Care should be taken to avoid coagulating against surrounding neural elements. Pitfalls in the use of bipolar coagulation include attempts to get by with an inadequate supply of forceps, the use of voltage settings that are too high, and the application of uninsulated forceps that promote heat and electrical transmission to surrounding neural tissue.

REFERENCES

1. Bailey G. Introduction to the microscope. In: Williams, McCulloch, Young; eds. *Microsurgery of the lumbar spine.* Aspen Publishing, 1990.
2. McCulloch JA. *Principles of microsurgery for lumbar disc disease.* New York: Raven Press, 1989.
3. Yasargil MG. *Microsurgery applied to neurosurgery.* Georg Thieme Verlag, 1969.

CHAPTER 6

Anterior Microdiscectomy for Soft Disc Protrusions

Paul H. Young

The anterior approach for disc extrusions or sequestrations was developed in the late 1950s (2) as an alternative to the classical laminectomy approaches. The difficulty and danger encountered in these early attempts to remove disc fragments and spurs anterior to the spinal cord or nerve roots from the posterior approach encouraged the development of anterior approaches (1–12).

INDICATIONS

The indications (Fig. 1) for an anterior microdiscectomy in the setting of soft disc herniations include the following: the presence of major neurological deficits (such as occur in spinal cord compression) due to central or paracentral disc protrusions, extrusions, or sequestrations; the presence of major motor and reflex loss in an appropriate radicular distribution from nerve root compression due to paracentral or foraminal disc protrusions, extrusions, or sequestrations; the persistence or recurrence of radicular pain not relieved by an adequate attempt at conservative treatment with or without abnormal neurological signs due to documented compression by an extruded or sequestered soft disc fragment; and radiographic evidence of severe spinal cord or radicular compression due to extruded or sequestered soft disc fragments.

INITIAL EXPLORATION OF THE PREVERTEBRAL SPACE

See Chapter 2.

EXPOSURE OF THE DISC SPACE

Using the operating microscope, the anterior longitudinal ligament is sharply incised parallel to the disc space 1 cm cranial and caudal to its firm attachment to the anterior annulus. The ligament is incised laterally to the uncovertebral joint or medial portion of the costal horn of the transverse process (Fig. 2). Hemostasis is obtained using bipolar coagulation and/or bone wax and extensive monopolar cauterization is avoided. The location of the vertebral artery just posterior to the costal horn of the transverse process should be kept in mind particularly at C7 where the artery may be in an even more superficial location.

Using a number 15 blade, the anterior annulus is incised across its attachments to the bordering vertebral body endplate (Fig. 3). In the absence of cervical traction, this disruption of the annulus will produce a degree of spontaneous disc protrusion anteriorly. The anterior annular incision is completed laterally near the medial borders of the uncinate process (easily identified as the disc space turns obliquely cranialward). This incision of the annulus is done under direct vision with care not to penetrate into the disc space more than 1 cm.

The operating microscope is angled rostrally in the direction of the plane of the disc space to improve the stereoscopic visualization of the anterior discal fragments. Loosened superficial fragments of annulus and nucleus are removed with a straight disc forceps and small straight or angled curettes (Fig. 4). All instruments placed into or near the intervertebral space are kept under constant direct visualization. Downward

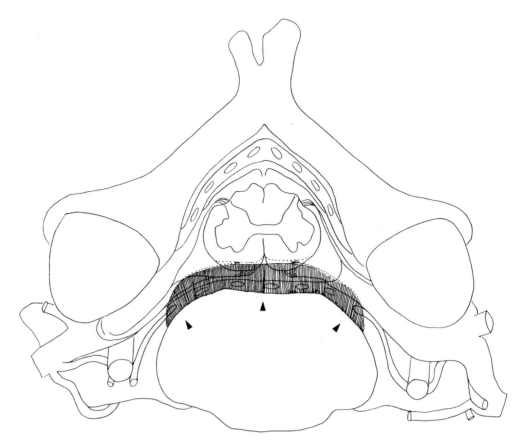

FIG. 1. Indications for anterior microdiscectomy.

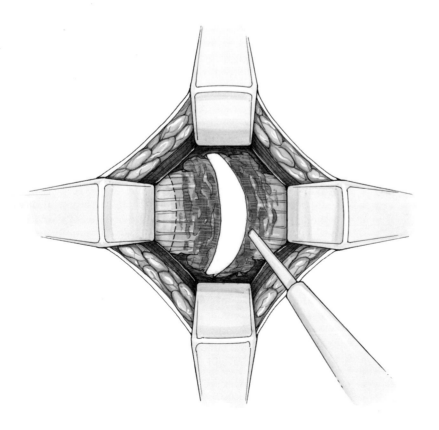

FIG. 2. Self-retaining retractors are placed beneath the freed margins of the longus colli muscles. Sharp dissection is used to incise the anterior longitudinal ligament immediately adjacent to the disc space. Coagulation is secured with mono- or bipolar cautery.

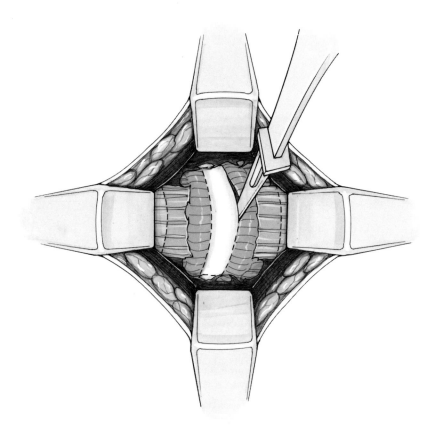

FIG. 3. The margins of the disc space are incised.

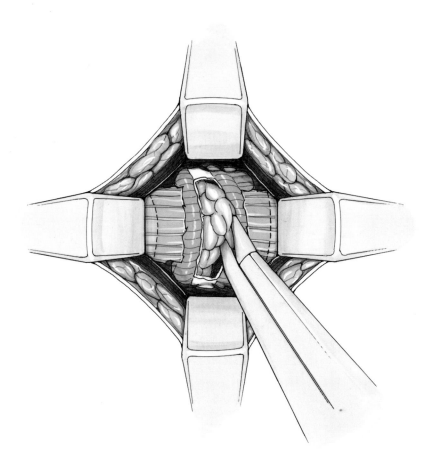

FIG. 4. The larger fragments of disc material are removed.

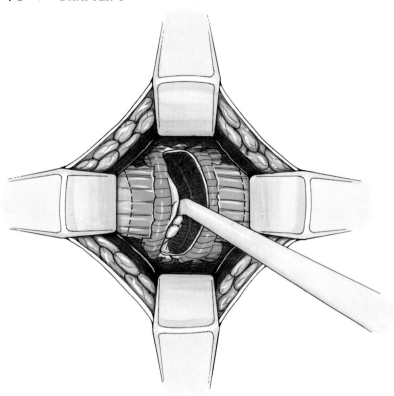

FIG. 5. The more posterior and lateral remnants of disc material are removed with a small angled curette.

pressure is never applied against the disc fragments pushing in a posterior direction. This maneuver could lead to the inadvertent further retropulsion of protruded or extruded disc fragments into the spinal canal.

Disc removal continues in this fashion until the entire interspace has been cleared of loose disc fragments (Fig. 5). Side-to-side angulation of the operating microscope is helpful in isolating and removing lateral fragments sometimes hidden in the lateral margins of the interspace (especially where it curves rostrally). Adequate lateral disc removal is varified when the uncovertebral joints can be clearly visualized. In addi-

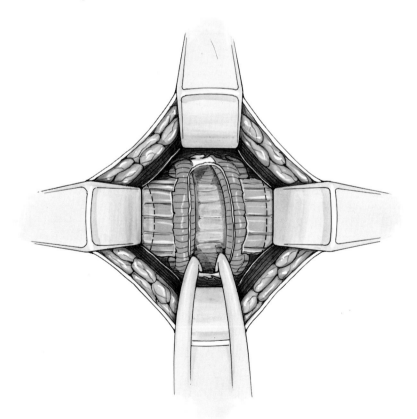

FIG. 6. The interspace spreader is positioned as far lateral as possible to preserve vision into the entire interspace while distracting.

tion, adequate posterior disc removal is accomplished when the glistening white vertical fibers of the posterior longitudinal ligament are clearly seen.

Special caution is applied in the use of instruments in the posterior and lateral aspects of the disc space as the inadvertent passage of an instrument through a hole in the posterior annulus and posterior longitudinal ligament into the spinal canal can be catastrophic. Disruption of the posterior annulus and posterior longitudinal ligament make sudden, unexpected penetration of instruments (especially small ones) into the spinal canal particularly easy.

Using an angled curette, the cartilaginous endplates are likewise completely removed. The attachments of the nuclear and annular disc components to the cartilaginous endplate and subchondral bone are firmest along the periphery and frequently the cartilaginous endplate is removed in conjunction with disc removal. All remnants of cartilaginous endplate, however, that remain following disc extirpation should be carefully retrieved, avoiding deep penetration into the subchondral bone.

An interspace spreader is placed laterally within the interspace just medial to the uncinate process (Fig. 6). Upon opening, the spreader produces distraction of the adjoining vertebral bodies and enlarges the surgeon's working area within the interspace. In addition, the uncovertebral joints are opened and the posterior longitudinal ligament tensed permitting improved identification and exploration of these structures (to ensure complete disc removal). Distraction of the interspace is particularly helpful when an element of associated segmental spondylosis is present. In addition to the use of the interspace spreader, it is helpful to remove anterior and posterior spurs (if present) as described in Chapter 7 before proceeding with further exploration of the spinal canal.

REMOVING EXTRUDED OR SEQUESTERED FRAGMENTS

Using preoperative radiographic studies as a guide, the precise position of extruded and sequestered disc fragments is appraised. Perforations of the posterior longitudinal ligament can be clearly identified using magnifications of 8–12 on the operating microscope. Disc fragments extruding through a ligamentous hole and obscuring further exploration are removed. The orifice of a perforation is enlarged slightly using a fine sharp hook, small blade, or 1-mm Kerrison rongeur.

The central three-fourths of the posterior longitudinal ligament is considerably thicker than the lateral margins bordering the foramen such that disc penetrations through the posterior longitudinal ligament are much more likely to occur laterally. Perforations of the posterior longitudinal ligament are generally parallel to the direction of the fibers (vertical). Once through the posterior longitudinal ligament, extruded disc fragments tend to sequester paracentrally or along the foramen although sequestered fragments may be found anywhere within the epidural space. In addition, epidural fragments travel caudally (rather than rostrally) most often. To explore these possibilities, it is important to widely open the posterior longitudinal ligament ipsilateral to the penetration (Fig. 7).

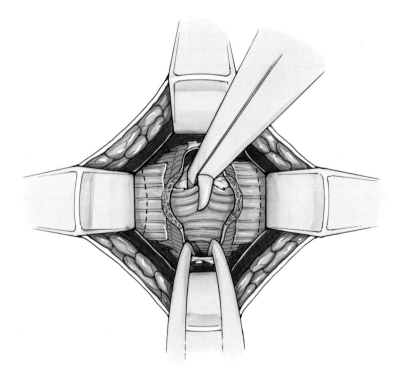

FIG. 7. The posterior longitudinal ligament is removed using an angled rongeur in order to better visualize ruptured disc fragments.

The ligament can be opened in either direction but this is generally easier from medial to lateral as it progressively thins along the proximal roots and medial foramina. Dilatation of the epidural space by disc fragments simplifies this opening. Particular attention is directed at the proximal root gutter where the posterior longitudinal ligament and epidural space thin considerably as the nerve roots pass obliquely anterior to enter the foramina. In addition, the narrow epidural space in this area is packed with epidural veins and loose areolar tissue surrounding the root as it enters the foramen.

EXPLORATION OF THE FORAMEN

The ipsilateral lateral exploration of the epidural space bordering the disc space of a sequestered fragment should include visualization of the proximal exiting nerve root to the lateral margin of the uncovertebral joint. This will expose ~5 mm of nerve root dural sleeve. The posterior longitudinal ligament overlying the uncovertebral joint varies in thickness from a thick band to only a few fibrous strands.

This lateral exploration along the nerve root should be accomplished with great care. Frequent anomalies such as duplications of dural nerve root sleeves may exist. Exploration in these situations will reveal two exiting roots. In addition, as the nerve root travels laterally it ascends anteriorly at a strikingly rapid pace. It is essential that clear stereoscopic visualization of the root(s) be obtained by dissection of the venous

areolar tissue encompassing them. The blind passage of probes, curettes, or rongeurs in this area is to be condemned. The looping of these instruments around roots may produce root avulsion. A small angled-mirror or ball dissector are helpful to fully explore this area.

By avoiding the use of paralyzing agents, thorough exploration of the paracentral and lateral zone can be accomplished without fear of root injury. A rapid depolarization of the nerve root(s) occurs with retraction, stretch or compressive forces or by the application of bipolar electrical current. This provides the surgeon with immediate physiological feedback similar to that obtained with evoked potential monitoring.

In most situations, it is not necessary to remove the thick medial portions of the posterior longitudinal ligament unless fragments of disc have migrated medially. Free disc fragments positioned directly behind the ligament are easily accessible. Those sequestering rostrally or caudally behind the adjoining vertebral bodies pose a more difficult problem. In these situations, removal of the medial posterior longitudinal ligament and adjacent vertebral bodies to an extent necessary to clearly identify and remove sequestered fragments is essential (Fig. 8).

Adequate epidural exploration generally requires visualization (and not just blind palpation) of the epidural disc cavity which in chronic sequestrations may be thick-walled or even calcified. It is unnecessary (and unwise) to attempt removal of these fibrous tissue lined cavities that may be densely adherent to the surrounding dura.

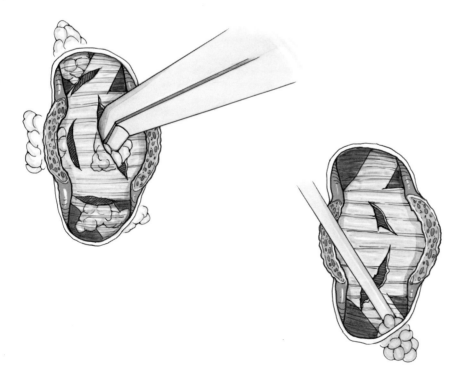

FIG. 8. Sequestered fragments of disc can be found in almost any location. These are removed by thoroughly exploring the epidural space after widely opening the initial site of ligament perforation.

LOCATIONS OF DISC EXTRUSIONS OR SEQUESTRATIONS: SUMMARY

For central disc extrusion/sequestration, open the medial posterior longitudinal ligament surrounding the fragment, explore the epidural space and/or fragment cavity, and perform partial corpectomy to the extent necessary to fully identify and completely remove all sequestered fragments.

For paracentral disc extrusion/sequestration, enlarge the perforation of the posterior longitudinal ligament around the fragment, explore the lateral epidural space, remove the adjoining posterior vertebral body margins to enlarge the epidural space, and identify and remove sequestered fragments.

For foraminal disc extrusion/sequestration, open the uncovertebral joint with removal of the posterior one-third of the uncinate process of the caudal vertebra, localize the pedicle beneath the uncinate process, excise the thin posterior longitudinal ligament overlying the most medial part of the nerve root of the foramen, and explore completely the foramen, with identification of the root(s) and the removal of all sequestered fragments.

NEED FOR FUSION

Following the satisfactory resolution of all radiographic abnormalities as confirmed by direct vision under the operating microscope, the need for bone stabilization is determined. This is based on the amount of adjoining vertebral body uncinate process and posterior longitudinal ligament removed. When the integrity of the adjoining vertebral bodies and posterior longitudinal ligament has been preserved and no associated foraminal osteophytic compression exists, no fusion may be necessary. If a wide excision of the posterior longitudinal ligament and uncovertebral joint has been necessary, a rectangular tricortical plug should be considered. On the other hand, if generous vertebral body resections or partial corpectomies were necessary to achieve complete sequestered fragment removal, then large (14–18 mm) dowels or even strut grafts may be necessary. (This topic is covered in detail in Chapter 8.)

HEMOSTASIS

Epidural bleeding is frequently encountered laterally along the nerve root particularly superiorly and anteriorly as the root enters the foramen through a maze of epidural and perivertebral vessels. Hemorrhage from these vessels or from the paravertebral venous plexus interferes with far lateral and foraminal exploration. The bleeding can be easily controlled with the placement of a small piece of gel-foam in contact against the venous plexus. This, however, limits further visualization or exploration. As a result, if bleeding ensues, it is a good idea to attempt control with bipolar coagulation under direct vision with caution against coagulation too close to the nerve root or vertebral artery. Frequently, the completion of the lateral and foraminal exploration is accomplished with mild oozing permitted as a slight aggravation. Once the exposure has been completed and adequate exploration of the foramen accomplished, then a gel-foam stamp is packed in the lateral zone and foramen to secure immediate hemostasis.

Epidural bleeding beneath the margins of the adjoining vertebral bodies can also be a nuisance. Generally, bipolar coagulation of the rim of the posterior longitudinal ligament or the epidural vessel itself is all that is necessary to achieve control. On occasion, it may be necessary to insert a small piece of gel-foam beneath the adjoining vertebral body rim in the epidural space.

CLOSURE

See Chapter 2.

REFERENCES

1. Clark WK. Anterior operative approaches for benign extradural cervical lesions. In: Youmans JR, ed. *Neurological surgery*. 2nd ed. Philadelphia: WB Saunders, 2613–2628, 1982.
2. Cloward RB. The anterior approach for removal of ruptured cervical discs. *J Neurosurg* 15:602–617, 1958.
3. Dunsker SB. Anterior cervical discectomy with and without fusion. *Clin Neurosurg* 24:516–521, 1977.
4. Hankinson HL, Wilson CB. Use of operating microscope in anterior cervical diskectomy without fusion. *J Neurosurg* 43:452–456, 1975.
5. Manabe S, Tateishi A. Epidural migration of extruded cervical discs and its surgical management. *Spine* 11:873–878, 1986.
6. Martins AN. Anterior cervical discectomy with and without interbody bone graft. *J Neurosurg* 44:290–295, 1976.
7. Murphy MG, Gado M. Anterior cervical discectomy without interbody bone graft. *J Neurosurg* 37:71–84, 1972.
8. Robertson JT. Anterior removal of cervical disc without fusion. *Clin Neurosurg* 20:259–261, 1973.
9. Seeman PS, Mager F, Grob D. Anterior interbody fusion with transdiscal decompression. In: *The cervical spine I*. Springer-Verlag, 273–277, 1987.
10. Tew JM, Mayfield FH. Proceedings Society of British Neurological Surgeons. Anterior cervical disectomy—a microsurgical approach. *J Neurol Neurosurg Psychiatry* 38:413, 1975.
11. Tribolet N, Zander E. Anterior discectomy without fusion for the treatment of ruptured cervical discs. *J Neurosurg Sci* 25:217–220, 1981.
12. Wilson DH, Campbell DD. Anterior cervical discectomy without bone graft. *J Neurosurg* 47:551–555, 1977.

CHAPTER 7

Anterior Microsurgical Approach for Central and Lateral Compression Related to Spondylosis

Paul H. Young

The original anterior approaches to the cervical spine (1–15) were designed primarily for spondylotic disease. Hoping to avoid the risk of worsening a myelopathy associated with posterior approaches, no attempt was made to decompress neural structures. The prime benefits of the anterior fusion for spondylosis were thought to be associated with the restoration of disc space height and motion segment stabilization. Symptoms improved due to the elimination of instability and the subsequent long-term resorption of osteophytic compression. The recent addition of the operating microscope to the anterior cervical decompression has resulted in improved anatomical visualization and has enhanced the cervical spine surgeon's ability to safely remove anterior compressive pathology in addition to effecting a fusion.

INDICATIONS FOR ANTERIOR DECOMPRESSION

Indications for anterior decompression are shown in Fig. 1. They are myelopathic signs or symptoms related to primarily anteriorly directed spinal cord compression by spurs, bars, ridges, OPLL, or vertebral body subluxation; marked radiculopathic signs and symptoms related to spondylotic compression of the nerve root(s) either laterally in the spinal canal or within the intervertebral foramina; radiculopathic symptoms alone related to spondylotic compression of the nerve root(s) in patients failing an adequate course

of conservative treatment; and asymptomatic but significant canal compromise and cord compression due to anterior spondylosis, motion segment instability or anterior canal masses.

EXPOSURE OF THE PREVERTEBRAL SPACE

See Chapter 2.

REMOVING ANTERIOR SPURS

Peridiscal spurs protruding anteriorly into the prevertebral space and concealing the disc space to the level of the anterior cortex of the adjoining vertebral bodies are removed using the high speed drill with a cutting burr under the operating microscope. Frequently, the removal of large converging anterior spurs will suddenly open the anterior aspects of what initially appeared to be a very narrow disc space (Fig. 2). The anterior spurs should not be removed below the plane of the anterior vertebral body surface. This osteophytectomy is carried laterally to the costal horn of the transverse process but not beyond at this point for fear of vertebral artery injury. It is important to preserve as much of the anterior cortex of the adjoining vertebral bodies as possible to avoid weakening the anterior support column at the subsequent fusion site. The anterior longitudinal ligament and adjacent anterior annulus are intimately connected to the base of

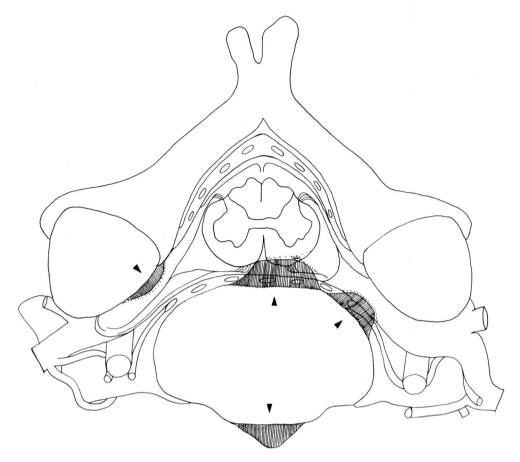

FIG. 1. Indications for anterior decompression of central and lateral spondylosis.

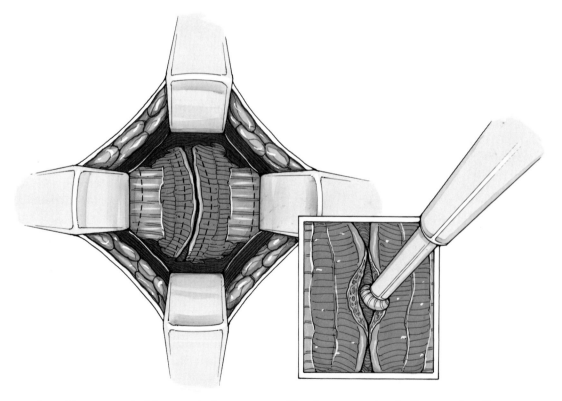

FIG. 2. The removal of large anterior spurs resulting in an opening in the anterior disc space.

the osteophytic spurs, and end up being removed with the spurs.

The anterior aspects of the disc space are cleared of soft annular and nuclear remnants using angled curettes to loosen and a disc forceps to retrieve the fragments (Fig. 3). It is important to emphasize that the working ends of all instruments placed into the disc space should be under constant visualization to avoid inadvertent intrusion into the spinal canal. The amount of disc found and removed will vary depending on the degree of spondylosis (and associated spontaneous disc resorption) present.

Following the total removal of soft disc remnants, particularly those in the anterior two-thirds of the disc space, the high-speed drill (Midas Rex M-8 or cutting burr) is used to create a small intervertebral trough in the lateral aspect of the disc space just medial to the uncovertebral joint for placement of an interspace spreader. This can be initially accomplished on either side, and, not infrequently, it is helpful especially when performing bilateral foramenotomies to alternate the interspace spreader from one side to the other. The depth of this trough should be 50% of the adjacent vertebral body height for adequate placement of the spreader blades. Inadequate insertion of the spreader tips either too superficially into the disc space or too laterally against the uncinate process will result in un-

necessary fractures of the adjacent vertebral body margins.

With mild to moderate distraction tension on the spreader, the adjoining vertebral bodies are displaced, thereby opening the disc space for better visualization of its deeper elements. The use of large amounts of force on the distraction device may result in fracture of the cortical bone adjacent to the spreader tips with penetration into the cancellous medullary zones of the adjacent vertebral bodies, producing venous bleeding and the potential for increased instability of the fusion mass. In addition, very large amounts of distraction can result in apophyseal capsular and ligamentous injury with significant increased postoperative pain and motion segment instability. Many of these pitfalls involved in the use of the intervertebral spreader can be avoided by the use of the Caspar distraction system (see Chapter 10).

With advanced spondylosis, no sizable disc space or disc material may be present. In this instance, it is necessary to use the high-speed drill to recreate the interspace from an anterior to a posterior direction. Initially, a small, 5-mm, horizontally rectangular or cylindrical opening is produced with removal of adjoining vertebral body endplates and osteophytic irregularities (Fig. 4). Frequently, in the most advanced spondylotic disc spaces, only a white band of cartilaginous tissue

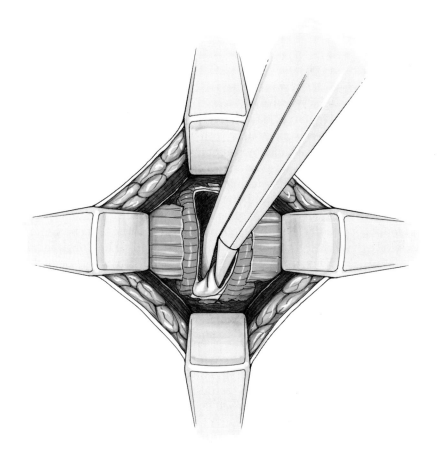

FIG. 3. Opening the lateral disc space in preparation for placement of the intervertebral spreader.

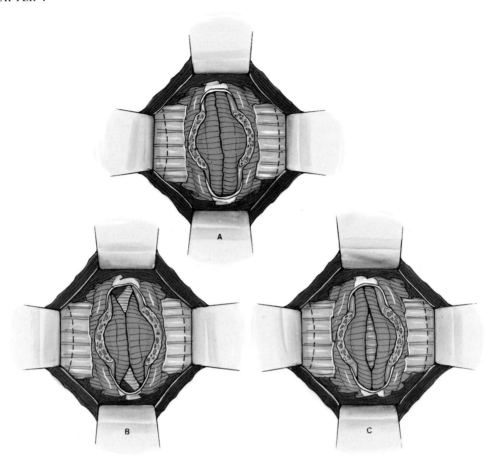

FIG. 4. Cylindrical decompression through intervertebral space with visualization of posterior spondylosis. **A:** Medial and lateral. **B:** Medial only. **C:** Lateral only.

remains to provide identification of the previous intervertebral space (Fig. 5). Equal amounts of the adjoining vertebral bodies surrounding this band are progressively removed as an intervertebral space is reformed. This removal is continued posteriorly until the posterior margins of the adjoining vertebral bodies and posterior osteophytes are encountered.

Based on preoperative radiographic studies, the rostral-caudal extent of spondylotic compression can be estimated. For medial canal compression, the amount of interspace widening and associated adjacent vertebral body removal should correspond to the rostral-caudal extent of canal compromise. For posterior osteophytic spurs localized to the disc space, a small (14–16 mm) parallelepiped or cylindrical decompression may be all that is necessary. More moderate amounts of compression with spurs, bars or ridges extending somewhat beyond the disc space demand a larger (16–18 mm) parallelepiped or cylindrical decompression. Multisegmental compression extending rostrally and/or caudally along the posterior surface of the adjoining vertebral bodies or between adjacent motion segments may require a partial or total corpectomy for adequate decompression.

The lateral extent of canal spondylotic compromise can also be estimated on preoperative radiographic studies. Most commonly, significant central osteophytosis is associated with at least some narrowing of the lateral canal by osteophytes arising from the posterior-medial base of the uncinate process (Fig. 4). At the base of the uncinate process, the central convexity of the spinal cord dural envelope flattens horizontally to gradually slope slightly anterior as the root dural sleeve enters the foramen. This flattened lateral zone can be easily identified even with the posterior longitudinal ligament intact. This marks the proximal portion of the nerve root(s) at the medial aspect of the pedicles as the roots enter the foramena—a keen anterior intracanal landmark identifying the lateral margin of the spinal canal.

The final extent of bone removal is dictated by the need for adequate canal decompression. The posterior ostephytes generally must be completely removed regardless of their rostral-caudal and lateral extent. This is best accomplished using the high-speed drill (Midas-M8 or diamond burr) to progressively remove it (Fig. 6). When only a thin remnant of osteophyte remains embedded in and adherent to the posterior longitudinal

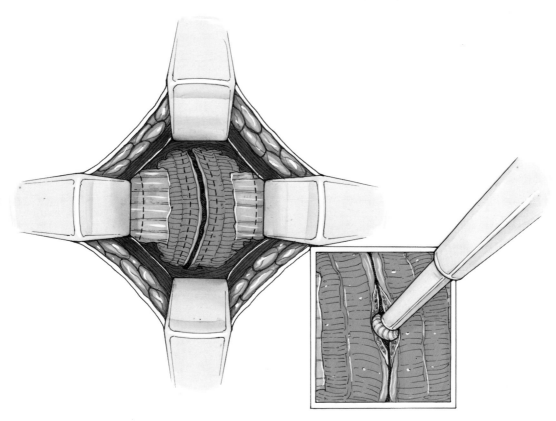

FIG. 5. Marked spondylotic narrowing with near complete disappearance of the disc space. Gradual intervertebral space widening using the high-speed drill.

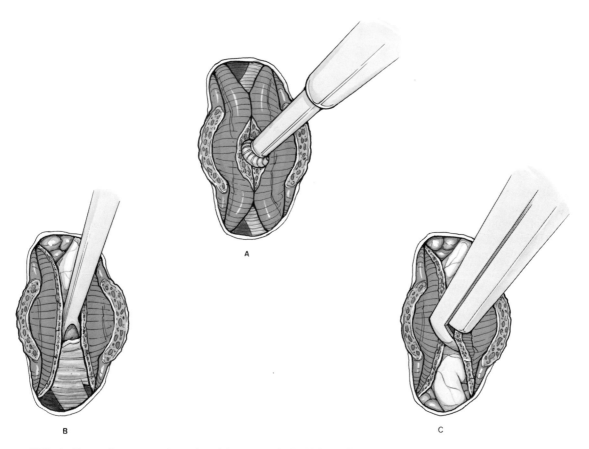

A

B

C

FIG. 6. Posterior osteophytosis with removal. **A:** Using high-speed drill. **B:** Using small angled curette with portion of the posterior longitudinal ligament preserved. **C:** Using small rongeur.

ligament, a small angled curette can be used to carefully displace it anteriorly into the interspace, or a small (1–2 mm) Kerrison rongeur can be used to gently bite it away (Fig. 6). The larger and more canal compromising an osteophyte, the greater its adherence to the posterior longitudinal ligament and the more of the ligament that is necessarily removed in conjunction with the osteophyte. Generally, remnants of the posterior longitudinal ligament will remain even after extensive osteophyte removal (Fig. 6). Fortunately, in spondylosis, the posterior longitudinal ligament is not significantly adherent to the anterior dural surface making osteophyte and associated ligament removal much easier. In ossification of the posterior ligament, on the other hand, significant dural adhesions are frequent, often resulting in a much more difficult excision.

In the removal of large midline spurs, bars, or ridges, it is sometimes helpful to thin the spur to a small remnant with the high-speed drill and then to incise the posterior longitudinal ligament adjacent to the spur and to remove both with a small angled curette or rongeur working within the epidural space. This permits an easier dissection plane (between the posterior longitudinal ligament and dura in the epidural space) than between the layer of the posterior longitudinal ligament behind the spur. In all patients, but especially those with very narrow spinal canals, a great deal of care must be exercised in the placement of instruments behind posterior spurs. In this setting, it is certainly safer to remove the osteophytic projections in a progressive fashion utilizing the high-speed drill with a small diamond burr, thereby avoiding any intrusion into the spinal canal.

On occasion, a large posteriorly projecting spur may become displaced from its attachments to the adjacent vertebral body margin, leaving it suspending within the posterior longitudinal ligament. Attempts to remove such displaced and free-floating spur may prove somewhat difficult. Certainly, downward posteriorly directed pressure to try and grasp an edge of the spur should be totally avoided as forces will be transmitted directly onto an already compromised spinal cord. These can be safely removed using the high-speed drill (diamond burr) to progressively shave them away. In addition, not infrequently, a spur or bar is encountered that seems to project behind the vertebral body of origin into the spinal canal. When detached, these spurs disappear from vision when approached with an angled curette or rongeur. In this setting, it is advisable to remove adjoining vertebral body using the high-speed burr to the extent necessary to regain visualization in order to prevent any possibility of spinal canal compromise.

Clearly, the end point of vertebral body and osteophyte removal is the thorough decompression of the spinal canal as adequate spinal cord decompression is crucial for optimal functional recovery. Attempts to limit the decompression to less than adequate in order to accommodate an inaccurately predesigned bone graft (too small) will limit the success of this approach. In addition, enlarging a decompression to fit a larger than necessary bone graft increases both immediate instability and the risk of graft failure. In all anterior decompressions, regardless of extent, the size and shape of the decompression should be related to the location and extent of the pathology rather than the size and shape of the intended bone graft material. In other words, the bone graft should be molded to fit the decompressive opening; the decompression should not be limited or expanded to accommodate the graft.

Foraminal Stenosis

Generally, the posterior longitudinal ligament weakens paracentrally and laterally, and as a result the surgeon must avoid not only any tension posteriorly on the posterior longitudinal ligament but also any postero-lateral pressure as this may result in sudden intrusion into the lateral spinal canal or foramen. The same basic techniques as described under the removal of central spurs are applicable to foraminal spurs. In general, it is easier to work from a lateral to medial direction beginning at the base of the uncinate process as the spurs generally are more prominent medially with firmer attachments to the posterior longitudinal ligament. If, however, the osteophytosis is more prominent paracentrally or laterally at the base of the uncinate process, a medial to lateral removal may be advantageous.

The high-speed drill is used with the diamond burr to remove the posterior one-half of the uncinate process of the caudal vertebra. This opens the posterior aspect of the uncovertebral joint and allows direct visualization of the proximal nerve root. Only a small amount of posterior longitudinal ligament may be present laterally at the foraminal orifice.

The foraminal osteophytic decompression is accomplished with interspace distraction using the interspace spreader. Frequently, it is necessary to rotate the spreader from one side to the other to obtain maximal lateral visualization of each foramen.

As with medial spurs, it is possible to either remove the posterior bone entirely with the diamond burr or leave a small sheet which can then be removed with an angled curette or rongeur. The removal of caudal uncinate process and rostral uncinate groove bone is carried out until the intervertebral foramen can be widely identified and the nerve root followed under direct vision. It may be necessary to remove further anterior portions of the uncinate process to further en-

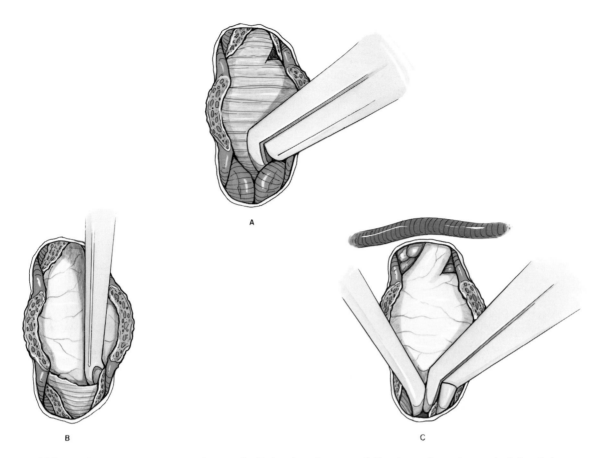

FIG. 7. Foramenotomy techniques. **A:** Enlarging foramen following adequate contralateral decompression. **B:** Removal of final spur origin tissue along the base of the uncinate process. **C:** Adequate visualization of nerve root in foramen with superior retraction and further foraminal decompression.

large the foramen (Fig. 7). On occasion, it may even be necessary to carry this bone removal through the entire uncinate process down to the pedicle. Under no circumstances should an instrument be forced blindly into a tight foramen, a maneuver that can lead to further root compression or avulsion. Depending on the nature of the osteophytic process, the foramen may need to be further opened anteriorly (uncinate process), posteriorly (apophyseal joint), or inferiorly (pedicle), using a combination of drilling with the diamond burr or using angled curettes and rongeurs under direct vision around the root(s). Following adequate foraminal decompression with visualization of the root, a small ball-nerve hook can then be easily passed around the nerve root into the distal foramen. During this process, the caudal pedicle should be located in order to better gauge the foraminal size.

The foraminotomy should not be considered complete until the proximal 10–12 mm of nerve root can be clearly identified. The frequent presence of cervical root dural duplications such that both motor and sensory roots possess separate dural sleeves should be anticipated. In this situation, the motor root will be located anterior or inferior, with the sensory root posterior or superior in the foramen. It is imperative that the surgeon be on the lookout for this common anomaly to prevent inadvertent root injury.

HEMOSTASIS

As decompression proceeds laterally epidural bleeding may ensue. The paravertebral plexus and radicular vessels travelling through the foramen may bleed making the combination of absolute hemostasis and excellent visualization during the decompression difficult. In general, it is better to permit a small amount of venous oozing, controlling it with gentle suction during the decompression rather than attempting to secure absolute hemostasis at each step along the way, which interferes with adequate visualization. Gel-foam placed under a cottonoid and held gently in place immediately secures hemostasis but also totally obscures further vision.

Medial and paracentral bleeding from epidural veins or posterior longitudinal ligament vessels can be accomplished using bipolar cauterization. On occasion, small strips of gel-foam may need to be inserted beneath the vertebral body margins to tamponade the epidural space. The liberal use of bone wax especially in the bone graft bed should be avoided as it may interfere with the eventual fusion.

Following adequate decompression and resolution of all preoperative radiographic defects, an appropriate bony fusion is performed as described in Chapter 10.

CLOSURE

Closure is accomplished following adequate hemostasis and irrigation with antibiotic solution as indicated in Chapter 2.

REFERENCES

1. Bailey RW, Badgley CE. Stabilization of the cervical spine by anterior fusion. *J Bone Joint Surg [Am]* 42A:565–594, 1960.
2. Bohlman HH. Cervical spondylosis with moderate to severe myelopathy—report of 17 cases treated by Robinson anterior cervical discectomy and fusion. *Spine* 2:151, 1977.
3. Bohlman HH, Eismont FJ. Surgical techniques of anterior decompression and fusion for spinal cord injuries. *Clin Orthop* 13:57–67, 1981.
4. Cloward R. The anterior approach for removal of ruptured cervical discs. *J Neurosurg* 15:602–617, 1958.
5. Dunkser SB. Anterior cerivcal discectomy with and without fusion. *Clin Neurosurg* 24:516–521, 1977.
6. Fang HSY, Ong GB, Hodgson AR. Anterior spinal fusion: the operative approaches. *Clin Orthop* 35:16–33, 1964.
7. Galera GR, Tovi D. Anterior disc excision with interbody fusion in cervical spondylotic myelpathy and rhizopathy. *J Neurosurg* 28:305–310, 1968.
8. Hankinson H, Wilson CB. Use of the operating microscope in anterior cervical discectomy with fusion. *J Neurosurg* 43:452, 1975.
9. Hoff J, Hood T. Anterior operative approaches for benign extradural cervical lesions. In: Youmans JR, ed. *Neurological surgery*. 3rd ed. Philadelphia; WB Saunders, 2923–2936, 1990.
10. Lunsford LD, Bissonette DJ, Jannetta PJ, et al. Anterior surgery for cervical disc disease. *J Neurosurg* 53:1–19, 1980.
11. Mann KS, Khosla VK, Gulati DR. Cervical spondylotic myelopathy treated by single stage multilevel anterior decompression. *J Neurosurg* 60:81–87, 1984.
12. Martins AN. Anterior cervical discectomy with and without interbody bone graft. *J Neurosurg* 44:290–295, 1976.
13. Smith G, Robinson R. The treatment of certain cervical spine disorders by anterior removal of the intervertebral disc and interbody fusion. *J Bone Joint Surg [Am]* 40A:607, 1958.
14. White AA III, Southwick WO, DePonte RJ et al. Relief of pain by anterior cervical spine fusion for spondylosis: a report of sixty-five cases. *J Bone Joint Surg* 55A:525, 1973.
15. Senegas J, Guerin J, Vital JM, Duplan B, Dols JM. Treatment of myelopathy in cervical spondylosis by extensive anterior decompression of the cord. *Rev Chir Orthop* 71:291–300, 1985.

CHAPTER 8

Principles of Bone Fusion in Anterior Cervical Spine Microsurgery

Paul H. Young

The eventual success (or failure) of an anterior vertebral body fusion in the cervical spine depends on three key factors: (a) the choice of *grafting material*, (b) the *preparation of the fusion site*, and (c) the effects of *local and systemic factors*.

GRAFT MATERIAL

Ideal Graft Material

The ideal graft material should promote the following essential properties that have been shown to enhance the bone healing process: osteogenesis, osteoscaffolding, and osteoinduction.

Osteogenesis is the production of new bone by living osteocytes within and around the fusion site. *Osteoscaffolding* is the ability of bone graft material to provide a framework or scaffold for the ingrowth of new bone. *Osteoinduction* refers to the promotion of immature osteoblastic cell differentiation into mature bone producing osteoclasts.

Available Graft Material

Presently available graft material includes autogenous bone, allograft bone, xenograft bone, bone marrow, and synthetic grafting material.

Autogenous Bone (Autograft)

A cervical autograft is bone transplanted from some part of the patient's own body (iliac crest, fibula tibia,

rib, etc.) (1–7). Its major advantages over other grafting materials include its sterility, histocompatability and resultant nonreactivity, possession of osteocytic cells and associated vessels that may survive the transplantation process, and ability to provide a multitude of osteoinductive substances (including bone collagens, minerals and bone morphogenic protein, etc.).

A fresh autograft is presently the best bone graft material. The use of autografts, however, for cervical anterior fusions is limited on occasion by its lack of availability and commonly by the morbidity associated with its harvesting.

A variation of the autogenous graft is the free vascularized cervical autograft in which bone with a vascular pedicle is utilized and microanastomoses are performed with a superior, middle, or inferior thyroid artery and vein (8–17). The use of a vascular pedicle improves the success rate of fusion, but the long operative time and increased technical difficulty related to this procedure make its application possible only in special situations (such as fusion beds effected by radiation, diminished vascularity or induced fibrosis, or when postoperative radiation therapy is planned) (6).

Allograft Bone

A cervical allograft is bone transplanted from another person with different genetic characteristics (1–7). Allografts essentially provide only a scaffold for bone remodeling and a weak osteoinductive matrix. In most applications, allograft bone is a less ideal fusion material than autograft due to its immunogenesity and complete lack of functioning cells as no living cells survive the transplant process. When used as a cervical interbody graft material, however, allograft bone may be as good as autogenous bone due to the large surface area of contact between donor and recipient bone inherent in this application (12).

Allograft bone is currently processed for preservation and to reduce its immunogenesity by removing nearly all the cells from the bone. This processing may include freezing (to −20°C) or freeze-drying followed by sterilization with ethylene oxide, radiation, or chemicals. Freeze-drying is the more effective method of removing protein immunogenesity, but it also tends to reduce the mechanical strength of the bone.

The major advantage of cervical interbody allograft is that it avoids the morbidity associated with the harvesting of autograft. Its major disadvantage is its potential (theoretical more than practical) for the transmission of infectious diseases.

Xenograft (Heterograft)

Cervical xenograft is bone transplanted from another animal species (18–20). Xenograft bone has up to the present witnessed only a very limited application in the cervical spine as it generally evokes a tremendous immune response with graft absorption and provides no advantages over the use of allograft bone.

Bone Marrow

Autogenous bone marrow can be used as an adjunctive graft material to enhance the osteogenetic and osteoinductive properties of other cervical graft materials (21–40). Due to its lack of supportive substrate, marrow cannot be used as a sole agent. A similar material, demineralized bone matrix, is a form of alloimplant bone that possesses low immunogenesity yet has a large amount of bone morphogenic protein (BMP) and other bioactive proteins.

Bone morphogenic protein is a bioactive substance that induces undifferentiated stem cells into cartilage and bone forming cells. Autogenous bone marrow and allogenic bone morphogenic protein can be used to enhance the biological fusion potential of cervical allografts.

Synthetic Materials

Tricalcium phosphate (TCP) and hydroxylapatite are ceramic implants that are presently being investigated for use in cervical spine fusions (41–54). These are biocompatible and bioabsorbable substances that permit the rapid ingrowth of bone and promote bone modeling essential for optimum mechanical bone strength. At present, these materials alone cannot be used as reliable bone substitutes for cervical interbody fusions.

NEW ADVANCES

Composite grafts consisting of fresh autogenous cancellous bone marrow and cortical allograft likely will yield more new bone formation than presently obtained by either alone. In addition, the combination of bone morphogenic protein to promote osteoinduction and a cortical-cancellous allograft to provide a supportive framework will likely be the next major advances in cervical spine bone transplantation.

Methyl Methacrylate

Methyl methacrylate has been used as a stabilizing agent particularly in patients harboring metastatic or unresectable primary tumors with a limited life-span (87–90). To obtain stability with the use of methyl methacrylate, it is necessary that it be anchored to adjacent vertebrae by screws, wires, or other devices, which clearly places its use in a disadvantageous position.

FUSION SITE: General Principles

If not already accomplished as part of the interbody graft site opening, the fusion site must be prepared by carefully decorticating all lining cartilage surfaces to promote local osteoblastic potential. This should be accomplished with the high-speed burr using copious irrigation to prevent thermonecrosis of local, living bone-forming cells. The surface area of contact between the intervening vertebral bodies and graft should be maximized to improve the initial mechanical bone and increase the adjacent population of osteoblastic cells. In addition, the longus colli muscles and prevertebral soft tissues should be preserved, including their vascularity to promote the influx of nutritional and systemic factors essential for the bone healing process.

Positive factors in the bone healing process include a well-vascularized graft bed; a small hematoma to transmit healing factors to graft bed; a local inflammatory response; an increase in the quantity of osteogenetic cells present in local bone marrow; a large surface area for graft-vertebral body interface for improved immediate mechanical stability; the presence of bone morphogenic protein, local growth factors, and angiogenetic factors; proper amounts of insulin, insulin-like growth factors, testosterone, estrogen, growth hormone, thyroxin, PTH, calcitonin, vitamin A, vitamin D, and anabolic steroids; and the use of electrical stimulation which increases osteoblastic activity (56–61).

Negative factors in the bone healing process include the presence of devascularized traumatized longus colli and prevertebral tissue; local bone disease including osteoporosis; the presence of a radiation scar or radiation denervation; tumor infiltration into the graft bed; infection at the graft site; excessive mechanical motion and ongoing motion segment instability; the presence of bone wax; the use of cortical steroids; the use of nonsteroidal antiinflammatory drugs; the presence of malnutrition disorders, including vitamin D deficiency, iron deficiency, negative nitrogen balance, calcium deficiency, vitamin D intoxication, and vitamin A intoxication; chemotherapy; preexisting rheumatoid arthritis, inappropriate ADH, or castration; and cigarette smoking.

BIOLOGY OF BONE HEALING

The biology of bone healing is described here (62–65). Two types of bone that are present in varying proportions depending upon graft material can be identified: compact or cortical bone; and spongy, trabeculated, or cancellous bone.

Cortical bone is dense and solid, whereas *cancellous bone* is composed of a mesh-work of medullary spaces. Most of the individual skeletal bones contain hard compact cortical bone surrounding soft medullary cancellous bone. Marrow cells that are both hematopoietic and osteogenetic are found within the trabeculae of the cancellous bone. The trabeculae of cancellous bone are oriented in relation to the direction of stresses, whereas cortical bone is composed of lamellae. The basic organization of cortical bone is that of the osteon with constantly absorbing and remodeling the bony substrate.

The acute inflammatory response associated with the grafting process hastens the arrival of macrophages clearing cellular debris and mesenchymal cells acting as osteoprogenitor cells. The living bone cell in the osteon is the osteocyte. Activated osteoblasts deposit osteoid on bony substances, and activated osteoclasts remove bone debris.

The ideal interbody graft should consist of the proper proportion of cortical and cancellous components—the compact part providing immediate strength to the fusion site and the spongy part providing both bone progenitor cells as well as a scaffold for rapid bone ingrowth. Failure of sufficient mechanical strength or lack of adequate osteoblast and osteoclast activation may result in bone graft failure with collapse, resorption or nonunion.

CHRONOLOGY OF BONE HEALING: Autograft Versus Allograft

The time sequence of the bone healing process for cervical intervertebral body graft differs depending on the use of autograft or allograft material (Table 1). Though the autograft healing process is clearly more rapid than that surrounding the use of allograft, the final mechanical result in the cervical intervertebral body application may not be significantly different.

TABLE 1. *Time sequence of the healing process in autograft and allograft*

Time	Autograft	Allograft
0–3 days	Acute inflammatory response Initiation of infiltrating vascular beds into the graft from surrounding muscle and soft tissue	Increased inflammatory response
3–7 days	Arrival of mesenchymal and pleuri-potential cells Surviving graft osteoclasts produce bone resorption	Initiation of infiltrating vascular beds into the graft from surrounding muscle and soft tissue
7–14 days	Infiltrating osteoclasts from host appear producing bone resorption and cavity formation Osteoinductive substances are released	Arrival of mesenchymal and pleuri-potential cells Infiltrating osteoclasts from host appear producing bone resorption and graft necrosis Osteoinductive substances are released
2–4 weeks	Increased vascularization of the graft Osteoid deposited (new bone) Progressive mineralization of new bone	Progressive graft resorption
4–8 weeks	Bone reformation and remodeling with increase in mechanical strength	Increased vascularization of the graft Osteoblasts appear—osteoid deposited (new bone) Progressive mineralization of new bone
8–16 weeks	Progressive deposition of organic bone matrix	Bone reformation and remodeling with increase in mechanical strength

TABLE 2. *Time sequence of the healing process in cancellous and cortical bone*

Time	Cancellous bone	Cortical bone
0–3 days	Infiltration of vascular beds into the graft medullary cavities	
3–7 days	Arrival of mesenchymal and pleuri-potential cells	
7–14 days		Infiltration of vascular beds into Volkmann's canals
4–8 weeks		Arrival of mesenchymal cells especially osteoclasts with the production of resorptive cavities

Similar differences can be seen between the healing processes of cancellous and cortical bone (Table 2).

Clearly the final decision concerning the proportions of cancellous and cortical bone components in a particular cervical intervertebral graft should take into account these marked healing differences. For most applications, a medullary center of cancellous bone surrounded on the nonfusion surfaces by cortical bone is most ideal.

TECHNIQUES OF ANTERIOR CERVICAL SPINE FUSION

The pioneers of anterior cervical bone fusion and the distinctive types of motion segment stabilization each advocated are Smith and Robinson rectangular plug (69); Bailey and Badgley rectangular strut (73); and Cloward cylindrical dowel (75).

It is clear that anterior interbody fusion is not always necessary following one-, two-, or three-level anterior microdiscectomies for disc extrusion without associated spondylosis, as in most situations a spontaneous fusion will occur by 6 months if the cartilaginous endplates and osteophytes have been completely removed. For those patients not undergoing fusion following discectomy, it is clear that significant interscapular, neck, and shoulder pain are considerably more frequent postoperatively than if a fusion is accomplished. Fortunately, even without a fusion these symptoms generally resolve within 6–12 weeks, and long-term no difference in clinical outcome or fusion rate occurs (91–101).

The need for fusion should be pre- and intraoperatively based on the following variables: the presence of significant preoperative motion segment instability from spondylotic disruption of supporting structures (degenerative subluxation) at neighboring disc spaces; the need for multilevel exposures; the necessity of complete disc excision with partial or total removal of the annulus, anterior longitudinal ligament and posterior longitudinal ligament; the extensive operative removal of one or both uncovertebral joints for foraminal decompression; and the need for immediate stabilization.

ANTERIOR INTERBODY FUSIONS

Rectangular Plug Graft (Smith-Robinson)

The rectangular plug graft (Smith-Robinson) is described here (66–72) (Fig. 1).

Advantages

The total surface area of a full width-horizontal rectangular graft is nearly 30% more than that of the cylindrical graft of a comparable size, suggesting that the immediate stability of this type of graft is greater than that with the dowel graft.

Graft Site Preparation (Wolfhard Caspar, M.D., and Haynes Harkey, M.D.)

The vertebral body subchondral endplates are prepared to accept the rectangular graft using a high-speed drill (either the Midas Rex with M-8 dissecting tool or another drill with a cylindrical or conical bit). When used with a gentle "sweeping action" along the plane of the disc space, these bits will shape the endplates so that they become perfectly parallel to each other. It is important that the underlying cancellous bone not be exposed by complete removal of the cortical plates since this will decrease the intrinsic supporting capacity of the vertebral body and predispose the sturdy graft to penetrate the weakened vertebral bodies. The endplates can be shaved with this "sweeping action" until punctate hemorrhages become visible leaving ample cortical bone to support the graft yet promoting adequate bone healing.

Due to the different shape of the upper and lower ends of the vertebral bodies, production of parallel surfaces for grafting requires selective drilling of the anterior and posterior one-third of the caudal endplate

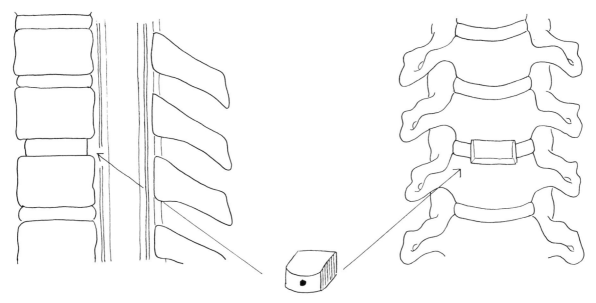

FIG. 1. Rectangular plug fusion (Smith-Robinson).

and the posterior one-third or one-half of the rostral endplate (Fig. 2). When performed correctly, the graft site has parallel surfaces with sufficient cortical bone remaining to support the graft. A common error is failure to remove enough anterior and posterior bony lip thus leaving a central gap between the bone graft and vertebral endplate (Fig. 3). A more serious error is the "ramp effect" resulting from excessive bone removal from the anterior two-thirds of the lower vertebral body. This produces a graft site that is taller anteriorly than it is posteriorly and encourages forward dislocation of the graft (Fig. 4).

Determining Graft Dimensions: (Wolfhard Caspar, M.D., and Haynes Harkey, M.D.)

A tight fitting "gapless" graft requires an appropriately sized, well-formed bone plug as well as a meticulously prepared graft site. It is important to *accurately measure the graft site* to determine the proper size of the bone plug. A micrometer and depth gauge greatly improve accuracy when measuring the height and depth of the graft site. In this manner, the optimal graft can be harvested, which will produce a snug fit under moderate compression and will not compromise the spinal or root canals.

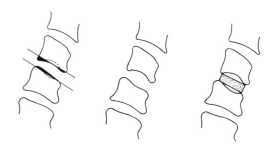

FIG. 3. Inadequate bony resection results in gaps between the vertebral endplates and the block graft, which may increase the chance of pseudoarthrosis.

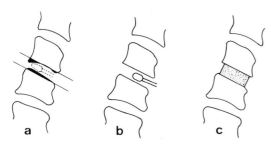

FIG. 2. The proper graft site is produced by drilling of the anterior and posterior one-third of the caudal endplate, and the posterior one-third or one-half of the rostral endplate. **A:** Operative site after disc removal; *shaded area* represnts extent of bony resection. **B:** Prepared graft site. **C:** Precise graft fit due to parallelism of graft site and graft.

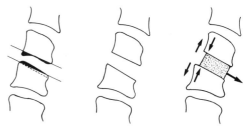

FIG. 4. If too much bone is resected from the anterior portion of the inferior vertebral body (correct resection shown as *shaded area* and *dotted line* illustrating excessive resection), the graft will more likely be extruded.

The depth of the graft site is measured in the midline of the vertebral body from the posterior cortex to the anterior cortex. Since the osteophytes and irregularities have been previously removed, this measurement will reflect the true depth of the vertebral body. The height of the graft site (i.e., the distance between the vertebral endplates) is measured in the maximum distracted condition. In an average single level fusion with an intact posterior longitudinal ligament, the thickness of the graft should equal the height of the distracted graft site. A graft of this size will produce the desired snug fit. If two levels are fused with an intact intervening vertebral body, the measurement should be made in the nondistracted position. Each bone plug should be 1–1.5 mm taller than these measurements in order to generate the appropriate compressive forces. Unfortunately, the ligaments and joint capsules are frequently ruptured in trauma, resulting in a hyperlax segment. Under these conditions, the maximum recommended graft size is 10 mm. This size of graft will not produce overdistraction of the joint or stretch the spinal cord.

The depth of the graft should measure 3 mm less than the anterior-posterior diameter of the prepared interspace—generally, ~15 mm in depth. This allows a sufficient margin of safety anterior to the spinal cord once the bone plug is seated into place. The appropriate length can be more easily and accurately cut using the guillotine graft cutter with integrated depth control (Aesculap Instrument Co., Burlingame, CA, U.S.A.).

The graft impactor is attached to the bone block after a hole is drilled through the center of the anterior cortical surface using the distraction screw drill bit. A cutting burr can be used to further shape the graft (Fig. 5). If the height needs to be reduced, the cortical bone should be drilled away, leaving the cancellous bone a bit thicker. Upon insertion, this excess cancellous bone will be compacted forming a more dense bone graft. The posterior edges of the graft cortex can be slightly rounded to assist insertion into the graft site and provide further protection against root injury.

Graft Placement: (Wolfhard Caspar, M.D., and Haynes Harkey, M.D.)

Once the shaping has been completed, the vertebral bodies are maximally distracted and the graft is inserted with the impactor and tapped into position (Fig. 6). This step can be done under fluoroscopic control, which gives a real-time image of the process. The graft should slide into a snug position without requiring excessive force or hammering. The anterior graft surface should be countersunk 1–2 mm beneath the anterior ridges of vertebral cortical bone. A blunt right angled probe can generally be slipped lateral to the graft, allowing the surgeon to palpate its posterior surface and judge the margin of safety anterior to the cord. Again, this can be done with fluoroscopy since the radiopaque probe will demonstrate the exact position of the posterior graft surface relative to the cord. If the graft does not fit satisfactorily, it can be removed and further shaped or repositioned. Excessive manipulation, however, tends to weaken the graft and care should be taken not to split the cortical graft surface.

After the bone plug has been seated, a spongioplasty is performed. The residual spaces lateral to the graft are filled with cancellous bone as if filling a smoking pipe. Tiny chips of spongiosa (may be mixed with fibrin glue if available) are loosely placed at the depths and more tightly compacted towards the surface. This will further enhance the potential for fusion.

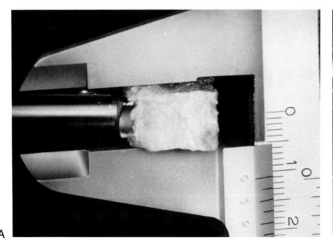
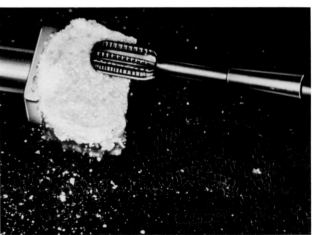

A   B

FIG. 5. A: Calipers are used to confirm parallelism and thickness of the graft. **B:** A cutting burr can be used to further shape the graft if necessary.

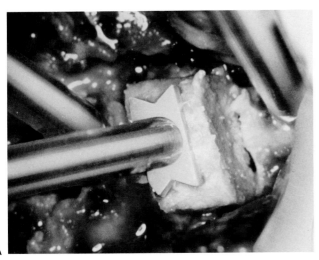
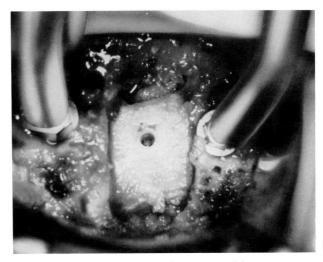

A

B

FIG. 6. The graft is inserted with the vertebral bodies fully distracted **(A)** and then tamped into place **(B)**.

Rectangular Strut (Bailey and Badgley)

On occasion, for adequate decompression, it may be necessary to remove a larger amount of subchondral bone resulting in the requirement of a rectangular block of bone 2–3 cm in height (73,74) (Fig. 7). In this situation, compressive forces alone cannot be used to maintain graft position as some graft penetration into the soft cancellous bone always occurs.

To compensate for this, it is helpful to anteriorly notch the rectangular graft on its cancellous cranial and caudal surfaces. Similarly shaped and positioned troughs are created in the adjoining vertebrae, subchondral cortical, or cancellous bone above and below. This increases the surface area of graft vertebral body contact. Then, with the interspace distracted, the graft is wedged into place and the traction released, thereby locking the graft firmly in position and maintaining fixed distraction and stabilization across the motion segment.

Bone Dowel Fusion (CLOWARD)

The popularity of the cylindrical disc space exposure and dowel graft fusion is based primarily on the relative ease of this anterior fusion technique (75–80) (Fig. 8). Comparable results to the rectangular plug or strut can be obtained with the dowel graft but immediate postoperative stability is less and the potential graft collapse is greater.

Using a high-speed drill (Midas-M8 or conical burr),

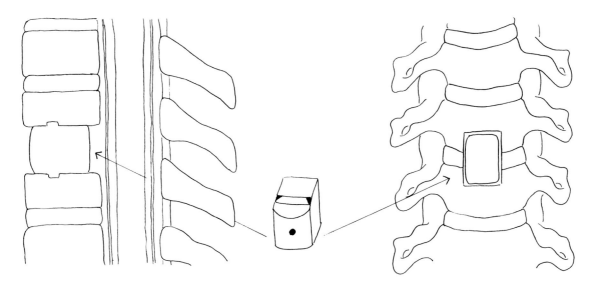

FIG. 7. Rectangular strut fusion (Bailey and Badgley).

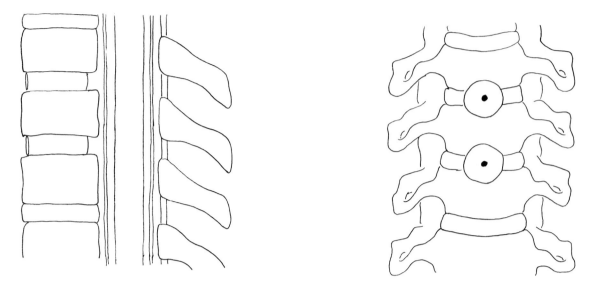

FIG. 8. Bone dowel fusion (Cloward).

a semicircular opening is created along both adjoining vertebral body subchondral junctions large enough to accommodate a 12–18 mm bone dowel. The dimension of the opening should be kept as small as possible, enlarging it only to provide decompression of posterior osteophytic spurs, bars, or ridges, or to uncover sequestered fragments of discs. The interspace spreader is used as the opening proceeds towards the posterior surface to provide better estimation of the eventual size. The shape of the opening is repeatedly checked during drilling to be certain that the horizontal alignment remains in the midline and the vertical alignment

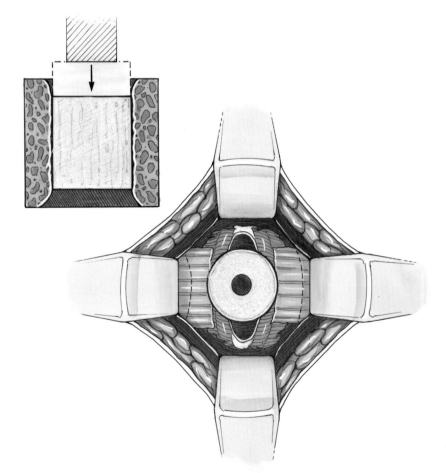

FIG. 9. Bone dowel countersunk below the anterior margin of the surrounding vertebral bodies.

encompasses equal amounts of each adjoining vertebral body. In addition, it is important not to make the opening too large for the size of the bone dowel available.

The opening is carried posteriorly in a symmetrical fashion all the way to the posterior longitudinal ligament. Bone bleeding is controlled with coagulation (mono- or bipolar) or minute amounts of bone wax. The generous application of bone wax to the vertebral body bone margins should be absolutely avoided as this certainly at least delays if not prevents eventual bone fusion.

The depth of the cylindrical opening is precisely measured with calibers and the bone dowel prepared accordingly. The length of the bone dowel should be 1 mm less than the depth of the opening. If the diameter of the bone dowel is too large to fit the opening, the bone dowel should be shaped with a rongeur or high speed burr to fit the opening rather than enlarging the opening to fit the bone dowel.

During placement of the bone dowel, the interspace displacement is slightly increased. The bone dowel is inserted into the opening and gently tapped into position. The bone dowel should be countersunk 1 mm below the anterior margin of the vertebral bodies (Fig. 9). Upon removal of the interspace spreader, the adjoining vertebral body compression should provide stabilization of the dowel.

If available, remnants of the bone dowel (removed during sizing) are used to fill in the openings in the disc space lateral to the bone dowel. Only those fragments able to be secured in position should be applied. Smaller fragments of bone that fall freely into the intervertebral space should be discarded for fear of migration into the epidural space.

For multiple-level cylindrical fusions, the residual vertebral body between adjacent spaces should be kept long enough (at least 1 cm) to avoid complete collapse of the remaining cancellous bone due to avascular necrosis.

Other Applications

It may at times be necessary to correct an exaggerated cervical kyphosis or lordosis. In this setting, an oval or trapezoid-shaped graft may be utilized. This can be constructed from the normal rectangular or cylindrical graft by removing bone from its anterior or posterior surface as may be required. Following distraction, the graft is wedged with the slightly larger surface anteriorly to correct kyphosis or posteriorly to correct lordosis.

CORPORECTOMY FUSIONS

Partial or complete vertebral body resection may be indicated for spondylotic processes extending between two motion segments behind a vertebral body; sequestered discs migrating well beyond the disc space to lie behind the midportion of a vertebral body; single or multisegments affected by opacification of the posterior longitudinal ligament (OPLL); vertebral body fractures with retropulsed fragments; and vertebral body tumors (81–86).

PARTIAL MIDLINE CORPORECTOMY

Procedure

A midline trough is cut using a high-speed drill progressively through the cancellous bone of the vertebral body(ies) between adjoining disc spaces (Fig. 10). The

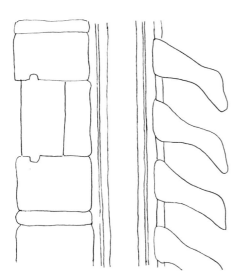 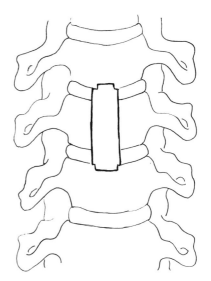

FIG. 10. Partial midline corporectomy fusion.

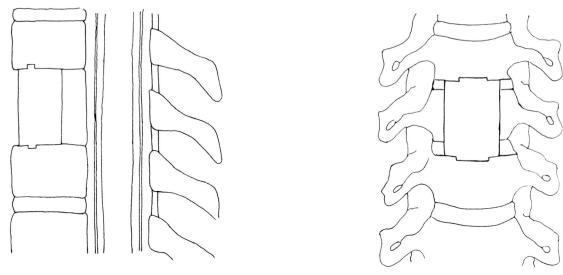

FIG. 11. Complete corporectomy fusion.

bordering discs are removed completely, and the cartilaginous plates on the inferior and superior aspects of the adjoining vertebral bodies removed. To improve stability, it is helpful to notch the cancellous end graft and trough the vertebral body subchondral bone as previously described. A tri-cortical cancellous iliac graft that corresponds in shape to the size of the trough is utilized.

COMPLETE CORPORECTOMY FUSION

Procedure

The anterior two-thirds of the involved vertebral body(ies) is(are) removed, keeping the bony removal medial enough as not to disrupt the pedicles (Fig. 11). Troughs are cut into the superior and inferior vertebral bodies subchondral cortical bone. It is important not to penetrate this cortical bone layer during graft site preparation so as not to destabilize the eventual strut compression by passage into the adjoining cancellous vertebral body bone.

Full-thickness anterior iliac crest (tri-cortical) or fibular, tibial, or rib strut grafts are used for bony fusion (13). When harvesting the strut, it is prudent to include several extra millimeters to allow for the formation of notches and reshaping. The use of a tibial or fibular bone strut is most ideal when attempting to precisely shape the curvature of the cervical spine over several segments.

Following proper graft and gap shaping the opening is enlarged by either skull traction or vertebral body distraction. In applying the graft, the strut must be inserted against the vertebral body subchondral bone with maximum contact along all surfaces. The cortical bone of the strut should be aligned according to stress forces. The upper graft notch is first introduced into the trough of the vertebral body above, and then an impactor is used to countersink the inferior portion of the graft into the underlying trough. The superior notch is slightly larger than the inferior notch allowing for easier insertion. The anterior cortical bone portions of the vertebral bodies surrounding the troughs are preserved so that the strut graft notches can be locked into place. This serves as a secure barrier against dislodgement.

Re-Do Fusions

The reexploration of a failed anterior cerival fusion may be necessary following the development of a symptomatic pseudoarthoris. The regrafting procedure is generally easy, although the initial identification of the site of the pseudoarthrosis may be difficult. In addition, the drilling of a new graft bed through the failed fusion mass must be accomplished carefully to maintain the correct orientation between the adjoining vertebral bodies.

HARVESTING ILIAC CREST BONE GRAFTS: (Wolfhard Caspar, M.D., and Haynes Harkey, M.D.)

In choosing a graft site, it is important to remember that the iliac crest can provide both tri-cortical and cortical-cancellous struts; the fibula (or fibia) primarily provides long and strong cortical struts, whereas the rib produces similar strut with a vascular pedicle.

Overall, the iliac crest is the ideal donor site for obtaining the greatest variety of bone grafts for anterior cervical fusions since blocks of bone with three cortical surfaces and ample cancellous matrix can be harvested over a wide range of dimensions.

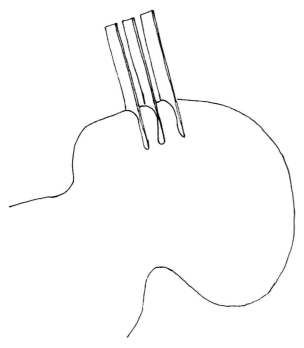

FIG. 12. Corticocancellous iliac crest rectangular grafts.

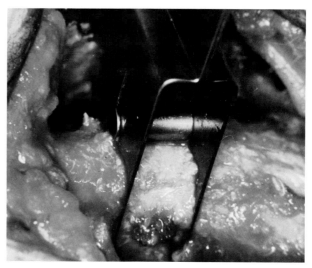

FIG. 13. Double-bladed oscillating saw produces a parallel graft of the appropriate dimensions.

When immediate strength and stability is important, a primarily cortical autograft is ideal, although cancellous bone generally supplies more viable cells and is more quickly vascularized and incorporated.

Prior to cutting the graft, all soft-tissue attachments should be dissected from the iliac crest using a vertical splitting incision of the muscle and fascia. This is more easily accomplished before attempting to remove bone particularly as remaining soft tissue can interfere with graft healing.

For obtaining rectangular plugs or small struts, the iliac crest osteotomies should be at right angles to the surface of the crest and parallel to each other. Grafts at oblique angles produce bone that is too soft predisposing to collapse (Fig. 12). It is important to use both the inner and outer cortices of the iliac crest plus the vertical bone of the iliac ridge. The cortices of iliac bone in this region are 7–9 mm thick. Grafts are accurately cut and less likely to be fractured if an oscillating saw is used and a recently developed double-bladed oscillating saw[1] ensures that the surfaces will be parallel (Fig. 13). If a single-bladed oscillating saw is used, the second cut should be made after carefully determining the correct distance from the first cut thereby avoiding loss of graft height due to the width of the blade (Fig. 14). Similarly, this loss of graft height should be considered when taking multiple grafts with the double-bladed saw (Fig. 15). Of course, it is always preferable to cut an over-sized graft that can be further shaped than to try and use a graft that is too small.

The dowels for the cylindrical opening should be cancellous in the midportion with cortical bone on both ends (K). These are best obtained across the back of the ilium just beneath the iliac crest.

Graft Failures

Graft failure may occur up to 30% of the time due to extrusion, bone resorption, fatigue, collapse, fracture, nonunion (pseudoarthrosis), or infection (102–106). Graft extrusion after single-level fusion is four

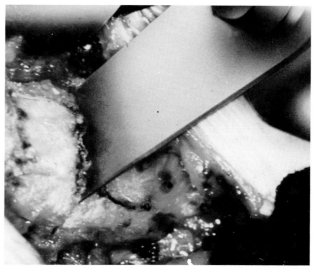

FIG. 14. Single-bladed oscillating saw for harvesting grafts for subtotal and total body replacement and plating.

---

[1]Double-bladed oscillating saw by Aesculap available in five sizes between 6 mm and 10 mm at 1 mm increments.

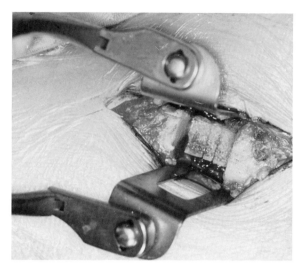

FIG. 15. Donor site after removing two bone plugs. Note the small "island" of bone left between the two donor sites. If the double-bladed saw is used to harvest two or more block grafts, both blades should cut bone with each attempt. This ensures that the surfaces will be parallel and the graft will be the appropriate thickness.

times more common with the cylindrical graft than the rectangular strut or plug. There are several factors that appear to increase the chance of graft resorption, collapse or fracture, and subsequent risk of pseudoarthrosis: multilevel fusions, the use of allograft or xenograft over autograft, significant preexisting instability, insufficient post-operative immobilization during the healing phase, and choosing a graft with insufficient cortical bone for support.

The presence of a postoperative pseudoarthrosis is generally not related to the occurrence of a less than satisfactory clinical result. Patients with the most striking postoperative pain seldom have a radiographic pseudoarthrosis, whereas patients with the most significant pseudoarthroses many times have no significant symptomatology. It is clear that a good clinical result, i.e., pain relief, and a successful fusion (arthrodesis) are not always synonymous. In terms of the fusion rate, it is clear that autogenous bone is superior to allograft which is far superior to xenograft. However, it is not at all uncommon for an asymptomatic pseudoarthrosis to be an excellent clinical result.

REFERENCES

Allografts and Autografts

1. Brown MD, Malinin TI, Davis PB. A roentgenographic evaluation of frozen allografts versus autografts in anterior cervical fusions. *Clin Orthop* 119:231, 1976.
2. Malanin TI, Rosomoff HL, Sutton CH. Human cadaver femoral head homografts for anterior cervical spine fusions. *Surg Neurol* 7:249, 1977.
3. Malinin TI, Eismont FJ, Brown MD. Material used in spine stabilization. Chapter 3, Dunsker et al. (Eds): *The Unstable Spine.* Grune & Stratton, Inc, 25–43, 1986.
4. Nasca RJ, Whelchel JD. Use of cyropreserved bone in spinal surgery. *Spine* 12:222–227, 1987.
5. Schneider JR, Bright RW. Anterior cervical fusion using preserved bone allografts. *Transplant Proc 8 (Suppl 1):* 73, 1976.
6. Weiland AJ, Phillips TW, Randolph MA. Bone Grafts: A radiologic, histologic and biomechanical model comparing autografts, allografts and free vascularized bone grafts. *Plast Reconstr Surg* 74:368, 1984.
7. Vieira JM, Reis JJ, Freitas CT. Intersomatic athrodesis of the cervical spine with autologous bone graft. *Cervical Spine II.* Springer-Verlag, 118–123, 1989.

Vascularized Autografts

8. Bradford DS. Anterior vascular pedicle bone grafting for the treatment of kyphosis. *Spine* 5:318, 1980.
9. Dell PC, Burchardt H, Glowzewskie FP. A roentgenographic, biomechanical and histological evaluation of vascularized and nonvascularized segmental fibular canine autografts. *J Bone Joint Surg [Am]* 67A:105, 1985.
10. Doi K, Kykawai S, Sumiura S, Sakai K. Intercervical fusion using the free vascularized fibular graft. *Spine* 13:1239–1244, 1988.
11. Hartman JT, McCarron RF, Robertson WW. A pedicle bone grafting procedure for failed lumbosacral spinal fusion. *Clin Orthop* 178:223, 1983.
12. Hubbard LF, Herndon JH, Buonanno AR. Free vascularized fibula transfer for stabilization of the thoracolumbar spine. A case report. *Spine* 10:89, 1985.
13. McBride GG, Bradford DS. Vertebral body replacement with femoral neck allograft and vacularized rib strut graft. A technique for treating post-traumatic kyphosis with neurologic deficit. *Spine* 8:406, 1983.
14. Rose GK, Owen R, Sanderson JM. Transposition of rib with blood supply for the stabilization of spinal kyphosis. *J Bone Joint Surg [Br]* 57B:112, 1975.
15. Shaffer JW, Fields GA, Goldberg VM, Davy DT. Fate of vascularized and non-vascularized autografts. *Clin Orthop* 197:32, 1985.
16. Weiland AJ, Moore JR, Daniel RK. Vascularized bone autografts: experience with 41 cases. *Clin Orthop* 174:87, 1983.
17. Weiland AJ, Phillips TW, Randolph MA. Bone grafts: a radiologic, histology and biomechanical model comparing autografts, allografts and free vascularized bone grafts. *Plast Reconstr Surg* 74:368, 1984.

Xenografts

18. McMurray GN. The evaluation of Kiel bone in spinal fusions. *J Bone Joint Surg [Br]* 64B:101, 1982.
19. Salama R. Xenogeneic bone grafting in humans. *Clin Orthop* 174:113, 1983.
20. Siqueira EB, Kranzler LI. Cervical interbody fusion using calf bone. *Surg Neurol* 18:37, 1982.

Osteoinduction

21. Bolander ME, Balian G. The use of demineralized bone matrix in the repair of segmental defects. *J Bone Joint Surg [Am]* 68A:1264, 1986.
22. Burwell RC. Studies on the transplantation of bone. VII. The fresh composite homo-autograft of cancellous bone. An analysis of factors leading to osteogenesis in marrow transplants and in marrow containing bone grafts. *J Bone Joint Surg [Br]* 46B:110, 1964.

23. Burwell RG. The function of bone marrow in the incorporation of a bone graft. *Clin Orthop* 200:125, 1985.
24. Canalis E. Effect of growth factors on bone cell replication and differentiation. *Clin Orthop* 193:246, 1985.
25. Freidenstein AJ, Petrakova KV, Kurolesova AI, Frolova GP. Heterotopic transplants of bone marrow. Analysis of precursor cells for osteogenic and haemopoietic tissues. *Transplantation* 6:230, 1968.
26. Glowacki J, Kaban LB, Murray JE, et al. Application of the biological principle of induced osteogenesis for craniofacial defects. *Lancet* 1:959, 1981.
27. Glowacki J, Altobelli D, Mulliken JB. Fate of mineralized and demineralized osseous implants in cranial defects. *Calcif Tissue Int* 30:71, 1981.
28. Glowacki J, Mulliken JB. Demineralized bone implants. *Clin Plast Surg* 12:233, 1985.
29. Harakas NK. Demineralized bone matrix-induced osteogenesis. *Clin Orthop* 188:239, 1984.
30. Lindholm TS, Urist MR. A quantitative analysis of new bone formation by induction in composite graft of bone marrow and bone matrix. *Clin Orthop* 150:288, 1956.
31. Lovell T, Dawson EG. BMP augmentation of experimental spinal fusion. Presented at the Trans 32nd Orthop Res Soc Meeting, 1986.
32. Mulliken JB, Glowacki J. Induced osteogenesis for the repair and reconstruction of the craniofacial region. *Plast Reconstr Surg* 65:553, 1980.
33. Mulliken JB, Kaban LB, Glowacki J. Induced osteogenesis—the biologic principle and clinical applications. *J Surg Res* 37:487, 1984.
34. Muthukumaran N, Reddi AH. Bone matrix-induced local bone induction. *Clin Orthop* 200:159, 1985.
35. Nilsson OS, Urist MR, Dawson T, et al. Bone repair induced by bone morphogenetic protein in ulnar defects in dogs. *J Bone Joint Surg [Br]* 68B:635, 1986.
36. Takagi K, Urist MR. The role of bone marrow in bone morphogenetic protein-induced repair of femoral massive diaphyseal defects. *Clin Orthop* 171:225, 1982.
37. Tuli SN, Singh AD. The osteoinductive property of decalcified bone matrix. An experimental study. *J Bone Joint Surg [Br]* 60B:116, 1978.
38. Sato K, Urist MR. Induced regeneration of calvaria by bone morphogenetic protein (BMP) in dogs. *Clin Orthop* 197:301, 1985.
39. Urist MR. Bone: formation by autoinduction. *Science* 150:893, 1965.
40. Urist MR. New bone formation induced in post fetal life by bone morphogenetic protein. In: Becker RD, ed. *Mechanisms of growth control.* Springfield, IL: Charles C. Thomas, 406, 1981.

Ceramics

41. Cook SD, Reynolds MC, Whitecloud TS, et al. Evaluation of hydroxyapatite graft materials in canine cerivcal spine fusions. *Spine* 11:305–309, 1986.
42. Cook SD, Whitecloud TS, Reynolds MC, et al. Hydroxylapatite graft materials for cervical spine fusions. In: *Cervical spine I* Springer-Verlag, 257–262, 1987.
43. Ferraro JW. Experimental evaluation of ceramic calcium phosphate as a substitute for bone grafts. *Plast Reconstr Surg* 63:634, 1979.
44. Flatley TJ, Lynch KL, Benson MD. Tissue response to implants of calcium phosphate ceramic in rabbit spine. *Clin Orthop* 179:246, 1983.
45. Holmes RE, Bucholz RW, Mooney V. Porous hydroxyapatite as a bone graft substitute in diaphyseal defects: a histometric study. *J Orthop Res* 5:114, 1987.
46. Jarcho M. Calcium phosphate ceramics as hard tissue prosthetics. *Clin Orthop* 157:259, 1981.
47. Lesoin F, Bouasakao N, Krivosic I, DuPont A, Jomin M. Use of acrylic prosthesis for a giant-cell tumor of the cervical spine. *Surg Neurol* 17:358–362, 1981.

48. Moore DC, Chapman MW, Manske D. The evaluation of a biphasic calcium phosphate ceramic for use in grafting long-bone diaphyseal defects. *J Orthop Res* 5:356, 1987.
49. Muschler GM, Lane JM, Werntx J, et al. The use of composite bone graft materials in a segmental femoral defect model in the rat. Presented at the Inaugural Meet Internal Soc Fracture Repair, Helsinki, September 2, 1987.
50. Patka P. *Bone replacement by calcium phosphate ceramics: an experimental study.* Amsterdam: Free University Press, 1984.
51. Rejda BV, Peelen JGJ, deGroot K. Tricalcium phosphate as a bone substitute. *J Bioeng* 1:93, 1977.
52. Scoville WB, Palmer AH, Samra A, Chong G. The use of acrylic plastic for vertebral replacement or fixation in metastic disease of the spine. Technical note. *J Neurosurg* 17:274–279, 1967.
53. Senter HJ, Kortyna R, Kemp WR. The anterior cervical discectomy with hydroxylapatite fusion. *Neurosurgery* 25:39–43, 1989.
54. Waisbrod H, Gerbershagen HU. A pilot study of the value of ceramics for bone replacement. *Arch Orthop Trauma Surg* 105:298, 1986.

Electrical Stimulation

55. Bassett CA, Pilla AA, Pawluk RJ. A non-operative salvage of surgically resistant pseudoarthroses and nonunion by pulsing electromagnetic fields. *Clin Orthop* 124:128, 1977.
56. Bassett CAL, Mitchell SN, Gaston SR. Pulsing electromagnetic field treatment in ununited fractures and failed arthrodeses. *JAMA* 247:263, 1982.
57. Bassett CAL. The development and application of pulsed electromagnetic fields (PEMF's) for united fractures and arthrodeses. *Orthop Clin North Am* 15:61, 1984.
58. Crock HV. *Practice of spinal surgery.* Springer-Verlag, 179–218, 1983.
59. Kane WJ. Direct current, electrical bone growth stimulation for spinal fusion. *Spine* 13:363–365, 1988.
60. Kane WJ. Electrical stimulation of spinal fusions. In: Cotler, ed. *Spinal fusion.* Springer-Verlag, 33–44, 1990.
61. Nerubay J, Marganit B, Bubis JJ, Tadmor A, Katznelson A. Stimluation of bone formation by electrical current on spinal fusion. *Spine* 11:167–169, 1986.

Physiology/Biology of Bone Fusion

62. Kaufman HH, Jones E. The principles of bony spinal fusion. *Spine* 24:264–270, 1989.
63. McCulloch JA. *Principles of microsurgery for lumbar disc disease.* New York: Raven Press, 1989.
64. Muschler GF, Lane JM, Dawson EG. The biology of spinal fusion. In: Cotler, ed. *Spinal fusion.* Springer-Verlag, 9–21, 1990.
65. Prolo DJ, Rodrigo JJ. Contemporary bone graft physiology I and surgery. *Clin Orthop* 200:322, 1985.

Rectangular Plug Fusion

66. Aronson NI, Filtzer DL, Bagan M. Anterior cervical fusion by the Smith-Robinson approach. *J Neurosurg* 29:397–404, 1968.
67. Aronson NI. Management of soft disc protrusions using the Smith-Robinson approach. *Clin Neurosurg* 20:253, 1973.
68. Kehr P, Lang G. Transdiscal osteophytectomy and fusion according to Robinson's method. In: *Cervical spine I.* Springer-Verlag, 304–307, 1987.
69. Robinson RA, Smith GW. Anterolateral cervical disc removal and interbody fusion cerivcal disc syndromes. *Johns Hopkins Hospital* 96:223–224, 1955.
70. Robinson RA. Anterior and posterior cervical fusions. *Clin Orthop* 35:34–62, 1964.

71. Robinson RA, Riley LH. Anterior interbody fusion of the cervical spine. *The craft of surgery*. 2nd ed. Boston: Little, Brown, 1873–1881, 1971.
72. Smith GW, Robinson RA. The treatment of certain cervical spine disorders by anterior removal of the intervertebral disc and interbody fusion. *J Bone Joint Surg [Am]* 40A:607–624, 1958.

Rectangular Strut Fusion

73. Bailey RW, Badgley CE. Stabilization of the cervical spine by anterior fusion. *J Bone Joint Surg [Am]* 42A:565–594, 1960.
74. Jones AA, Rothman RH, Balderston RA. Fusion technique for degenerative disease. In: Cotler JM, Cotler HB, eds. *Spinal fusion*. Springer-Verlag, 1990.

Bone Dowel Fusion

75. Cloward RB. The anterior approach for removal of ruptured cervical disc. *J Neurosurg* 15:602, 1958.
76. Cloward RB. New methods of diagnosis and treatment of cervical disc disease. *Clin Neurosurg* 8:93–132, 1962.
77. Cloward RB. Lesions of the intervertebral disc and their treatment by interbody fusion methods. *Clin Orthop* 27:51–77, 1963.
78. Dohn DF. Anterior interbody fusion for treatment of cervical disk conditions. *JAMA* –900, 1966.
79. Espersen JO, Buhl M, Eriksen FF, et al. Treatment of cervical disc disease using Cloward's technique I: general results, effects of different operative methods and complications in 1,106 patients. *Acta Neurochir (Wien)* 70:97, 1984.
80. Gruninger W, Gruss P. The influence of Cloward fusion operation on the motility of the cervical spine. In: Grote W, ed. *Advances in neurosurgery 8*. New York: Springer-Verlag, 291–294, 1980.

Corporectomy and Strut Fusion

81. Hanai K, Fujiyoshi F, Kamei K. Sub total vertebrectomy and spinal fusion for cervical spondylotic myelopathy. *Spine* 11:310–315, 1986.
82. Senegas J, Guerin J. Technique de decompression medullaire anterieure dans les stenoses canalaires etendues. *Rev Chir Orthop* 61(suppl 2):219–223, 1975.
83. Senegas J, Gauzere JM. Plaidoyer pour la chirurgi anterieure dans le traitement des traumatismes graves des cinq dernieres vertebres cervicales. *Rev Chir Orthop* 62(suppl 2):123–128, 1976.
84. Whitecloud TS III, Larocca SH. Fibular strut graft in reconstructive surgery of the cervical spine. In: Cotler, ed. *Spine Fusion*. Springer-Verlag, 33–44, 1990.
85. Whitecloud TS III. Cervical spondylotic myelopathy: the results of anterior decompression and stabilization. In: *Cervical spine I*. 278–281, 1987.
86. Whitehill R, Wilhelm CE, Moskal et al. Posterior strut fusions to enhance immediate postoperative cervical stability. *Spine* 11:6, 1986.

Methyl Methacrylate

87. Bryan WJ, Inglis AE, Sculco TP, Ranawat CS. Methylmethacrylate stabilization for enhancement of posterior cervical arthrodesis in rheumatoid arthritis. *J Bone Joint Surg [Am]* 64A:1045, 1982.
88. Clark CR, Keggi KJ, Panjabi MM. Methylmethacrylate stabilization of the cervical spine. *J Bone Joint Surg [Am]* 66A:40, 1984.
89. McAfee PC, Bohlman HH, Ducker T, Eismont FJ. Failure of stabilization of the spine with methylmethacrylate a retrospective analysis of 24 cases. *J Bone Joint Surg [Am]* 68A:1145, 1986.
90. Whitehall R, Barry JC. The evolution of stability in cervical spinal constructs using either autogenous bone graft or methylmethacrylate cement: a follow-up report on canine in vivo model. *Spine* 10:32, 1985.

No Fusion

91. Brown CW, Orme TJ, Richardson HD. The rate of pseudarthrosis (surgical non-union) in patients who are smokers and patients who are non-smokers. *Spine* 11:942, 1986.
92. Dunsker SB. Anterior cervical discectomy with and without fusion. *Clin Neurosurg* 24:516–521, 1977.
93. Hankinson HL, Wilson CB. Use of the operating microscope in anterior cervical discectomy without fusion. *J Neurosurg* 43:452–456, 1975.
94. Hirsch C. Cervical disc rupture. Diagnosis and therapy. *Acta Orthop Scand* 30:172–186, 1960.
95. Martins An. Anterior cervical discectomy with and without interbody bone graft. *J Neurosurg* 44:290–295, 1976.
96. Murphy MG, Gado M. Anterior cervical discectomy without interbody bone graft. *J Neurosurg* 37:71–74, 1972.
97. Riley LH, Robinson Ra, Johnson KA, et al. The results of anterior interbody fusion of the cervical spine. Review of ninety-three consecutive cases. *J Neurosurg* 30:127–133, 1969.
98. Robertson JT. Anterior removal of cervical disc without fusion. *Clin Neurosurg* 20:259–261, 1973.
99. Robertson JT. Anterior operations for herniated cervical disc and myelopathya. *Clin Neurosurg* 25:245–250, 1978.
100. Tew JM Jr, Mayfield FH. Surgery of the anterior cervical spine: prevention of complications. In: Dunsker SB, ed. *Cervical spondylosis*. New York: Raven Press, 191–208, 1981.
101. White AA, Southwick WO, Deponte RJ, et al. Relief of pain by anterior cervical-spine fusion for spondylosis. A report of sixty-five patients. *J Bone Joint Surg [Am]* 55A:525–534, 1973.

Graft Extrusion or Collapse

102. Burchardt H. Biology of bone transplantation. *Orthop Clin North Am* 18:187–196, 1987.
103. Lunsford LD, Bissonette DJ, Jannetta PJ, et al. Anterior surgery for cervical disc disease. Part 1: Treatment of lateral cervical disc herniation in 253 cases. *J Neurosurg* 53:1–11, 1980.
104. Lunsford LD, Bissonette DJ, Zorub DS. Anterior surgery of cervical disc disease. Part 2: Treatment of cervical spondylotic myelopathy in 32 cases. *J Neurosurg* 53:12–19, 1980.
105. Simmons EH, Bhalla SK. Anterior cervical discectomy and fusion. A clinical and biomechanical study with eight year follow up. *J Bone Joint Surg [Br]* 51B:225–237, 1969.
106. Tew JM Jr, Mayfield FH. Complications of surgery of the anterior cervical spine. *Clin Neurosurg* 23:424–434, 1976.

CHAPTER 9

Anterior Microsurgery for Degenerative Cervical Disc Disease

Overall Results

Paul H. Young

PRESENT SERIES

From September 1984 until September 1989, 250 consecutive microsurgical procedures from the anterior approach for degenerative cervical disc disease were performed by the author. The following is a detailed analysis of these cases.

PATIENT PROFILE

Fifty-six percent of these patients were male and 44% were female (Table 1). The patients ranged in age from 15 to 82, with 14% of the patients between the ages of 20 and 35, 46% between the ages of 35 and 50, 34% between 50 and 70, and 6% over the age of 70. Overall, 80% of the patients were between the ages of 35 and 70. Fifty-six percent of the patients were office workers (white collar), whereas 30% were laborers (blue collar). Ten percent of the patients were retired, whereas only 4% were unemployed at the time of surgery.

Six percent of the patients had undergone one or more prior operative procedures consisting of either a decompressive cervical laminectomy of discectomy (with or without fusion), whereas 7% of the patients in this series had undergone a previous lumbar procedure.

CLINICAL STATUS

Eighty-eight percent of the patients presented with both neck and arm pain of varying proportions (Table 2). Ten percent underwent surgery for neck pain alone, whereas only 1% presented with arm pain exclusively. In addition, 1% of patients were operated upon in the absence of any complaint of pain.

Neurological findings including muscle weakness and reflex changes were present in 55% of the patients. Radicular numbness was found in 67%, and only 3% of the patients had myelopathic signs prior to surgery.

Surgical Decision Making

The patient's clinical status was the single most important factor in determining the role and timing of surgical intervention. Those patients without radicular pain or positive radiological findings were treated with at least 2 or 3 months of conservative treatment before surgery was even considered. Patients with radicular pain but no neurological findings generally underwent a month of physical therapy (including traction) in combination with medical treatment. Those individuals with marked radicular or moderate myelopathic symptomatology and appropriate neurological deficits were considered for surgery after only a brief period

103

TABLE 1. *Patient profile: September 1, 1984, to September 1, 1989*

Characteristic	n (%)
Sex	
Male	141 (56%)
Female	109 (44%)
Total	250
Age (years)	
15–20	1 (<1%)
21–34	35 (14%)
35–49	116 (46%)
50–70	84 (34%)
Over 70	14 (6%)
Occupation	
Office worker	140 (56%)
Laborer	75 (30%)
Retired	25 (10%)
Unemployed	10 (4%)
Previous surgery	
Decompressive laminectomy or discectomy	16 (6%)
Lumbar spine surgery	17 (7%)

of therapy lasting 2–4 weeks. Finally, patients with severe arm pain and marked neurologic findings or patients with severe or progressive myelopathy underwent surgery without delay.

RADIOGRAPHIC EVALUATION

All patients in this series was evaluated by either computed axial tomography (CAT), magnetic resonance imaging (MRI), and/or myelography prior to surgery. Most recently, patients are evaluated initially with MRI alone, this modality completely eliminating the use of CAT and significantly diminishing (by 75%) the role of myelography.

On the basis of radiographic evaluations and surgical morphology, intervertebral discs and spinal canal pathology is divided into six categories (Table 3): (a) disc extrusion, (b) disc sequestration, (c) midline osteophytic canal stenosis, (d) lateral canal or foraminal stenosis, and (e) disc extrusion in association with osteophytic midline or lateral canal stenosis, or (f) foraminal stenosis.

TABLE 2. *Clinical status*

Characteristic	n (%)
Pain	
Neck and arm	219 (88%)
Neck only	26 (10%)
Arm only	3 (1%)
No pain	2 (1%)
Neurological change	
Motor/reflex loss	138 (55%)
Radicular numbness	168 (67%)
Myelopathy	8 (3%)

TABLE 3. *Surgery*

Characteristic	n (%)
Disc pathology	
Extrusion	145 (58%)
Sequestered	75 (30%)
Midline spondylosis	80 (32%)
Lateral spondylosis	70 (28%)
Extrusion and spondylosis	63 (25%)
Level	
C3–C4	9 (4%)
C4–C5	20 (8%)
C5–C6	76 (30%)
C6–C7	56 (22%)
C7–T1	1 (<1%)
C3–C4/C4–C5	3 (1%)
C4–C5/C5–C6	14 (6%)
C5–C6/C6–C7	58 (23%)
C3–C4/C5–C6	1 (1%)
C4–C5/C6–C7	1 (1%)
C3–C4/C4–C5/C5–C6	2 (1%)
C4–C5/C5–C6/C6–C7	8 (3%)
C3–C4/C5–C6/C6–C7	1 (<1%)
Length of surgery (hr)	
<1	84 (34%)
1–1½	109 (44%)
1½–2	40 (16%)
>2	17 (6%)
Procedure	
Microdiscectomy	13 (5%)
Microdiscectomy with iliac crest fusion	15 (6%)
Microdiscectomy with allograft	222 (89%)
Blood loss (ml)	
0–50	150 (60%)
51–100	72 (28%)
100–200	24 (10%)
>200	4 (2%)

Disc Extrusion

Cervical disc extrusions involve significant herniation of annular and/or nuclear material beyond the confines of the intervertebral space. These extrusions must be located in a midline, paracentral, or foraminal location. Frequently, disc extrusions deform the posterior longitudinal ligament and are associated with osteophytic spurs. Extruded discs were identified in 58% of the patients either exclusively or in combination with a sequestered disc.

Sequestered Discs

Sequestered discs involve the herniation of nuclear material through the annulus and posterior longitudinal ligament with migration of fragmented fragments in the epidural space or foramen. Sequestered discs were found to migrate into the epidural space rostrally or caudally behind the vertebral body or laterally into the foramen inferior or superior to the nerve root. With time, sequestered discs are covered by a glistening white fibrotic capsule, which is densely adherent to the dura. Sequestered discs were identified in 30% of the patients.

Midline Spondylosis

Midline spondylosis involves the protrusion into the spinal canal by a centrally located osteophytic bar or ridge. Midline spondylosis was identified in 32% of the patients in this series at either a single level or multiple levels.

Lateral or Foraminal Spondylosis

Lateral spondylosis involves spondylotic compression in the lateral gutter of the intervertebral foramen, whereas foraminal stenosis involves the actual narrowing of the foramen by osteophytes protruding from the uncovertebral or facet joints. This was identified as probably related to symptomatology in 28% of the patients either unilaterally or bilaterally at one or more levels.

Disc Extrusion in Association with Stenosis

A combination of disc extrusion and either midline or foraminal stenosis was identified in 25% of the patients.

SURGERY

The anterior approach was utilized in all patients (Table 3). A single-level anterior microdiscectomy was performed in 64% of patients, a two-level procedure in 32%, and a three-level procedure in 4%. Bone grafts, either iliac crest autograft (6%) or freeze-dried allograft (89%), were used in 95% of the patients; 5% underwent no fusion. The total operative blood loss was <50 cc in 60% of patients, <100 cc in 88%, and <200 cc in 98% of the patients in this series. In 34% of patients, the operating time was <1 hr, in 78% it was <1½ hr, and in 94% <2 hr.

POSTOPERATIVE RESULTS

Ninety-two percent of patients were able to ambulate on the first postoperative day, and 100% were ambulating by the third postoperative day (Table 4). Eighty-two percent of patients were discharged on the first postoperative day, and 94% before the second postoperative day. The 15 patients hospitalized 2 days were for the most part older individuals with preoperative ambulatory difficulties who required physical therapy or other medical treatment prior to discharge.

TABLE 4. *Postoperative results*

Characteristic	n (%)
Ambulation (days)	
1	230 (92%)
2	18 (7%)
3	2 (1%)
Discharge (days)	
1	206 (82%)
2	29 (12%)
3	15 (6%)
Full home activity (weeks)	
1	69 (28%)
1–2	109 (44%)
2–4	52 (20%)
4	20 (8%)
Return to work (months)	
1	64 (26%)
2	105 (42%)
3–4	66 (26%)
>5	15 (6%)
Complications	
Neck pain	
Persistent	31 (12%)
Recurrent	10 (4%)
Arm pain	
Persistent	22 (9%)
Recurrent	7 (3%)
Dysphagia (>1 week)	2 (1%)
Hoarseness (>2 weeks)	4 (2%)
Disability	2 (1%)
Subcutaneous infection	4 (2%)
Subluxation	1 (<1%)
Death	1 (<1%)
Repeat surgery	0

Seventy-two percent of patients had resumed full home activity by 2 weeks, and 92% by 1 month. Twenty-six percent of the patients were able to return to work before 1 month, 68% before 2 months, and 94% by the fourth postoperative month. Two percent of the operative patients who had previously worked were unable to return to work after surgery and requested permanent disability.

COMPLICATIONS

The most frequent postoperative complication was persistent (12%) or recurrent (4%) neck pain and/or persistent (9%) or recurrent (3%) arm pain (Table 4). In these patients, the pain was severe enough to interfere with the patient's ability to return to rigorous or strenuous physical activity, and in 8% of patients overall it was significant enough that it was necessary to proceed with additional diagnostic tests (MRI and/or myelography). Recurrent pain in patients who had become asymptomatic postoperatively occurred in a total of 12 patients (5%). No patient in this series had significant enough postoperative clinical findings to warrant repeat surgical exploration.

Four patients in this series (2%) had a subcutaneous postoperative infection. In all cases, the infection cleared completely with a short course of oral antibiotics and no patients experienced a disc space infection. No patients suffered a cerebrospinal fluid leak postoperatively.

Two patients complained of dysphasia lasting 1 week, but both resolved before 1 month. Four patients (2%) complained of hoarseness lasting 2 weeks, and in two of these patients the hoarseness was permanent, requiring ENT evaluation and treatment. One patient suffered clinically significant postoperative subluxation, requiring short-term collar use and traction. One patient succumbed on the second postoperative day of a previously uncomplicated postoperative recovery from a sudden cardiac arrest.

Two patients experienced significant increase in neurological deficits postoperatively. Both had recognized motor root avulsion, and both suffered brief C7 radicular weakness, which resolved almost completely over 6 months.

REPORTED RESULTS AND COMPARISONS

The overall reported good results for both posterior (1–23) and anterior (24–63) approaches in treating root compression due to a bony spur are comparable. For spondylotic radiculopathy, long-term success using the anterior approach can be expected in an average of 76% of patients, whereas the posterior approach is successful in 68%. There is no statistical difference between these results, suggesting that the issue of the need for osteophyte removal versus performing a simple nerve root decompression will remain a controversial point of discussion depending on the surgeon's personal perspective. In addition, overall there is a 90–92% chance that the patient will receive at least a satisfactory outcome and only a 2–5% chance that the outcome will be less than satisfactory with either procedure.

For soft disc herniations, the anterior and posterior approaches yield similarly good short-term results in 74–100% of cases (average, 82%). Long-term good results (after 1 year) vary from 63% to 71% (average, 68%), with a recurrence rate of 10–18% (average, 14%) for the anterior approach, and from 0% to 11% (average, 6%) for the posterior approach. Generally, better results are obtained in patients undergoing surgery at one level only.

For spondylotic myelopathy, 40–84% of patients show significant improvement (average, 50%) using the anterior or posterior approach, with the duration and severity of the myelopathy and the patients' age being important prognostic factors. In OPLL patients, anterior decompression yields good results in an average of 82% of cases, laminectomy in 66%, whereas 80% improved after a laminoplasty procedure.

It can be simply stated that reported results suggest that satisfactory improvement can be expected utilizing either the anterior or posterior approach for radiculopathy secondary to spur formation or disc herniation. In addition, somewhat poor but still satisfactory results can be obtained for myelopathic processes utilizing either the anterior or posterior decompressive approaches. If the risk of serious complications can be kept to a minimum, it is clear that surgical approaches for both radiculopathic and myelopathic processes are a clear improvement over the natural history of these disorders.

The present series documents the benefits of the anterior approach in a variety of cervical spine degenerative conditions causing radiculopathy and myelopathy. Good results combined with a minimum of complications make this approach a safe, effective means of dealing with neurologic disability as a result of cervical spondylosis.

REFERENCES

Posterior Procedures

1. Alsharif H, Ezzat SH, Hay A, Motty NA, Malek SA. The results of surgical treatment of spondylotic radiculomyelopathy with complete cervicallaminectomy and posterior foramen magnum decompression. *Acta Neurochir (Wien)* 48:83, 1979.
2. Bishara SN. The posterior operation in the treatment of cervical spondylosis with myelopathy: a long-term follow-up study. *J Neurol Neurosurg Psychiatry* 34:393–398, 1971.
3. DalleOre G, Vivenza C. Cervical spondylotic myelopathies—long-term results of surgical treatment. In Grote W, et al., eds. *Advances in neurosurgery 8.* New York: Springer-Verlag, 1988.
4. Ehni G. *Cervical arthrosis diseases of the cervical motion segments.* Chicago: Yearbook Medical Publishers, 1984.
5. Epstein J, Carras R, Levine LS, et al. Importance of removing osteophytes as part of the surgical treatment of myelo radiculopathy in cervical spondylosis. *J Neurosurg* 30:219, 1969.
6. Epstein JA, Janin Y, Carras R, Lavine LS. A comparative study of the treatment of cervical spondylotic myeloradiculopathy. *Acta Neurochir (Wien)* 61:89–104, 1982.
7. Fager CA. Results of adequate posterior decompression in the relief of spondylotic cervical myelopathy. *J Neurosurg* 38:684–692, 1973.
8. Fager CA. Management of cervical disc lesions and spondylosis by posterior approaches. *Clin Neurosurg* 24:488–507, 1976.
9. Fager CA. Posterior surgical tactics for the neurological symptoms of cervical disc and spondylitic lesions. *Clin Neurosurg* 25:218–244, 1978.
10. Guidetti B, Fortuna A. Long term results of surgical treatment of myelopathy due to cervical spondylosis. *J Neurosurg* 30:714, 1969.
11. Haft H, Shenkin HA. Surgical end results of cervical ridge and disc problems. *JAMA* 186:312–315, 1963.
12. Henderson CM, Hennessy RG, Shuey HM, Shackelford EG. Posterolateral foraminotomy as an exclusive operative technique for cervical radiculopathy: review of 846 consecutively operated cases. *Neurosurgery* 13:504–512, 1983.
13. Hukuda S, Mochizuki T, Ogata M, Shichikawa K, Shimomura Y. Operations for cervical spondylotic myelopathy: a comparison of the results of anterior and posterior procedures. *J Bone Joint Surg [Br]* 67B, 609–615, 1985.
14. Hukuda S, Ogata M, Mochizuki T, Shichikawa K. Laminectomy versus laminoplasty for cervical myelopathy: brief report. *J Bone Joint Surg [Br]* 70B:325–326, 1988.
15. Jenkins DHR. Extensive cervical laminectomy: long-term results. *Br J Surg* 60:852, 1973.

16. Murphy F, Simmons JCH, Brunson, B. Surgical treatment of laterally ruptured cervical disc. Review of 648 cases 1936–1972. *J NSG* 38:679–683, 1973.

17. Nurick S. The natural history and results of surgical treatment of the spinal cord disorder associated with cervical spondylosis. *Brain* 95:101–108, 1971.

18. Odom GL, Finney W, Woodhall B. Cervical disk lesion. *JAMA* 166:23–28, 1958.

19. Rothman RH, Simeone FA. *The spine. Vol. 1.* 2nd ed. Philadelphia: WB Saunders, 1982.

20. Scoville WB. Cervical spondylosis treated by bilateral facetectomy and laminectomy. *J Neurosurg* 18:423–428, 1961.

21. Scoville WB, Dohrmann GT, Corkill G. Late results of cervical disc surgery. *J Neurosurg* 45:203–310, 1976.

22. Sunder-Plassmann M, Farenbauer F. Long-term follow-up after surgery for spondylogenous myelopathy. In: Grote W, et al., eds. *Advances in neurosurgery 8.* New York: Springer-Verlag, 83–85, 1980.

23. Tezuka A, Yamada K, Ikata, T. Surgical results of cervical spondylotic radiculomyelopathy observed for more than five years. *Tokushima J Exp Med* 23:9, 1976.

Anterior Procedures

24. Aronson N, Bagan M, Filtzer DL. Results of using the Smith-Robinson approach for herniated and extruded cervical discs. Technical note. *J Neurosurg* 32:721–722, 1970.

25. Boni M, Denaro V. The cervical stenosis syndrome with a review of 87 patients treated by operation. *Int Orthop* 185:195, 1982.

26. Boni M, Cherubino P, Oenaro V, Benazzo.F. Multiple subtotal somatectomy: technique and evaluation of a series of thirty-nine cases. *Spine* 9:358, 1984.

27. Bernard TN Jr, Whitecloud TS III. Cervical spondylotic myelopathy and myeloradiculopathy: anterior decompression and stabilization with autogenous fibula strut graft. *Clin Orthop* 221:149, 1987.

28. Bertalanffy H, Eggert H-R. Clinical long-term results of anterior discectomy without fusion for treatment of cervical radiculopathy and myelopathy. A follow-up of 164 cases. *Acta Neurochir (Wien)* 90:127–135, 1988.

29. Cherubino P, Ceciliani L, Benazzo F, Borromeo U. Long-term clinical and radiographic evaluations of cervical herniated discs operated by Cloward's Technique. In: *Cervical Spine II.* Springer-Verlag, 203–207, 1989.

30. Chirls M. Retrospective study of cervical spondylosis treated by anterior interbody fusion in 505 patients performed by the Cloward technique. *Bulletin of the Hospital Joint Dis* 39:74, 1978.

31. Cloward RB. The anterior surgical approach to the cervical spine—the Cloward procedure, past, present and future. *Spine* 13:823–827, 1988.

32. Connolley EA, Seymour RJ, Adams JE. Clinical evaluation of anterior cervical fusion for degenerative cervical disc disease. *J Neurosurg* 23:431–437, 1965.

33. Crandall P, Batzdor U. Cervical spondylotic myelopathy. *J Neurosurg* 25:57, 1966.

34. Cuatico W. Anterior cervical discectomy without interbody fusion. An analysis of 81 cases. *Acta Neurochir (Wien)* 57:269–274, 1981.

35. Depalma AF, Rothman RH, et al. Anterior interbody fusion for a severe cervical disc degeneration. *Surg Gynecol Obstet* 134:755, 1972.

36. Dereymaeker A, Ghosez JP, Henkes R. Surgical treatment of the cervical disc, comparing results from a posterior decompression laminectomy and from the anterior fusion approach. *Neurochirurgie* 9:13, 1963.

37. Dohn DF. Anterior interbody fusion for treatment of cervical disc conditions. *JAMA* 197:175–178, 1966.

38. Espersen JO, Buhl M, Eriksen EF, et al. Treatment of cervical disc disease using Cloward's technique. 1. General results, effect of different operative methods and complications in 1106 patients. *Acta Neurochir (Wien)* 70:97–114, 1984.

39. Galera R, Tovi D. Anterior disc excision with interbody fusion in cervical spondylotic myelopathy and rhizopathy. *J Neurosurg* 28:305–310, 1968.

40. Grisoli F, Graziani N, Fabrizi A, Peragut JC, Vincentelli F, Diaz-Vasquez P. Anterior discectomy without fusion for treatment of cervical lateral soft disc extrusion. Follow-up with 120 cases. *Neurosurgery* 24:853–859, 1989.

41. Guarnaschelli JJ. Anterior cervical discectomy without fusion: a comparison study of 500 cases. Presented at the Neurosurgical Society of America, Charleston, South Carolina, May 19–22, 1985.

42. Guidetti B, Fortuna A. Long-term results of surgical treatment of myelopathy due to cervical spondylosis. *J Neurol* 30:714–721, 1969.

43. Hanai K, Fujiyoshi F, Kamei K. Subtotal vertebrectomy and spinal fusion for cervical spondylotic myelopathy. *Spine* 11:310, 1986.

44. Hicks DS, Whitecloud TS, Cracco A, et al. Cervical spondylotic myelopathy: results of anterior decompression and stabilization. *Orthop Trans* 4:44, 1980.

45. Husag L, Probst C. Microsurgical anterior approach to cervical discs. Review of 60 consecutive cases of discectomy without fusion. *Acta Neurochir (Wien)* 73:229–242, 1984.

46. Kojima T, Waga S, Kubo Y, Kanamaru K, Shimosaka S, Shimizu T. Anterior cervical vertebrectomy and interbody fusion for multilevel spondylosis and ossification of posterior longitudinal ligament. *Neurosurgery* 24:864–872, 1989.

47. Lunsford LD, Bissonette DJ, Jannetta PJ, et al. Anterior surgery for cervical disc disease. Part 1: Treatment of lateral cervical disc herniation in 253 cases. *J Neurosurg* 53:1–11, 1980.

48. Lunsford LD, Bissonette DJ, Zorub DS. Anterior surgery of cervical disc disease. Part 2: Treatment of cervical spondylotic myelopathy in 32 cases. *J Neurosurg* 53:12–19, 1980.

49. Martins AN. Anterior cervical discectomy with and without interbody bone graft. *J Neurosurg* 44:290, 1976.

50. Murphy F, Simmons JCH, Brunson B. Ruptured cervical disc. 1939–1972. *Clin Neurosurg* 20:9–17, 1973.

51. Mosdal C. Cervical osteochondrosis and disc herniation. Eighteen years' use of interbody fusion by Cloward's technique in 755 cases. *Acta Neurochir (Wien)* 70:207–225, 1984.

52. O'Laoire SA, Thomas DGT. Spinal cord compression due to prolapse of cervical intervertebral disc (herniation of nucleus pulposus): treatment in 26 cases by discectomy without interbody bone graft. *J Neurosurg* 59:847–853, 1983.

53. Phillips DG. Surgical treatment of myelopathy with cervical spondylosis. *J Neurol Neurosurg Psychiatry* 36:879–884, 1973.

54. Raaf JE. Surgical treatment of patients with cervical disc lesions. *J Trauma* 9:327–338, 1969.

55. Riley LH, Robinson RA, Johnson KA, et al. The results of anterior interbody fusion of the cervical spine. Review of ninety-three consecutive cases. *J Neurosurg* 30:127–133, 1969.

56. Robinson RA, Walker AE, Ferlic DC, Wiecking DK. The results of anterior interbody fusion of the cervical spine. *J Bone Joint Surg [Am]* 44A:1569–1587, 1962.

57. Robertson JT. Anterior cervical discectomy without fusion: long term results. *Clin Neurosurg* 27:440–449, 1979.

58. Simmons EH, Bhallia SK. Anterior cervical discectomy and fusion. Clinical biomechanical study with 8 year follow-up. *J Bone Joint Surg [Br]* 51(B):225, 1969.

59. Stuck RM. Anterior cervical disc excision and fusion—report of 200 consecutive cases. *Rocky Mountain Med J* 60:25, 1963.

60. White AA, Southwick WO, Deponte RJ, et al. Relief of pain by anterior cervical spine fusion for spondylosis—a report of 65 cases. *J Bone Joint Surg [Am]* 55(A):525, 1973.

61. Williams JL, Allen MB, Harkess JW. Late results of cervical discectomy and interbody fusion. Some factors influencing the results. *J Bone Joint Surg [Am]* 50A:277–286, 1968.

62. Wilson DH, Campbell DD. Anterior cervical discectomy without bone graft: report of seventy-one cases. *J Neurosurg* 47:551, 1977.

63. Yonenobu K, Fugi T, Ono K, Okada K, Yamamoto T, Harada N. Choice of surgical treatment for multisegmental cervical spondylotic myelopathy. *Spine* 10:710, 1985.

CHAPTER 10

Anterior Cervical Fusion

Caspar Osteosynthetic Stabilization

Wolfhard Caspar and Haynes Louis Harkey

The management principles for cervical spine fractures and fracture dislocations are well recognized: reduction, decompression, and stabilization. Over the years, many techniques have been devised in an attempt to adequately fulfill these principles. With the introduction of the *anterior approach,* the spectrum of operative therapeutic modalities for cervical spine trauma was considerably broadened. This approach was found to permit optimal *decompression of the anterior neural elements* but unfortunately tended to *further destabilize the fractured spinal segments.* The introduction of *plate osteosynthesis* to the anterior approach has overcome this main disadvantage while maximizing the advantages. With the currently available technology, it is now possible to successfully treat most, if not all, cervical spine trauma with a single operative procedure. Initial surgical trials suggest that the results of this approach with respect to *neurologic outcome,* as well as *spinal stability and function,* may be *superior* to previous techniques.

HISTORICAL PERSPECTIVE

The first anterior cervical decompressions and interbody fusions were performed in the 1950s for degenerative diseases (20,22,35,39,41). Bailey first reported the use of anterior fusion for trauma in the cervical spine in 1960 (2). The following year, Cloward (21) and Verbiest (42) published similar reports on anterior fusion for both acute and chronic traumatic cervical abnormalities, and, interestingly, each author

noted neurologic improvement in patients with long-standing deformities. In fact, Cloward (21) states that "this method of treatment can be expected to give far better results and a higher salvage rate in these serious injuries than we have been able to accomplish by therapeutic programs employed in the past." We consider this statement valid today, particularly with respect to the Caspar plating technique.

The first reported *cervical plating procedures* were for cervical spine fractures (3,33,41). Most of the earlier attempts at cervical spine plating made use of preexisting plates designed for other bony structures. Orosco (33), who was one of the earliest to attempt cervical plating, however, designed a plate specifically for this procedure. Variations of these techniques have been reported since these pioneering efforts (4,5,23, 26,27,30,34,36,37).

BIOMECHANICAL PRINCIPLES

Strong scientific evidence at this time suggested that anterior plate stabilization might yield results superior to those previously obtained by conservative measures or posterior stabilization. The scientific basis lay in two observations: neurologic recovery follows restoration of stability in experimentally produced cervical spine fractures, and bone healing is improved through plate osteosynthesis.

Using an experimental model to simulate spinal cord trauma, Ducker (24) found that immobilization of the spine affected neurologic outcome. Significantly larger weights were required to produce paraplegia in monkeys when the spine was immobilized following the experimental trauma. This was the first experimental demonstration of a dictum that had been well accepted by spinal surgeons for many years.

The theoretical principles of internal fixation of fractures are based on research and clinical applications construed in Germany and Switzerland during the first half of this century. The Organization for the Advancement of Osteosynthesis (AO) was established to foster research in internal fixation and to develop standardized instrumentation and techniques. The term *"osteosynthesis"* refers to the *concept of establishing a functionally stable fixation that allows early and painless active mobilization of the injured extremity, thereby minimizing the loss of joint mobility associated with prolonged immobilization.*

In Muller's comprehensive manual of AO theory and technique, three criteria for rigid internal fixation were outlined: anatomical reduction to the original shape, mechanical stability, and maintenance of blood supply (32). To obtain long-lasting stability, the *normal anatomical structure should be restored* to prevent unequal distribution of forces that could lead to delayed deformity or osteoarthritis of the adjacent joints. *Mechanical stability is obtained through compression of the bone fragments with screws or plates.* In addition, compression of fractured bone ends enhances osteogenesis resulting in extremely rapid ossification (primary bone healing) (19). When the elements are splinted with a plate, the extremity can be painlessly mobilized and healing will occur without callus formation. Callus formation is considered a sign of instability (32). If two necrotic bone ends are approximated or soft tissue is interposed, healing will be impeded and screw loosening will occur. However, if there is one devascularized bone fragment, healing will still occur particularly if the fragments are compressed. In addition, it is well known that a graft compressed between two viable bone ends will be incorporated into the healing process.

Although initially outlined for long bone fractures, AO objectives and principles can certainly be applied to the cervical spine as well (Table 1). *Early mobilization in cervical trauma* patients, especially those with complete paralysis, is intended more for the *prevention of pulmonary and skin complications* associated with prolonged bed confinement than the restoration of segmental spine mobility. Nonetheless, these advantages are well recognized and worthwhile. *Reduction and restoration of the normal bony alignment* in the cervical spine will relieve bony compression of the neural elements and decrease the likelihood of delayed kyphotic angulation. If nonunion occurs following anterior cervical fusion, there is a risk of recurrent subluxation and secondary spinal cord injury. Subsequent injury can be acute or slowly progressive due to repetitive trauma inflicted by an unstable segment. Even when a stable union forms, if it results in kyphotic angulation, friction or pulsation cord damage can result in delayed injury. This phenomenon is further aggravated by congenital spinal canal stenosis. Therefore, establishing and maintaining a *normal lordotic curvature* is highly important.

Despite these publications between 1971 and 1981, the anterior plate stabilization technique for unstable cervical spine injuries did not attain widespread use. This can probably be attributed to several factors, including a lack of suitable plating material, inadequate instrumentation for exposure and plate application, and failures due to surgical technique. Early attempts at cervical spine plating utilized plates that lacked the flexibility needed to satisfy all the possible conditions that might arise. An insufficient variety of plates and screws prevented a precise fit over a wide variety of vertebral body sizes. The available screw hole configurations limited the number, positioning, and angle of screw placement into the vertebral body. In addition, a wide view unobstructed by surrounding tissues and instruments is necessary for meticulous cord decompression and accurate placement of plates and screws. The instrumentation available for exposure of the anterior spinal column for decompression, grafting, and placement of osteosynthetic plates was inadequate. Finally, as a result of improper surgical technique, complications such as screw loosening, nonunion, esophageal and recurrent laryngeal injuries, and postoperative infections tended to deter further attempts at anterior plate stabilization.

At this point, it was clear that AO principles should be incorporated into the surgical treatment of cervical trauma. Noting the successes and failures of previous attempts at anterior cervical plating, a completely new concept was developed based on osteosynthesis in the cervical spine (6–18). To apply this concept, it was apparent that a new system of instrumentation which could fulfill the requirements of surgical decompression and rigid internal stabilization would be needed. The Caspar anterior cervical trapezial plate stabilization procedure and instrumentation was therefore designed. As with all new techniques, experience has led to continuous refinement of both the procedure and instrumentation.

TABLE 1. *Requirements for optimal fracture healing and neurologic recovery*

Anatomical realignment
Absolute immobilization
Bone to bone contact
Compression of fracture fragments

ANTERIOR STABILIZATION: ADVANTAGES AND DISADVANTAGES

Treatment Goals in Cervical Trauma

The objectives of surgical therapy for cervical trauma are to *restore the integrity of the spinal canal* and *reestablish stability.* The spinal cord and nerve roots have the greatest chance of recovery if these objectives are fulfilled. These goals can be achieved through the following steps: *realignment* by traction or distraction; operative cord and root *decompression* of space occupying lesions such as disc fragments, scar tissue, and bone; *bone graft fusion;* and rigid *internal fixation* with the Caspar trapezial osteosynthetic plate until fracture healing occurs. Anterior cervical stabilization can easily fulfill these goals and, in some cases, is the only approach that will.

Advantages of the Anterior Approach

Through existing tissue planes a wide, less bloody exposure of the cervical spine can be rapidly obtained with minimal operative trauma. By preserving intact posterior stabilizing elements (muscle, ligaments, joint capsule, bone), improved mobility and stability can be achieved with less postoperative pain. Decompression through the disc space or through the vertebral body allows *optimal exposure* of the anterior cord surface and nerve roots, which is frequently needed in cervical spine trauma. Although "locked" facets previously constituted a contraindication to the anterior approach, the new vertebral body distractor system in combination with a vertebral body spreader permits reduction of most acute subluxations. This obviates the need for a posterior or combined anterior-posterior approach except in cases of transpedicular fractures.

Advantages of Anterior Fusion

Anterior interbody fusion results in a block vertebra that resembles the "natural" fusion seen in congenital block vertebra and autofusions. This stabilizes the area

TABLE 2. *Technical advantages of anterior trapezial plate stabilization*

Easy and quick exposure
Less tissue injury
Minimal blood loss
Optimal decompression of the spinal cord and nerve roots
Stabilization at the area of greatest biomechanical stress
Correction and maintenance of lordotic curvature
Subtotal and total vertebral body replacement possible
Reduction of locked facets possible using a newly designed device.

TABLE 3. *Advantages from the patient's point of view*

Relief of pain
Fast recovery
Early rehabilitation
More favorable outcome
Less need for external stabilization

of maximum biomechanical stress. When vertebral body compression fractures are present, subtotal or total body replacements can be performed.

Advantages of Anterior Plating

Internal fixation produces *immediate stabilization* allowing early postoperative mobilization with less need for external bracing devices (Tables 2 and 3). This early stability establishes an optimal environment for healing of injured musculoskeletal and neural structures since microtrauma resulting from persistent instability can interfere with their recovery. Absolute immobilization plus compression of bone surfaces results in faster bone healing with reduced callus formation (1,32). Therefore less graft resorption tends to occur and hypertrophic scarring is avoided. Even when graft resorption does occur, fusion still ensues through lateral bony bridging.[1] Proper shaping of the plate yields restoration of the normal lordotic curvature correcting kyphotic angulation and axis deviation. Coupled with preservation of the posterior supporting elements, this prevents delayed swan neck deformities and persistent spinal cord trauma, which could limit functional recovery or result in delayed progressive neurologic deficits.

Disadvantages of Anterior Plating

Anterior cervical plating for trauma is an *aggressive surgical procedure* for a condition which has been treated adequately by conservative measures. It requires insertion of a foreign body with the associated risk and *complications common to all implantable materials* as well as those associated specifically with metal plates and screws implanted in the cervical region. Screw placement can be hazardous with resulting *spinal cord injury* if proper technique and extreme care are not utilized. Screw loosening can lead to failure of adequate segmental stabilization and the subsequent complications of *nonunion.* In addition, a migrating

---

[1] In the authors' experience of over 200 cervical plating procedures, there have only been six cases of delayed fusion. In each case, fusion was ultimately achieved within 1 year without adversely affecting the overall outcome. Incidentally, all these cases were operated upon for degenerative processes.

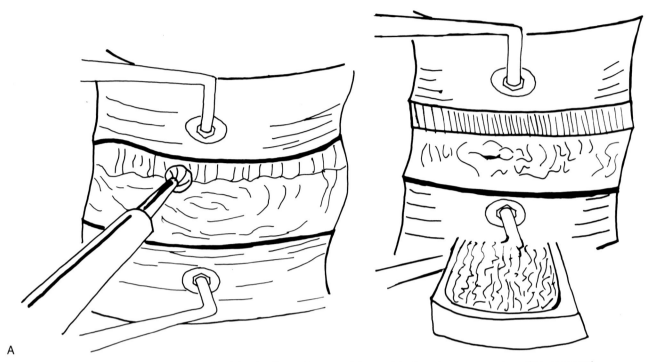

FIG. 1. The Caspar vertebral body distractor provides unhindered exposure for disc removal, graft site preparation **(A)**, and graft positioning **(B)**. A tricortical bone graft provides the most stable construct for intervertebral fusion.

screw can compromise or injure the soft tissue structures of the neck resulting in difficulty swallowing, or esophageal perforation.[2]

Most, if not all, of the complications experienced so far with Caspar trapezial plate osteosynthesis can be attributed to a surgeon's error or *failures in operative technique*. In our experience of over 400 plating procedures since 1980, plate related complications have been within a well tolerated minimum. We have found that the advantages far outweigh the disadvantages and combine to produce the most favorable overall outcome with the greatest economy of time and expense.

CONCEPTS IN INTERVERTEBRAL BONE GRAFTING

Anterior cervical plating provides *immediate but temporary stability* and must always be accompanied by *intervertebral bone graft fusion* to provide long-term stability. Proper fusion technique enhances the chance of rapid, solid bone healing. Plating across an intact disc or plating resulting in a pseudoarthrosis following unsuccessful bony fusion will be accompanied by subsequent micromotion that will ultimately result

in screw loosening and destabilization. Likewise, graft complications such as graft failure, graft penetration into the adjacent vertebral bodies, or graft dislocation that result in pseudoarthrosis, avascular bone necrosis, neural compression, or dysphagia can be avoided through proper preparation and placement of the graft. This becomes particularly true when dealing with cases of poor quality bone such as osteoporosis, diabetes, and rheumatoid arthritis in which screw torque is considerably reduced.

Iliac crest, tricortical, block graft as described by *Smith and Robinson* provides the best substrate for bony fusion (39). The three cortical surfaces provide a stout supportive structure more resistant to collapse than the dowel type graft (28,43), and this configuration has been shown to form a more stable construct (44). When correctly seated into place, a block graft provides a better contour for fixation of the trapezial plate. Unlike the Cloward technique, preparation of the graft site for a tricortical block graft leaves the vertebral endplates intact, avoiding penetration of the graft into the vertebral body (28). Similarly, when adjacent levels are fused, the intervening vertebral body has sufficient thickness to support the block grafts as opposed to the Cloward technique which results in significant resection of the intervening body when two adjacent levels are fused.

Using a conventional disc space spreader with either dowel or block graft technique creates a disc space

---

[2] The converging disposition of the screws in the Caspar plating system avoids esophageal perforation in the event of screw protrusion.

opening that is asymmetrical and partially obstructed, complicating graft placement. However, the Caspar distractor achieves a more effective, symmetric, and unobstructed opening of the interspace (Fig. 1). This exposure allows for a tight-fitting graft with as much bone-to-bone contact as possible. Calipers can be used for precise measurement of the graft site, and a dual-bladed oscillating saw can harvest the perfect-sized graft with parallel surfaces.

In cervical spine plating, there is a race between bone healing and hardware failure. Meticulous grafting technique gives the healing process an advantage. Once a solid bony union is achieved, the hardware is no longer biomechanically functional and, therefore, is no longer at risk of failure.

CONCEPTS IN SCREW PLACEMENT

Inadvertent injury to the spinal cord and screw loosening are two persistent concerns with respect to screw fixation in the cervical spine. To avoid screw loosening, bone-to-thread contact should be maximized to provide the greatest amount of holding power. The optimal transverse trajectory for cervical body screws is a slightly oblique, medially directed angle of ~15° and a sagittal trajectory that is parallel to the vertebral endplates (Figs. 2 and 3). This trajectory minimizes the extrusion vectors. The *screws should be placed through both anterior and posterior cortices* since the majority of the holding power of a screw is obtained from cortical bone as opposed to cancellous

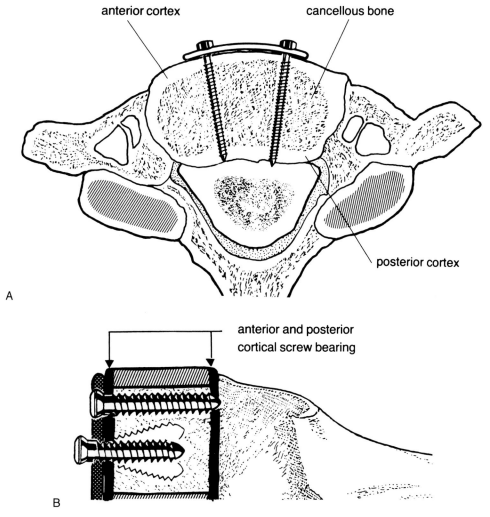

FIG. 2. The optimal transverse trajectory for screw placement is an oblique, slightly medially directed angle **(A)**, and the optimal sagittal trajectory is parallel to the vertebral endplates **(B)**. The screw tip should penetrate the posterior cortex to prevent screw loosening.

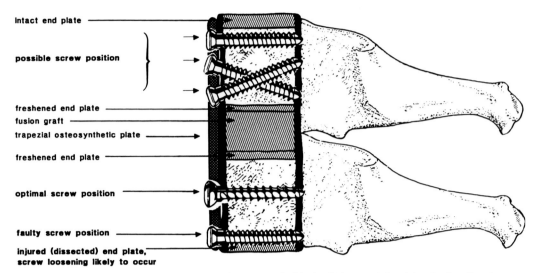

intact end plate

possible screw position

freshened end plate
fusion graft
trapezial osteosynthetic plate
freshened end plate

optimal screw position

faulty screw position

injured (dissected) end plate,
screw loosening likely to occur

FIG. 3. If screws cannot be placed in the central third of the vertebral body (*optimal screw position*), they can be angled (*possible screw positions*), but should avoid penetration of the endplate.

bone (29). Whenever possible, at least two screws should be placed into each vertebral body, not only for added holding power but also to prevent rotation around a single fixation point. This holds particularly true for the screws below the fusion which sustain the greatest biomechanical stress and are more likely to loosen.

Figure 4 demonstrates the space available between the posterior cortical surface and the spinal cord, which provides a margin of safety for screw placement. The posterior longitudinal ligament protects the dura from the screw tip, whereas the epidural space allows for some displacement. A converging trajectory directs the screw tip away from the anterior roots. Even considering this ample margin of safety, *precise bicortical placement requires the use of high resolution fluoroscopy.*

APPLICATIONS

The versatility of the system allows the surgeon to anteriorly decompress and stabilize the cervical spine under many clinical conditions (Tables 4 and 5).

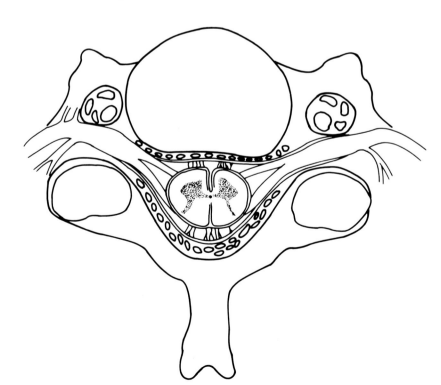

FIG. 4. Schematic in the axial plane of the spinal subarachnoid space. The epidural and subarachnoid spaces provide ample margin of error against slight screw tip penetration of the posterior cortex. In addition, the Caspar instrumentation automatically directs the screw holes in a medially converging course, which reduces the danger of injury to the roots.

TABLE 4. *Anterior fusion and stabilization techniques for cervical trauma*

Technique	Pathology
Single level fusion and plating	Instability (lig. disrupture with sublux./lux. including facet and/or pedicle/lamina fracture) *without* significant body fracture.
Multiple (two) level fusion and plating	Traumatic disc rupture (prolaps).
Subtotal body replacement and plating	Wedge/tear drop fracture. Posterior ½–⅓ of body and wall left intact.
Total body replacement and plating	Burst fracture (comminutive) with involvement of posterior wall (neuro-canal compromise due to dislocated body or fragments).

TABLE 5. *Anterior cervical spine: trapezial plate osteosynthesis: November 1980–1991*

Indication	No. of cases
Trauma	108
Myelopathy	99
Radiculopathy	143
Failed disc surgery	34
Tumor	14
Inflammatory process	2
Other	8
Total	408

Single or Multilevel Fusion

In simple fracture dislocations, the neural elements can be *decompressed through the disc space*, the *normal lordotic curvature reestablished*, and *stability obtained with bone grafting and trapezial plate appli-* *cation* (Fig. 5). This can be done for one or more unstable levels.

Subtotal Body Replacement and Plating

When tear-drop fractures or anterior body compression fractures accompany an unstable spine, the *bone fragments can be removed* along with the discectomies above and below the fractured body. The block graft is constructed to span the distance between the adjacent intact vertebral bodies. A plate is then applied with screws through both the anterior and posterior cortices of the intact vertebral bodies. Screws are also

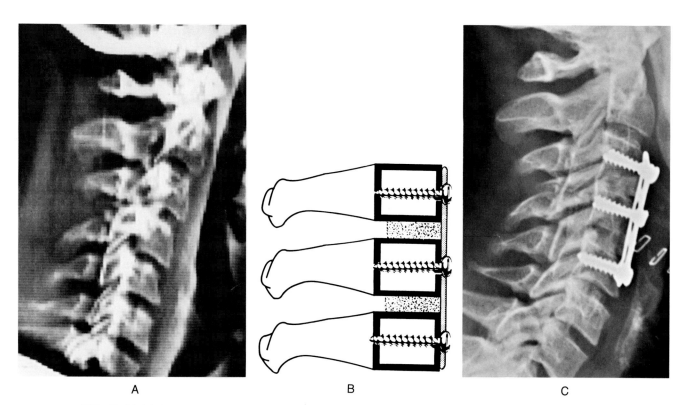

A   B   C

FIG. 5. Multiple level anterior fusion and plating. **A:** An unusual case of two level traumatic instability (functional studies not shown here demonstrated instability at the C4–C5 level). **B:** Schematic representation. **C:** Postoperative roentgenogram demonstrating the two-level interbody fusion and plating.

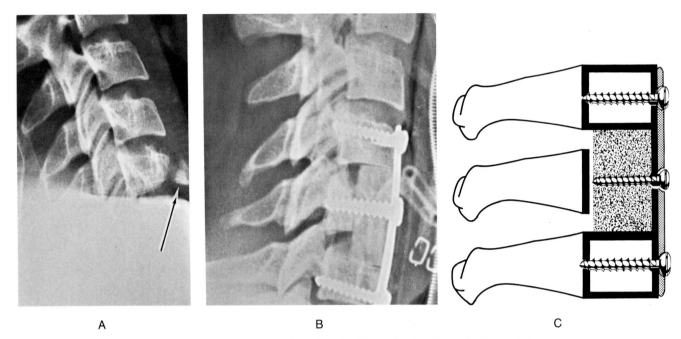

A   B   C

FIG. 6. Subtotal body replacement and plating. **A:** C5 wedge fracture. **B:** C5 partial corpectomy, anterior fusion, and C4–C6 plate stabilization. **C:** The middle pair of screws pass through the bone graft and into the posterior cortex of the remaining vertebral body thus binding the two together. A tear-drop (anterior wedge) fracture without bony canal compromise lends itself to subtotal body replacement. In this manner, vertebral body as well as disc space height is re-constituted and progressive angulation prevented. If the posterior aspect of the vertebral body is intact, this type of fusion is mechanically the strongest. If neural compression is demonstrated by radiographic studies, total corpectomy is the method of choice.

placed at the center of the plate through the graft and the posterior cortex of the partially resected vertebral body (Fig. 6).

Total Body Replacement and Plating

For severe compression fractures of the vertebral body, particularly when bony fragments are retro-pulsed and compromising the spinal cord, a *complete vertebrectomy* may be performed. A block graft is situated in the defect tightly abutting the adjacent vertebral endplates. The screws are applied through both the anterior and posterior cortices of the intact vertebral bodies. However, the central graft holding screws should penetrate only the anterior two-thirds of the graft thereby preventing posterior displacement of the graft (Fig. 7). This technique can be applied in other situations requiring corpectomy such as ossification of the posterior longitudinal ligament or vertebral body destruction secondary to tumor or infection.

INSTRUMENTATION[3]

Instruments for Operative Exposure

This system consists of a *set of four self-retaining retractors with a variety of blade sizes* that are easily interchangeable (Fig. 8). As a result, the instruments can be put together in such a fashion that optimal exposure of the anterior surface of the cervical spine is unhindered by the surrounding anatomy and instrumentation. The retractor blades for lateral spreading are now available in a radiolucent material that does not obstruct fluoroscopic imaging (Fig. 9).

Instruments for Spinal Realignment, Decompression, and Fusion

The cervial vertebral body distraction system (Fig. 11) consists of a vertebral body distractor, distraction

[3] Aesculap Instrument Co., Burlingame, CA, U.S.A., and Aesculap Werde AG, Tuttlingen, Germany.

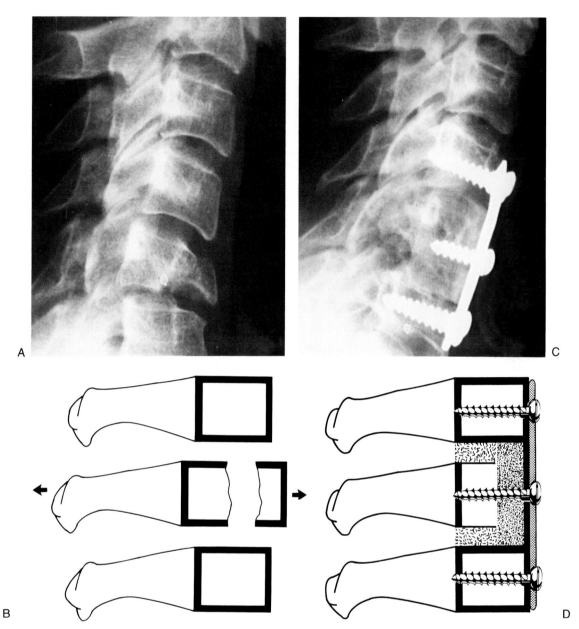

FIG. 7. Total body replacement and plating. **A:** Compression fracture of C5 with bony compression of the spinal cord. **B:** Schematic drawing of the bony injury. **C:** Total body replacement and plating. **D:** Schematic representation.

pins in four lengths (14, 16, 18, and 20 mm), a drill for the distraction screw-holes, drill-guide (used in conjunction with the distractor) for parallel positioning of the distraction pins, and a screwdriver. This system is based on a radically new concept of vertebral body distraction that relies on *forces applied outside the interspace* through distraction pins placed in the vertebral bodies above and below the disc space.

There are several advantages afforded by this system over conventional vertebral body distractors. Visualization within the disc space is improved since there are no distraction devices within the disc space ob-

structing the view. In addition, the vertebral bodies are distracted in a symmetrical fashion providing improved exposure in the posterior disc region. The distraction pins placed into the vertebral bodies avoid endplate damage and distractor slippage. The distractor can be placed so that it spans multiple disc spaces and the intervening vertebral body(s) enabling resection of vertebra destroyed by trauma or tumor. If three or more distraction pins are placed, distraction can be alternated between neighboring segments. Graft placement is facilitated by unhindered, parallel distraction allowing larger, stronger bone grafts to be placed.

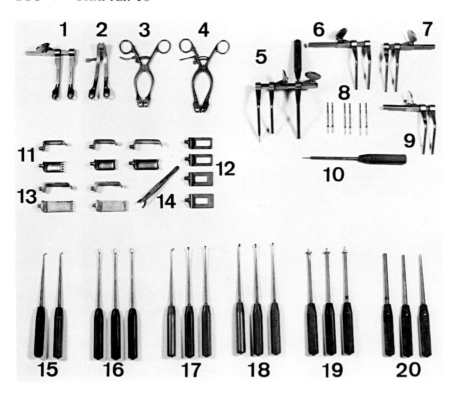

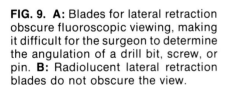

FIG. 8. Instruments for operative exposure. **1:** Hinged, toothed bar retractor (parallel opening). **2:** Hinged speculum retractor (conical opening). **3:** Straight spreader (semicircular opening). **4.** Hinged spreader (semicircular opening). **5:** Distractor left (extra long) with attached drilling case for parallel distraction pin placement. **6:** Distractor right (extra long). **7:** Distractor left (regular length). **8:** Three pairs of distraction pins with 14, 16, and 18 mm penetration depth. **9:** Distractor right (regular length). **10:** Distraction pin driver with inserted distraction pin 11–13 selection of various retractors blades. **11:** Three pairs of interchangeable retractor blades, toothed, pronged, and blunt (sea gull design). **12:** Two pairs of fenestrated retractor blades for iliac crest exposure. **13:** Pair of radiolucent retractor blades for transverse retraction in plating procedure. **14:** Blade extruding forceps. **15:** Single and double angle posterior ligament dissector and osteophyte remover. **16:** Fenestrated square-shaped toothed curettes. **17:** Curved curettes. **18:** Straight curettes. **19:** Small, large "butterfly type" graft holders and impactors. **20:** Graft and cancellous bone tappers.

FIG. 9. **A:** Blades for lateral retraction obscure fluoroscopic viewing, making it difficult for the surgeon to determine the angulation of a drill bit, screw, or pin. **B:** Radiolucent lateral retraction blades do not obscure the view.

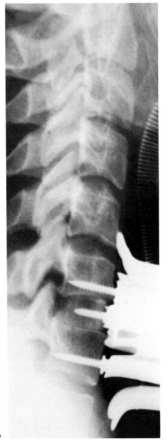

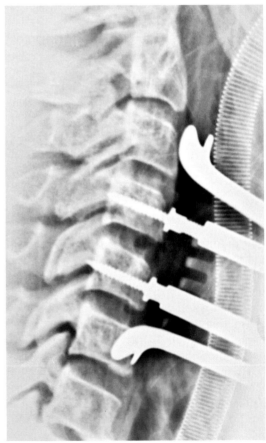

A

B

TABLE 6. *Trapezial cervical plates*

Type	Size
Single-level plates	26 mm
	28 mm
	30 mm[a]
	32 mm
C2/C3-plates ("Hangman plates")	34 mm
	36 mm
Two-level plates	42 mm
	44 mm
	46 mm
	48 mm[a]
	50 mm
	52 mm
Two/three-level plates	54 mm
	57 mm
	60 mm
Three-level plates	63 mm
	66 mm[a]
	69 mm
	72 mm
Three/four-level plates	75 mm
	78 mm
Four-level plates	81 mm
	84 mm[a]
	87 mm
	90 mm

[a] Mean standard.

Once in position, the graft can be compressed between the vertebral bodies by using the distractor in the reverse direction.

Vertebral body dissectors, angled singly or doubly, are used to manipulate and dissect the posterior longitudinal ligament, disc fragments, and osteophytes,

as well as exploring the root canal. Calipers aid measurement of the height, width, and depth of the graft site and the graft itself for precise fitting. Bone grafts are held for shaping and placement by dowel holders while tappers are used for final seating of the graft.

Instruments for Osteosynthetic Stabilization

The plates are manufactured from spring elastic implantation steel, which can be contoured to the desired lordotic curve with the plate bender (Fig. 10). Different trapezial plate lengths are available for stabilization of one or more cervical spine segments between C2 and T1 (Table 6). These plates, which are contoured specifically for the cervical spine, have several unique features relative to plates previously used in the cervical spine. Their special geometric design provides adequate stability without being too thick or heavy. Diverging longitudinal double-row screw holes allow for simple, secure, and exact screw placement while enhancing stability and preventing rotational dislocation. Single screw holes prevent plate translocation, whereas long screw holes allow two screws to be placed in a single hole if necessary to provide additional holding power. Two adjacent screws approximately double the thread surface area within the vertebral body but also tend to compact the surrounding bone increasing the holding power of the individual screws.

A special drill and dual drill-guide with fine depth adjustment for drilling the holes to fix the plates is used. The guide allows drilling of adjacent screw holes,

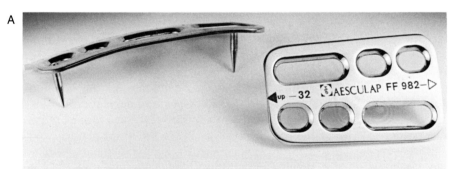
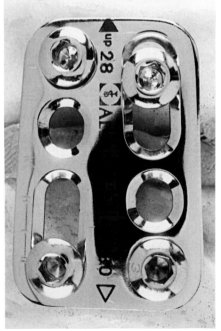

FIG. 10. **A:** Contoured cervical spine plates with recently added spikes to facilitate exact positioning during drilling and screw insertion. The plates will soon be manufactured with a pre-bent "normal lordotic curvature," which can be modified further by the surgeon. The plate will establish a normal lordotic curve in the spine upon tightening the screws if it is not already present. Once the plate is bent into position, the spikes go from a slight divergence to a roughly perpendicular position for ease in placement by tapping into the vertebral body. **B:** The plates are designed with two sizes of screw holes. Single screw holes prevent the plate from sliding relative to the screw. Oblong screw holes allow for adjacent screws and more variability for screw placement.

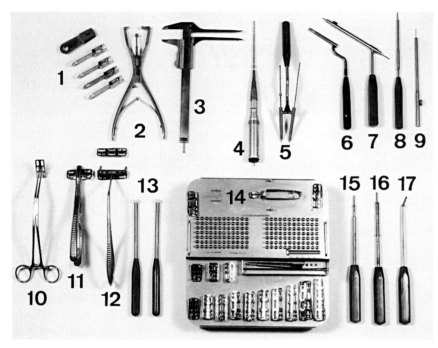

FIG. 11. Instruments for anterior plate stabilization. **1:** Twin saw blades for obtaining exactly parallel cuts. **2:** Iliac graft cutter and remover ("guillotine"). **3:** Calipers for obtaining exact disc space measurements. **4:** Microton motor and hand piece with inserted drill. **5:** Dual drill-guide with depth adjustment. **6:** Offset single drill-guide with depth adjustment. **7:** Offset screw driver guide for difficult positions. **8:** Screw threader. **9:** Depth gauge for determination of screw length. **10:** Plate holding and insertion forceps. **11:** Plate bender. **12:** Alternative plate holder with 90° offset. **13:** Graft holder for "spiked" plates. **14:** Assortment of plates and screws, drills, and K-wires in a sterilizing container. **15:** Screw holder and driver for number 7. **16:** Alternative holder and driver with removable holding sheath. **17:** "Ball" screw driver allows 30° of deviation in all directions inside the screw head's hex nut, specifically for use in the upper and lower spine (C2 and T1) for oblique insertion.

which are directed on a converging course towards the posterior vertebral cortex. In this manner, the optimal angle in the transverse plane is automatically achieved, obviating the need for anterior-posterior fluoroscopy. A single drill-guide with depth adjustment provides versatility for placing free handed single screw holes. A depth gauge determines the necessary length of screw which is a swiss pattern cortical screw. The plate is positioned with a plate holder for alignment and temporary plate fixation. Screw holes are tapped with the screw threader, and the screws are inserted with the screwdriver (Figure 11).

OPERATIVE TECHNIQUE

Pre-operative Medication

Foreign body implantation carries an *increased risk of infection*, with possibly more severe consequences than a similar operation without implants. Gram-positive bacteria, particularly staphylcoccus species, are the most common offending organisms in postoperative infections. Accordingly, the following *antibiotic regimen* is recommended: a first or second generation cephalosporin (2 g) plus gentamicin (80 mg) administered intravenously within 1 hr preceding skin incision followed by a second equivalent dose at the termination of the procedure or after 4 hr, whichever occurs first. Antibiotic coverage is continued for 36 hr at a reduced dose of cephalosporin (1 g) and gentamicin (1 mg/kg) every 8 hr with appropriate alterations for ab-

normal renal function, age or allergies. One author's (W.C.) infection rate for over 200 cases personally performed has been <0.5%.

High-dose steroids (Dexamethasone, 40 mg or equivalent) is administered intravenously prior to disc removal. This may provide some protection against inadvertent minor trauma to the neural elements during decompression.

Positioning

The patient is placed in the *supine position* with the *head of the table elevated 10–15°* relative to the feet (reverse Trendelenburg), providing a direct line of vision through the plane of the disc space. Additional adjustments of the neck position depend on the level of fusion. Upper and midcervical spine fusions require moderate *hyperextension*. In the lower cervical spine a neutral or very slightly hyperextended position is optimal. Cervico-thoracic fusions may require some flexion, which assists in fluoroscopic visualization of this area. A recently designed *neck/head rest* (Aesculap) facilitates the operative procedure by offering mechanisms for fine adjustments in positioning as well as firm cervical lordotic support (Fig. 12). It has the additional advantage of unhindered lateral access due to the slim design. A radiolucent neck support is available that allows anterior-posterior fluoroscopic visualization.

Skull traction (2–8 kg depending on pathology, level, and body weight) is applied along the axis of the cer-

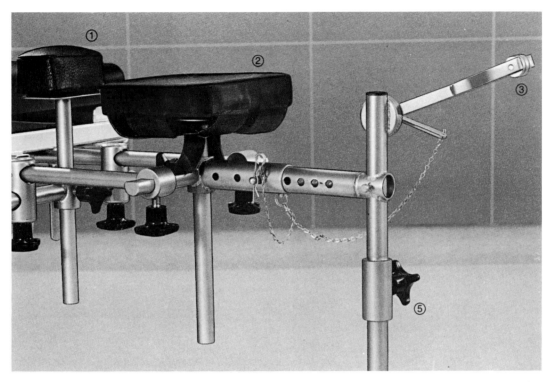

FIG. 12. Specially designed neck/head rest that provides adjustable neck support and allows for easy positioning of the fluoroscope. A radiolucent neck rest is available that allows anterior-posterior viewing.

vical spine while shoulder traction (1–2 kg/arm) is applied with padded wrist straps (Fig. 13). Traction stabilizes the spine in the longitudinal and rotational axis, limiting movement during the operative procedure and preventing plate stabilization in a malaligned position. An elastic chin strap further stabilizes the head and neck against unwanted rotation and flexion of the cranio-cervical junction. The skin has a tendency to

be tented by this elastic mandibular suspension, therefore, care should be taken to relax the skin prior to marking the incision.

At this point, the *fluoroscopy equipment* is positioned and fine adjustments are made in the neck support and traction (Fig. 13). This should be done prior to draping since fine adjustments are more easily made at this point when the true anatomical position is vis-

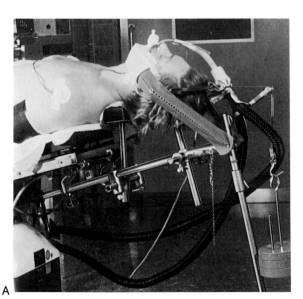

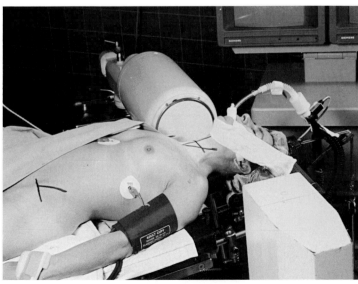

A

B

FIG. 13. A: Proper positioning with the head elevated 10–15°, neck extended, skull traction applied, and chin stabilized with the elastic chin strap. **B:** Fluoroscopy equipment in position.

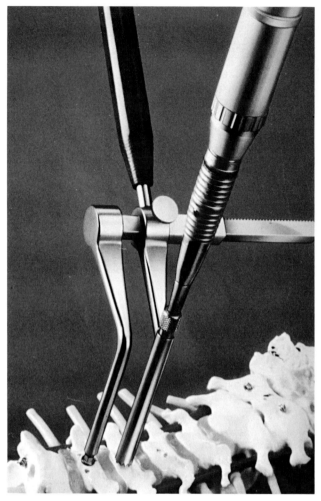

FIG. 14. Drilling the second distraction pin hole using the distraction drill-guide assembly.

ible.[4] The pelvis is supported by firm pads improving access to the iliac crest.

Meticulous care should be taken during draping to ensure a *sterile, water-proof field*. This is best achieved using a layer of adhesive-backed plastic drape over the prepared skin followed by cloth or paper drapes. A second plastic drape can be applied to secure the drape edges as well as any wires and cables that cross the sterile field.

Initial Exposure and Graft Site Preparation

Exposing the Spine

The anterior aspects of the vertebral bodies and disc spaces of interest are exposed, as described in Chapter 2.

Positioning the Vertebral Body Distractor

The level is unequivocally verified by fluoroscopy and the disc is partially resected prior to the insertion of the vertebral body distractor. The first distraction pin hole is placed free handedly in the inferior vertebral body. The guide is positioned in the center of the vertebral body under direct vision and is held with the

---

[4] The advantages of the modern digital image intensifiers are numerous, justifying the additional expense. Improved imagery assists in delicate decompression and precision screw placement while subjecting the patient, surgeon, and assistants to less radiation. Dual monitors providing a real-time image and a stored "last view" allow the surgeon to compare a current image to previous conditions. Of course, leaded aprons and radiation dosage meters should be worn by all personnel involved. Numerous intraoperative measurements with dosage meters attached to the unprotected arm have shown that the X-Ray exposure of the surgeon is within an acceptable range.

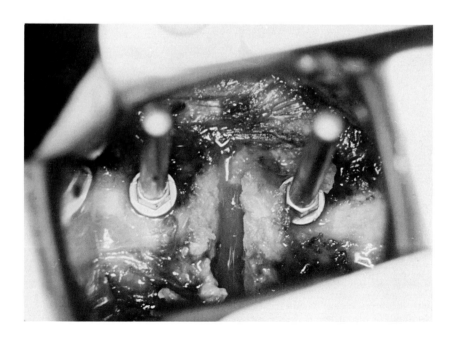

FIG. 15. Distraction pins should be inserted so that the base plate is flush with the vertebral body.

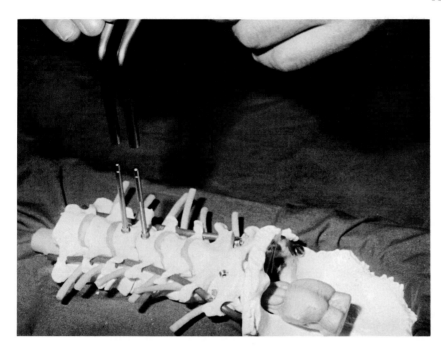

FIG. 16. Vertebral body distractor being inserted over the distraction pins.

handle pointing away from the surgeon to avoid subsequent interference with the crossbar assembly while drilling. The drill-guide is angled with a slight caudal inclination in a plane parallel to that of the adjacent vertebral endplate. The final trajectory is verified with fluoroscopy. The drill bit is constructed with a safety stop, which allows only an 8-mm penetration into the vertebral body thus preventing accidental injury to the spinal cord. The first distraction pin is seated into place.

The distraction drill-guide is assembled using both the immobile distractor arm (with the attached crossbar) and the drill-guide with the angled hand piece which was used for drilling the first hole. Slipping the fixed arm of the distraction drill-guide assembly over the first distraction pin, each subsequent drill hole is made in the center of the next cranial vertebral body

(Fig. 14). For operations involving two or three neighboring segments, three or four distraction pins can be used. This process ensures that all of the distraction pins will be parallel once they are inserted. The distraction pins must be completely inserted so that the base plates are flush with the vertebral body in order to prevent them from tearing out during distraction (Fig. 15). The vertebral body distractor is placed over the shafts of the distraction pins after exchanging the drill-guide for the movable distractor arm (Fig. 16). Distraction forces should be applied in a stepwise fashion to prevent rupture of intact elastic tissues surrounding the vertebral joints and to avoid dislodging the distraction pins. We usually open several notches on the ratchet and begin further clearing of the disc space returning to spread another notch or two after several minutes (Fig. 17).

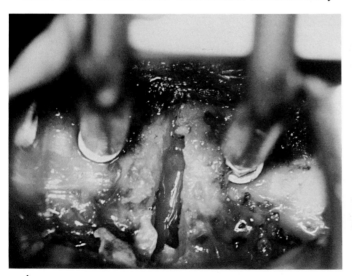 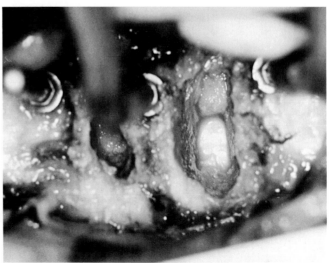

A **FIG. 17. A:** Operative site with distractor in place. **B:** Operative site after "step-wise" distraction. B

Discectomy and Bony Preparation

A total discectomy with Smith-Robinson type fusion is performed as illustrated in Chapter 8.

Graft Placement

Contrary to standard anterior fusion techniques, the bone plug is not countersunk for plating but is left flush with the anterior surface of the spine providing a more stable interface with the vertebral bodies and plate. The appropriate length can be more easily and accurately cut using the guillotine graft cutter with integrated depth control (Fig. 18) (Aesculap).

Once the graft is ideally positioned, the vertebral body distractor is used to compress the fusion by operating it in reverse fashion for ~5 min, a function unique to this type of distractor. Compressing the fusion site acts to condense the graft, increasing the cancellous bone density and closing small gaps between the endplates and the graft.

Plating

The *plating procedure is tailored* to the requirements of each individual case. Most frequently, a single-level fusion is all that is required in cervical trauma. On rare occasions when two or more adjacent levels are un-

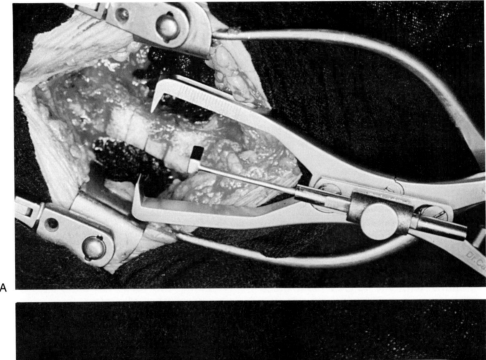

A

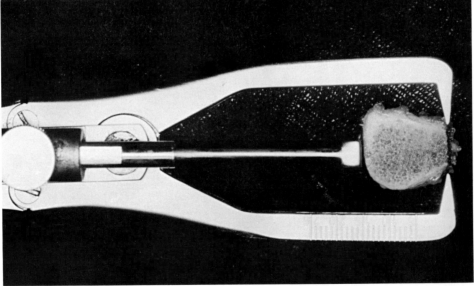

B

FIG. 18. Guillotine graft cutter with integrated depth control before **(A)** and after **(B)** harvesting the graft.

stable, a multilevel interbody fusion and plating is needed. In cases of vertebral body compression fractures when subtotal or total vertebral body replacements are required, the plate must span two or more disc spaces. Regardless of the situation, an appropriately sized plate should be available since a wide variety of plate lengths are manufactured.

Two very important points with regard to anterior cervical plating can not be overstated. The first point is that *fluoroscopic guidance throughout the procedure is absolutely mandatory*. Plate stabilization can not be properly or safely performed without using an image intensifier. Dispensing with roentgenographic guidance will very likely lead to faulty plate fixation and could lead to disastrous complications. The second point is to *never plate across an unfused disc space*. One should keep in mind that plate stabilization is merely a temporary internal splint which enhances the fusion process. It is the *ossification of the graft placed in the cleared disc space that provides the long-term stability*. If the plate crosses an intact disc space, screw loosening will eventually occur because of the micromotions that remain possible.

Selecting the Plate

The plate selected will bind the intact vertebral bodies above and below the level of instability. *For a single-level fracture subluxation, the plate should span the disc space plus the adjacent vertebral bodies.* For multilevel instability or vertebral body replacement procedures, the plate will span two or more disc spaces plus the intact vertebral bodies above and below the levels of instability. The ideally positioned plate should extend to within 1 mm of the next intact disc space. This allows for the expected settling that occurs due to graft resorption. Without this leeway, the plate could extend over a disc and may ultimately lead to screw loosening due to the repetitive leverage applied to the end of the plate. In addition, a plate that compromises an intact motion segment can lead to a chronic irritating condition. This may result in a long-lasting pain syndrome, formation of osteophytes and finally anterior autofusion. Symptomatic plate translocation should be treated by hardware removal after the plated level has fused.

The customized curvature that will be required to restore the best possible posture should be considered when selecting a plate. Although the final length can initially only be estimated, it is helpful to place the plate on the vertebral column and inspect its fit with fluoroscopy. Available plate lengths allow for a fairly accurate fitting, but it is better to have a plate that is slightly short and avoid approaching an intact disc.

Bending the Plate

To achieve a normal lordotic posture and obtain optimal facet alignment, the plate needs to be bent in a *convex fashion*. The degree of curvature required varies with the level of the spine being fused as well as the patient's normal shape. Generally speaking, the curve should be smoothly distributed along the length of the plate with the exception of C2–C3 instability. In this instance, the upper edge of the plate should be more sharply bent in order to conform to the ventral shape of the C2 vertebral body. Inadequate bending of the plate will result in an abnormally straight posture or, even worse, a kyphotic angulation. Overlordosis due to an excessively convex plate is generally prevented by the travel limitations of the facets; however, too much convexity could result in difficulty seating the central portion of the plate.

Once the bending is complete, the *plate should be positioned on the vertebral bodies and inspected with fluoroscopy*. The fit is judged appropriate when the ends of the plate rest ~2 mm from the upper and lower endplates and 5 mm of space exists between the center of the plate and the vertebral column. When this type of bowed configuration is achieved, tightening of the screws will shift the vertebral bodies into the appropriate lordotic curvature. The ends of the plate push and rotate the upper and lower points of contact posteriorly while pulling the central area forward. This is most easily appreciated when the plate spans three or more vertebral bodies. From past experience, a concave plate with the ends away from the vertebral body in the resting position produces too much force on the distal screws which then invariably loosen.

Fixing the Plate

By this point, the distraction screws have been removed and the ventral surface of the spine can be prepared to accept the plate. Any osteophytic spurs should be removed with a rongeur and overhanging lips should be burred flat. This produces a smooth surface so that the plate can be seated flush with the bone throughout its length. A plate that rests on ridges reduces the overall contact area and sacrifices structural stability. Do not assume that a protruding graft will be reduced when the plate is tightened into position. Attempting this will likely fail and may result in screw loosening. On the other hand, small cancellous bone chips (spongioplasty) can be used to fill gaps that remain around the block graft.

The plate should be positioned carefully prior to drilling the screw holes, and any adjustments in surface preparation and bending done at this time. Since the exposure is not truly midline, there is a tendency to position the plate slightly towards the side of the incision. The resulting oblique fixation could result in rotational malposture. This problem can be solved with an anterior-posterior fluoroscopic view. However, we have not found the anterior-posterior view necessary if meticulous attention is paid to patient positioning at the outset and the lateral vertebral borders are carefully identified throughout the region of fusion. This avoids cumbersome repositioning of the fluoroscope and allows the entire procedure to be performed with just the lateral view. When the surgeon is satisfied with positioning, the plate is tamped into place. It will be temporarily secured by the spikes at either end which are imbedded into the vertebral bodies (Fig. 10).

The approximate length of the drill hole to the posterior cortical surface can be estimated from the depth of the interspace which was measured prior to inserting the graft. The depth stop on the dual drill-guide should be adjusted prior to drilling. Holes should always be drilled with the plate in position, since the depth stop on the guide is designed to account for the thickness of the plate. In addition, the holes in the plate prevent the accidental alteration of the preset depth stop. The first drill hole is usually placed at the most easily accessible level since correct plate positioning is established by the initial screw holes. A blunt K-wire is placed through one of the drill casings to stabilize the casing tip while drilling. Holes are always drilled under fluoroscopic control to ensure that the drill tip does not penetrate too deeply. The surgeon is frequently able to feel when the posterior cortex is both reached and penetrated but relying on this alone is not recommended. A K-wire is then inserted into the freshly drilled hole under fluoroscopic vision. This allows palpation of the posterior cortex for evidence of penetration and visualization of the final trajectory of the screw. The K-wire is withdrawn 5 mm and left to stabilize the drill case for the second hole. The posterior cortex should be at least partially penetrated so that when the screw is tightened the threads will bite into the cortex rather than displace it. Use of the distraction screw holes should be avoided if at all possible because they tend to be enlarged during the distraction process and provide inadequate torque when securing the plate. Screw holes should be well within the ventral body, optimally within the central third of the body, when viewed from the lateral plane. *Certainly, the screw hole should not penetrate the vertebral endplate* (Fig. 3). If necessary, the single drill-guide can be used when the dual drill-guide does not correctly direct the drill. This is occasionally encountered when the first hole is not directed optimally or when the plate holes do not line up with the desired direction of drilling. Although diagonally directed holes are acceptable every attempt should be made to direct them perpen-

dicular to the plate or parallel to the body end plate. This is because angled screws require more torque to generate the same holding power against the plate (Fig. 3).

Preferably, *at least two holes are drilled into each vertebral body that is to be included into the fusion.* Holes should also be placed through the block graft and the posterior cortex of the remaining vertebral body in a subtotal vertebral body replacement (Fig. 6). However, in total vertebral body replacement, the holes should not completely penetrate the block graft (Fig. 7).

Problems visualizing the lower vertebrae may be encountered when fusing the lower cervical spine and cervico-thoracic junction. Additional traction on the arms can sometimes bring the lower vertebrae into view. Sometimes repositioning the C-arm in a more oblique fashion while forcing the shoulders towards the table will help. As long as the direction of drilling is visible, the hole can be placed semi-blindly. This requires drilling in small increments and palpating frequently with a stationary drill until the posterior cortex is partially penetrated.

Placing the Screws

Each screw hole should be measured with the depth gauge and a screw of correct length selected. If the posterior cortex has been countersunk but not completely penetrated, the measured length is used. If the posterior cortex is completely penetrated, the measured length minus 1 mm is most appropriate. This 1-mm difference compensates for the settling that occurs as the plate is tightened into position. Measurements should be made under fluoroscopy with the plate forced flush with the bone, eliminating the gap produced by the convex curvature. Each hole should be measured separately because of variability in body depth and hole angle. Likewise, each individual screw should be measured since the actual length may vary up to a millimeter from manufacturer's stated length, a problem inherent in the manufacturing process. Standard length is determined as an overall screw length including the head. For example, a 20-mm screw has 17 mm of available thread plus a 3-mm head. This discrepancy is accounted for when using the Caspar depth gauge.

Before the screws are placed, *each hole should be tapped to minimize heat production when the screw is tightened.* Heat produced during screw tightening can be quite high and has been shown to cause bone necrosis (32). When more than two levels are fused, the central screws should be tightened first followed by the distal screws. Initially, screws should be tightened one or two turns shy of their fullest extent to ensure

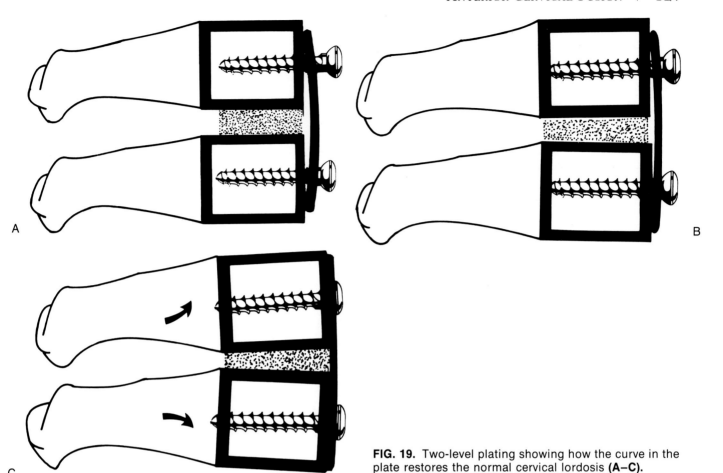

FIG. 19. Two-level plating showing how the curve in the plate restores the normal cervical lordosis **(A–C).**

that the plate will sit properly and that the selected screws are the correct length. As the screws are seated into place, the spine can be seen to shift into a lordotic curve if the plate is properly shaped (Figs. 19 and 20).

Ideally, the screw tips should completely penetrate the posterior cortex without extending into the spinal canal. Some penetration beyond the posterior cortex is allowed but no more than one thread width. This is tolerated because the posterior longitudinal ligament protects the spinal cord (Fig. 4). The posterior cortex provides a greater proportion of the overall screw torque than does the anterior cortex because it is usually slightly thicker. At any rate, *failure to bind the posterior cortex significantly reduces the overall torque obtained.* The authors have measured torques on >100 cases of cervical plating and have found that an average of 40–50 Ncm with ranges as high as 100 Ncm can be obtained in normal bone. Although no hard data exist, we believe that a torque of <25 Ncm is inadequate for long-term stabilization, and, in such cases, supplemental external bracing is recommended.

Repeated screw placement and removal should be avoided since each time a screw is replaced the torque is reduced. Successful fusion can be obtained with a single screw into a vertebral body, but several things can be attempted to salvage a stripped screw. The single drill-guide can be used to drill a new hole in a different direction. Alternatively, a second hole can be placed parallel and adjacent to the stripped hole (Fig. 21). With this technique, it is often difficult to achieve adequate torque with the new screw alone, but two screws are frequently sufficient. The proximity of the two screws tends to compact the intervening bone thereby increasing the torque of each individual screw. This type of screw is called a "locking screw." A less attractive option is to place small cancellous bone chips into the hole before reinserting the screw. Lastly, an oversized "rescue" screw that is 1-mm thicker in diameter than the standard screw is available (Fig. 22). Regardless, a completely stripped screw that cannot be salvaged by one of these methods should be removed because it will invariably come out and may cause trouble.

For subtotal vertebral body replacement, the screws should completely penetrate the graft and the posterior cortex of the remaining vertebral body. Significant torque can be obtained generating greater overall stability. The screws into block grafts for total vertebral

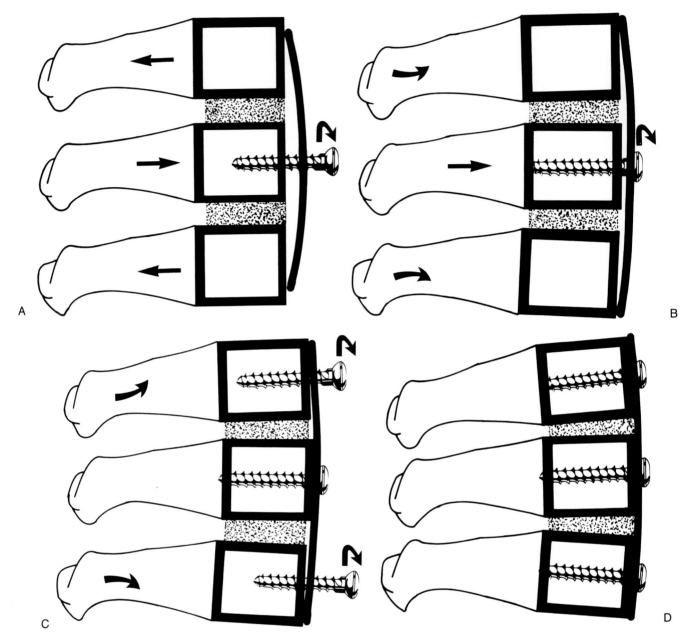

FIG. 20. Three-level fusion showing how the curve in the plate restores the normal cervical lordosis. The central screws should be tightened first **(A–D).**

body replacement should penetrate the anterior cortical surface and part of the cancellous bone. These screws merely prevent posterior dislocation and rotation of the bone plug and should not extend beyond the posterior surface of the graft.

Wound Closure

All instrumentation can be removed at this point. A small drain is placed anterior to the plate and exits the skin through a stab wound inferior to the incision. It is left for up to 36 hr postoperatively and then removed. The wound itself is closed as previously described (see Chapter 2).

Supplemental external immobilization is tailored to the individual case (see Chapter 19). Patients are monitored frequently with postoperative roentgenogram to evaluate the rate of fusion. Alterations in the type of collar and duration of wear are made based on the rate of fusion demonstrated by roentgenogram. For example, a young otherwise healthy patient will need only a soft collar for 4 weeks. An older patient or a patient with few risk factors for fusion will require a

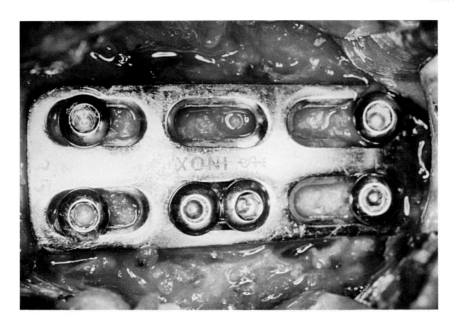

FIG. 21. Plate *in situ showing one possible method of screw placement.* Two screws can be placed adjacent to each other to increase torque.

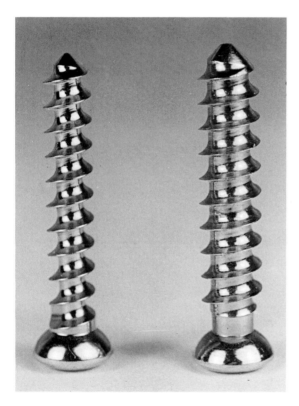

FIG. 22. Regular Swiss pattern cortical screw and oversized "rescue" screw. Care must be taken when using the rescue screw in holes placed too close to the vertebral endplate.

rigid collar for 8–12 weeks. An osteoporotic patient with combined posterior and anterior instability treated with a total body replacement will require a halo brace for 8–16 weeks.

Follow-up roentgenograms are performed in the operating room, on the first postoperative day, on discharge, and every 4 weeks until the fusion process is complete. Once fusion is achieved, external bracing is discontinued.

ILLUSTRATIVE CASES

Illustrative cases are represented in Figs. 23–33 and are fully described in the legends.

EXAMPLES OF TECHNICAL ERRORS

Examples of technical errors are represented in Figs. 34–40 and are fully described in the legends.

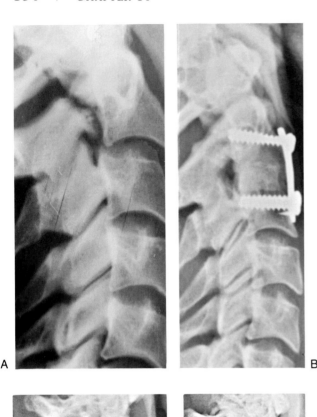

A
B

FIG. 23. A young male with a hangman's fracture following an automobile accident presented with neck pain and no neurologic deficit **(A).** Exposure of the upper cervical vertebra, particularly C2, requires hyperextension of the neck. The superior end of the plate must be custom bent to fit the contour of the C2 vertebral body. The extreme exposure frequently prevents the surgeon from placing screws perpendicular to the end plate so they usually must be angled through the vertebral body. Postoperative roentgenogram following plating **(B).** Although a hangman's fracture is often considered as a relative contraindication to anterior fusion, no additional posterior or external stabilization was required. From our experience with 12 hangman's fractures, anterior plating provides immediate postoperative stability and an optimal clinical result.

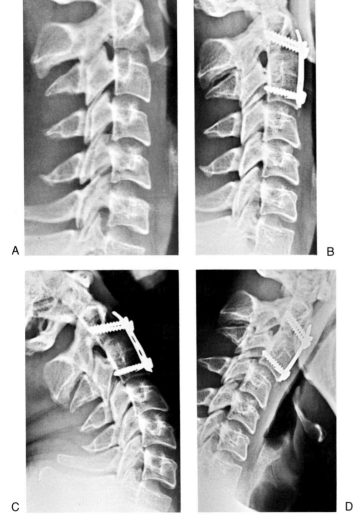

A
B
C
D

FIG. 24. This 30-year-old man suffered this unstable tear drop fracture in an automobile accident **(A).** He had no neurologic deficit but complained of dysphagia. He was treated initially with skeletal traction and then fused and stabilized with a plate. Postoperative functional studies at 1 year show remodeling of the posterior cortex **(B–D).**

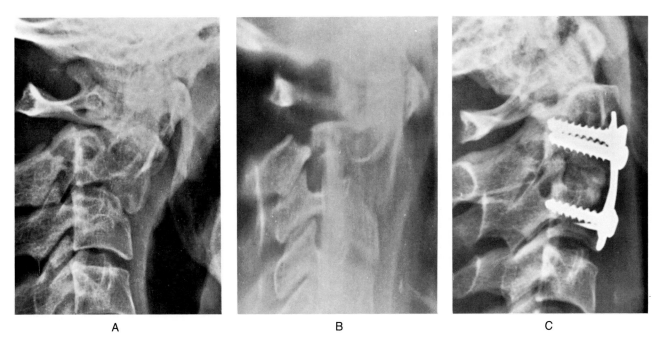

A   B   C

FIG. 25. A young man with neck pain but no neurologic deficit following an automobile accident and a complicated C2 fracture **(A).** Sagittal tomogram **(B).** The fractured C2 vertebral body was reduced and fixed with screws, and stability was reestablished with a graft and plate between the body of C2 and C3 **(C).**

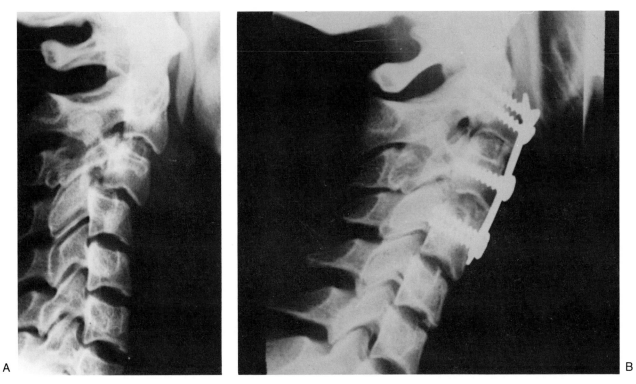

A   B

FIG. 26. This is an unusual case of multilevel instability in a young man after an automobile accident **(A).** There was subluxation at the C2–C3 and C3–C4 levels. Postoperative view **(B).**

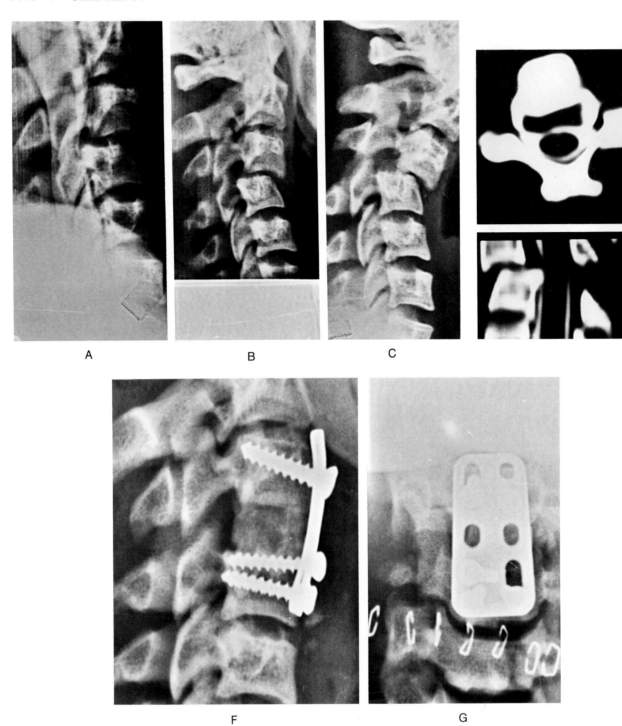

FIG. 27. This 20-year-old man was severely quadriplegic following an automobile accident. Realignment was achieved with skeletal traction, and he improved neurologically. He was stabilized with a plaster cast and did well until he fell. At this point, he deteriorated neurologically and had an attempted open reduction of a unilateral locked facet. The wrong facet was resected, which led to further instability. He was eventually reduced from an anterior approach and stabilized with a plate. **A:** Myelogram showing compression due to C3–C4 instability. **B:** Extension. **C:** Flexion. **D:** Axial CT showing persistent locked facet following resection of the facet on the opposite side. **E:** Sagittal CT reformat. **F:** Postoperative lateral roentgenograms showing a plate that is a bit too long and compromising the C2–C3 disc space. **G:** Postoperative anterior-posterior roentgenogram.

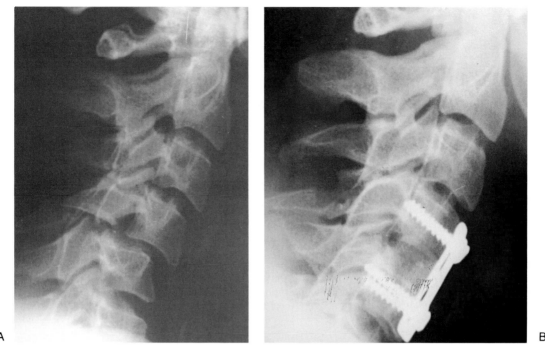

A   B

FIG. 28. This young man had severe quadriparesis after falling out of a tree. He had a C4–C5 subluxation without locked facets **(A)**. Postoperative view **(B)**.

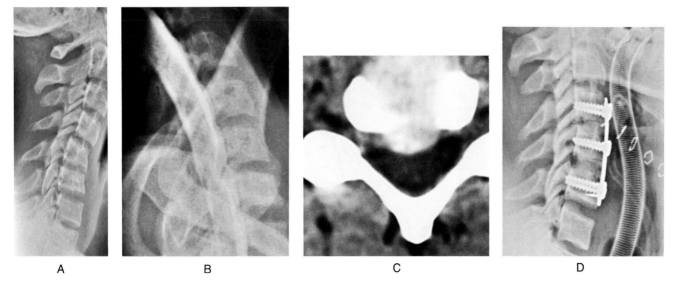

A   B   C   D

FIG. 29. This 22-year-old man had a C6 root deficit following an automobile accident. His roentgenograms, myelogram, and CT showed ligamentous instability at C4–C5 and a disc protrusion at C5–C6 **(A–C)**. This required a two-level plating procedure following C5–C6 discectomy **(D)**.

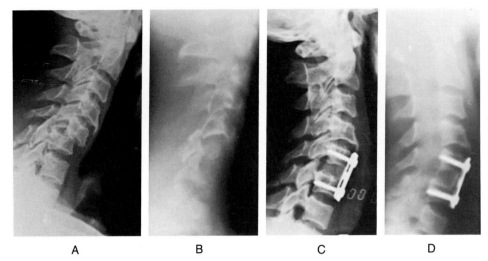

A   B   C   D

FIG. 30. After falling down stairs, this young man had a C5–C6 fracture subluxation with locked facets. Lateral roentgenogram **(A)** and lateral tomogram **(B)**. Fortunately, he only had a right C6 radiculopathy without any evidence of myelopathy. Lateral roentgenogram **(C)** and lateral tomogram **(D)** following plate stabilization. Note that the screws penetrate the posterior cortex of each vertebral body.

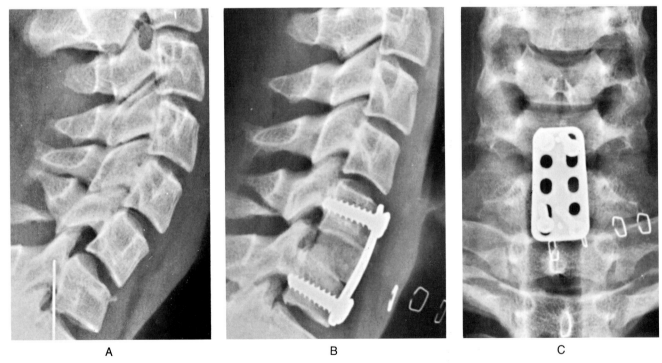

A   B   C

FIG. 31. This C6–C7 fracture subluxation with perched facets and fractured spinous process occurred after a diving accident in a 17-year-old man **(A).** He had neck pain but no neurologic deficit. Postoperative films **(B,C).**

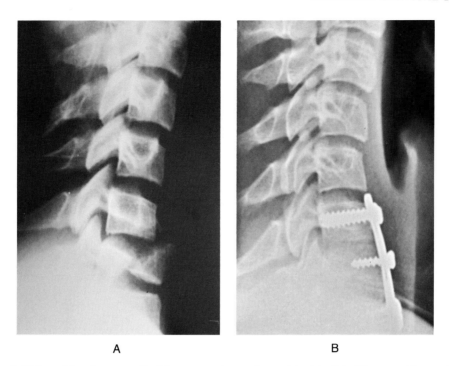

A   B

FIG. 32. A C7 burst fracture resulted from a motorcycle accident in this 24-year-old man **(A)**. He had complete loss of motor and sensory function in the legs and a weak grip bilaterally. He had conservative therapy for 6 weeks without any improvement in his neurologic function. He then underwent a delayed C7 total body replacement and plating with the hope of improvement in C8 root function **(B)**. In fact, he regained complete hand function as well as improved sensory function in his legs and improved sphincter control.

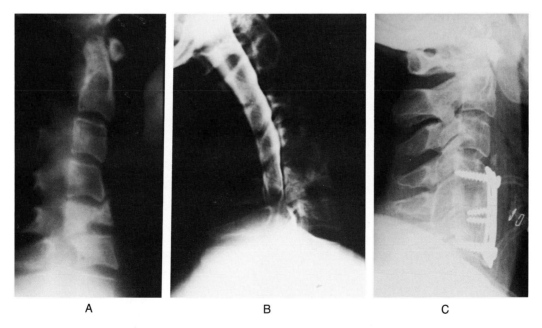

A   B   C

FIG. 33. This 40-year-old man suffered a C5 fracture at work resulting in quadriparesis which improved with conservative therapy. Six years later, he developed a progressive myelopathy due to the persistent spinal canal compromise and progressive kyphotic angulation **(A,B)**. He had excellent recovery of neurologic function after total body replacement and restoration of a normal stable cervical lordosis **(C)**.

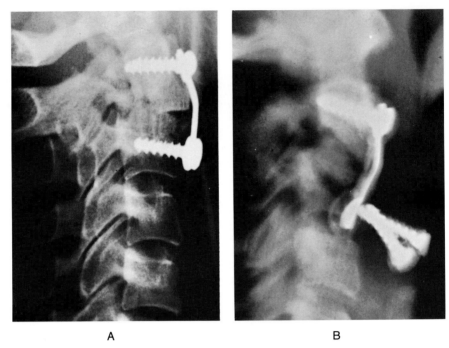

A

B

FIG. 34. Screw extrusion immediately postoperatively **(A)** and after total screw extrusion **(B)** resulting from poor surgical technique, including failure to realign the vertebral bodies, poor graft site preparation, poor graft placement, and failure to penetrate the posterior cortex with the screws.

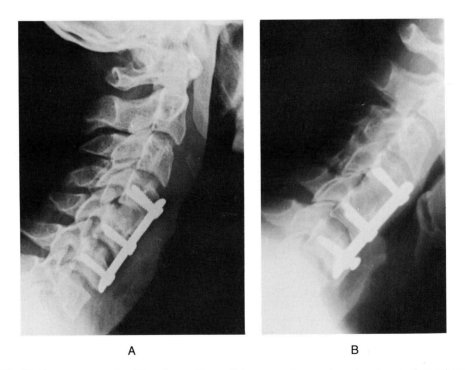

A

B

FIG. 35. Plating across a healthy disc will result in screw loosening due to persistently mobile segment which allows micromotion. Postoperative films **(A)** delayed screw loosening below the intact disc **(B).** Screw loosening is usually asymptomatic and self limiting but can precede screw extrusion.

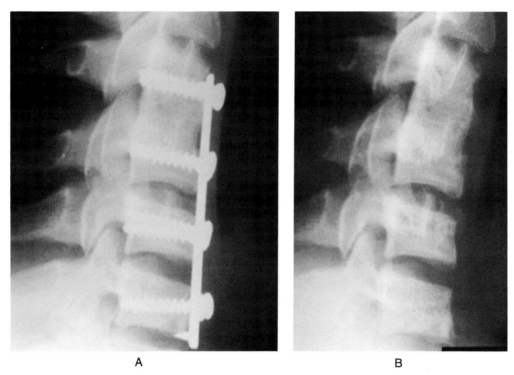

A   B

FIG. 36. This example of plating across healthy discs resulted in the unnecessary loss of function **(A).** The plate was subsequently removed and function was restored in the lower two levels **(B).**

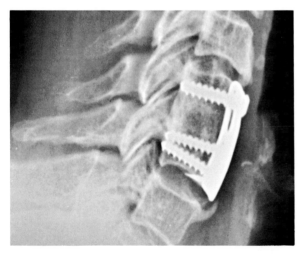

FIG. 37. Plates that are too long and compromise a healthy disc space can stimulate spur formation and subsequent loss of function.

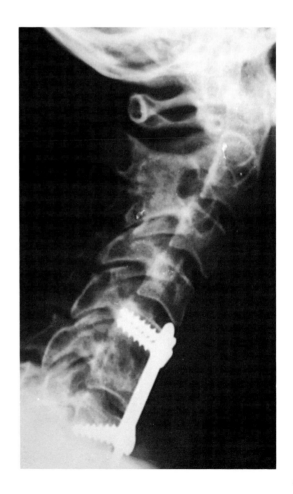

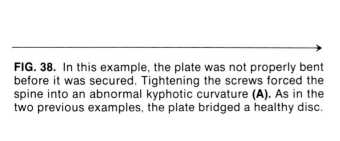

FIG. 38. In this example, the plate was not properly bent before it was secured. Tightening the screws forced the spine into an abnormal kyphotic curvature **(A).** As in the two previous examples, the plate bridged a healthy disc.

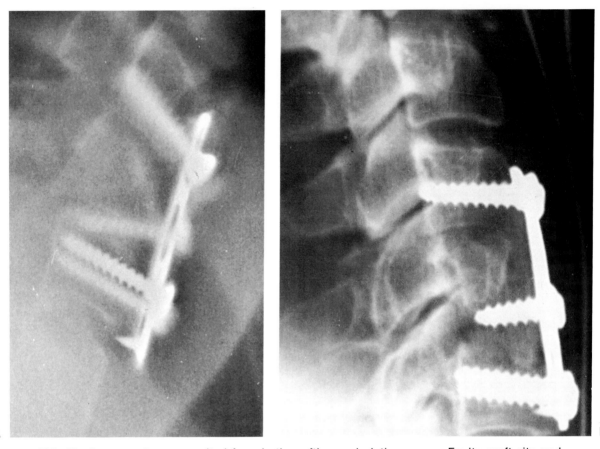

A

B

FIG. 39. A poor outcome resulted from both grafting and plating errors. Faulty graft site and graft preparation resulted in graft rotation and displacement upon screw tightening **(A).** The plate was not appropriately bent producing a kyphotic angulation and spinal canal compromise. In addition, the plate was too long so that the spike penetrated the disc. Following correction with proper technique **(B).**

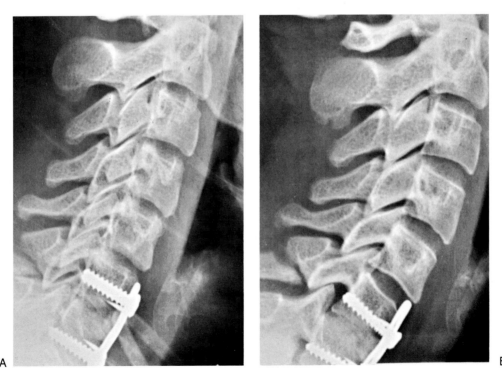

A

B

RESULTS

Clinical Material

The Caspar technique for anterior cervical trapezial plate stabilization has been used in 408 cases of varying pathology since it was first introduced in 1981 at the University of Saarland (Table 5). Since then, 108 traumatic cervical spine fractures have been treated using this technique. The first 60 cases have been reviewed in detail and the results are presented here.

The demographics of this group of patients were typical of most published series (Table 7). The neurological condition of each patient was classified into one of four groups (Table 8). Group I comprised 50% of the patients, all of whom had no neurologic deficit or only radicular findings without long tract signs. Five percent of the patients fell into Group II, having incomplete cord lesions but retaining useful motor function. Group III patients, consisting of 25% of the total, had incomplete cord lesions but no useful motor function. The remaining 20% of patients, all having complete cord lesions without any evidence of motor or sensory function below the level of injury, made up Group IV.

All the patients were evaluated radiologically with plain roentgenograms plus tomography, myelography, CT, CT myelography, and/or functional fluoroscopy as needed. All patients had unstabled cervical spine fractures or persistent spinal deformity with evidence of cord compression. The specific radiologic findings and level(s) of injury are summarized in Tables 9 and 10 respectively. For those patients admitted within 48 hr of their trauma, an attempt was made to realign persistent subluxation using skeletal traction.[6] Once maximum reduction had been obtained in these acute patients, myelography or CT myelography was performed. All acute trauma patients with evidence of persistent cord compression underwent operative decompression and fusion immediately following the studies. All other patients, including those with subacute injuries, chronic instability after conservative treatment, and stable but abnormal spinal deformities plus neurologic deficits, were operated upon within 48

---

[6] The University of Saarland is a tertiary care unit, and, therefore, fewer acute spinal cord injuries are seen than otherwise might be expected.

TABLE 7. *Cause of cervical spine injury*

Cause of injury	Cases	
	n	Percent
Vehicle accidents	31	51.7
Working place accidents	13	21.7
Sporting accidents	11	18.3
Suicide attempts	4	6.7
Assault	1	1.7
Total	60	100

TABLE 8. *Neurologic status at admission*

No cord lesion	
Group I (50%)	No minor clinically significant neurologic deficits
With cord lesion	
Group II (5%)	Showed an incomplete cord lesion with *useful* motor function
Group III (25%)	Showed an incomplete cord lesion with useless motor function
Group IV (20%)	Had complete sensory-motor-vegetative transverse lesion

TABLE 9. *Radiographic findings at admission (60 patients)*

Lesion	Cases	
	n	Percent
Vertebral body fracture	46	76.7
Compression fracture	27	45.0
Wedge fracture	19	31.7
Fracture of articular process and pedicles	18	30.0
Subluxation/dislocation	46	76.7
<⅓ of vertebral body	24	40.0
>⅓ of vertebral body	22	36.7
Instability, total posterior instability	36	60.0
	30	50.0

TABLE 10. *Location of injury*

Location	Cases	
	n	Percent
Upper cervical spine (C2–C3 and C3–C4)	12	20.0
Middle cervical spine (C4–C5 and C5–C6)	31	51.7
Lower cervical spine (C6–C7 and C7–T1)	17	28.3
Total	60	100

FIG. 40. Graft collapse may occur even with ideal technique. The previous plate design allowed the plate to move relative to the screws. In this case, the design fault allowed the plate to migrate across the adjacent disc space and could even penetrate the adjacent vertebral body. Immediately postoperative **(A)**. After plate migration **(B)**. The new design of plate has single screw holes that prevent this type of slippage (Fig. 13).

TABLE 11. *Time of operation after initial trauma (decompression and stabilization)*

	Cases	
	n	Percent
<48 hrs	5	8.3
2–7 days	24	40.0
8–14 days	7	11.7
2 weeks to 2 months	14	23.3
>2 months	10	16.7
Total	60	100

TABLE 12. *Surgical techniques for stabilization in 60 cases of cervical trauma*

Technique	n
Single-level fusion and plating	27
Multiple (2) fusion and plating	2
Subtotal body replacement and plating	17
Total body replacement and plating	14
Total	60

hr of admission. The timing of operative decompression and stabilization is summarized in Table 11.

The neurologic exam and radiologic studies determined the amount of decompression required in each case (Table 12). Stabilization was achieved by plating across a single segment in 27 cases. In two cases, two segments were incorporated into the fusion because of multilevel instability. Seventeen patients underwent subtotal body replacement and plating, whereas fourteen underwent total body replacement and plating.

Complications

The complications we have experienced with this procedure have been limited, and are listed in Table 13. There were no intraoperative deaths nor were there any major intraoperative injuries to vascular or neural structures. Four out of five postoperative deaths occurred >6 months following surgery, and, in each case, the deaths were unrelated to the surgery. The fifth death resulted from a postoperative pneumonia and heart failure in an elderly patient who had suffered a C3–C4 fracture without major neurologic deficit. Three cases required reoperation for persistent instability. In two cases, instability at a level adjacent to the fusion was not appreciated until after surgery. In the third case, a total body replacement failed due to a poorly shaped and inadequately secured block graft. In all three cases, a second operation resulted in a solid fusion without any additional complaints. There were three cases in which screws loosened to a minor degree (a distance of one to two threads), but each remained asymptomatic and no corrective procedure was required. The other complications noted in Tables 13 and 14 were all reversible except the pneumonia that resulted in death.

Fusion Rates

All patients including those requiring a second operation eventually obtained a solid bony union at the site of plate fixation. This finding was based upon fol-

TABLE 13. *Postoperative complications in 60 patients*

Complication	n	Comments
Technical complications		
Screw loosening (1–2 threads)	3	Asymptomatic. No functional significance, fusion stable.
Persistent instability	2	Instability in an adjacent segment primarily overlooked. Early reoperation, uneventful postoperative course.
Recurrent instability	1	Tilting of the inadequately shaped, placed, and not screw secured strut (total vertebral body replacement). Faulty plating. Early reoperation, fusion stable, spine in optimal posture.
Soft-tissue injury		
Vocal cord paresis	1	Reversible.
Dysphagia (>10 days)	1	Reversible.
Local infection	1	Patient with tracheostomy, wound infection, and septic bone graft necrosis. Conservative treatment with antibiotics and hard collar. Plate removed at 3 months, fusion stable.
General complications		
Pneumonia	4	
Gastric hemorrhage	2	
Deep leg vein thrombosis	1	
Neurologic worsening		
Early plus delayed	0	
Deaths	5	Unrelated to the operation. One death after 2 weeks on pneumonia and heart failure. Four deaths 6–12 months after hospital discharge.

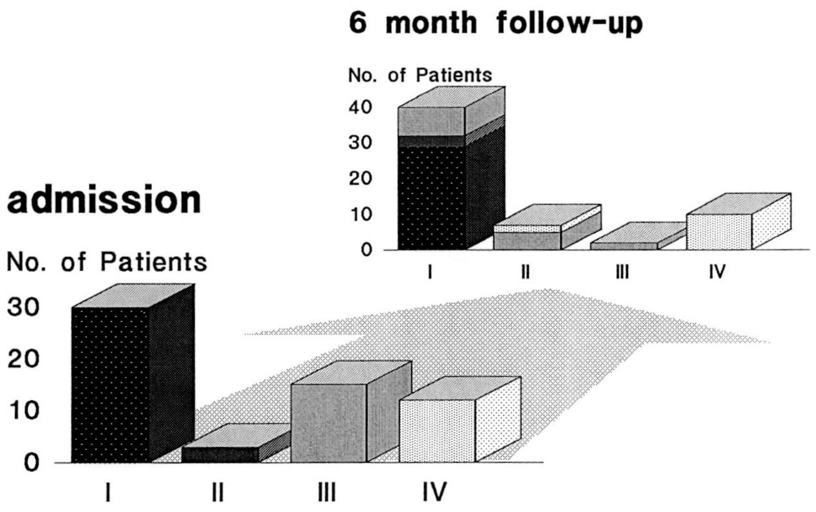

6 month follow-up

FIG. 41. Neurologic status.

low-up roentgenograms showing bone healing at the level of fusion without any evidence of a persistent "fracture" line. In addition, there was ultimately no instability demonstrated on dynamic roentgenographic studies, and there were no cases of delayed kyphosis observed within the follow-up period. Graft resorption of ~2 mm was frequently seen within the first few weeks following surgery, but this was never of any significance.

Neurologic Outcome

The neurologic status was assessed at 2 weeks, 6 months, and 1 year following the stabilization procedure. None of the 60 patients suffered either early or delayed neurologic deterioration. When neurologic improvement was observed, it was seen within 6 months of surgery without any significant change between 6 months and 1 year. Out of 47 patients presenting with neurologic deficits (radicular and/or long tract signs), 28 showed some improvement. Nearly 90% of the patients who presented with incomplete cord lesions showed good to excellent recovery, and 16% of patients with complete cord lesions showed some useful functional recovery. Neurologic outcomes are further summarized in Fig. 41.

These findings have been corroborated by several other surgeons applying the Caspar technique in cervical spine trauma (25,31,38,40). In nearly all the reported cases, immediate postoperative stability was obtained with acceptable complication rates. Goffin (25) and Levin (31) both reported high rates of improvement in patients with neurologic deficits following anterior plate stabilization. These authors all concluded that the Caspar technique is an excellent alternative, if not the procedure of choice, for stabilization of cervical spine fractures.

CONCLUSION

Based on our experience and that of others, it is obvious that Caspar trapezial plate stabilization is a safe procedure particularly if the technique is followed as described. A great deal has been learned since the first Caspar plate was applied, and, through trial and error, a freely applicable technique has been devised. At the risk of sounding dogmatic, the technique has been presented in great detail. It is hoped that this will help others to avoid some of the pitfalls and difficulties that we have encountered over the years.

Caspar plating technique is clearly a reliable method of stabilization in the cervical spine with many advantages. There is a higher rate of fusion in a shorter period of time and greater economic advantage due to a reduced overall treatment cost and an increased potential patient productivity. Although further studies are needed, preliminary evidence suggests that a better neurologic outcome can be obtained with this technique. In fact, this procedure may prove to be superior for all problems of the cervical spine requiring anterior decompression of the spinal cord and nerve roots. Studies are currently under way to evaluate its relative merits in degenerative diseases, especially cervical myelopathy, and modifications are being made to improve its suitability for neoplastic disease.

REFERENCES

1. Anderson LD. Compression plate fixation and the effect of different types of internal fixation on fracture healing. *J Bone Joint Surg [Am]* 47A:191–208, 1965.
2. Bailey RW, Badgley CE. Stabilization of the cervical spine by anterior fusion. *J Bone Joint Surg [Am]* 42A:565–624, 1960.
3. Bohler J. Sofort- und fruhbehandlung traumatischer querschnittlahmungen. *Zeitschor Orthopad Grenzgebiete* 103:512–528, 1967.

4. Bohler J, Gaudernak T. Anterior plate stabilization for fracture-dislocations of the lower cervical spine. *J Trauma* 20:203–205, 1980.

5. Bremer AM, Nguyen TQ. Internal metal plate fixation combined with anterior interbody fusion in cases of cervical spine injury. *Neurosurgery* 12:649–653, 1983.

6. Caspar W. Die ventrale interkorporale stabilisierung mit der HWS-Trapez-osteosyntheseplatte. Indikation, Technik, Ergebnisse. *Orthopade* 119:809–810, 1981.

7. Caspar W. Advances in cervical spine surgery. First experiences with the trapezial osteosynthetic plate and a new surgical instrumentation for anterior interbody stabilization. *Orthopaedic News* 4:7–8, 1982.

8. Caspar W. Advances in cervical spine surgery. First experiences with the trapezial osteosynthetic plate and a new surgical instrumentation for anterior interbody stabilization. In: *7th European Neurosurgical Congress*. Brussels: European Association Neurological Surgeons, 253, 1983.

9. Caspar W. Fortschritte bei der vorderen, cervicalen Plattenstabilisierung. Erste Erfahrungen mit der Trapezosteosyntheseplatte und einem neuen Instrumentarium fuer die Halswirbelsaeulenchirurgie. In: Hackenbroch MH, Refior HJ, Jaeger M, eds. *5th Munich Symposium for experimental orthopaedics, Biomechanik der Wirbelsaule, Ergbnisse praxisbozogener Grundlagenforschung.* Stuttgart and New York: Georg Thieme Verlag, 202–209, 1983.

10. Caspar W. A new plate and instrumentation for stabilization of unstable fractures and fracture dislocations of the cervical spine. In: *Traumatology of the spinal column. Proceedings of the First Viennese Workshop. International College of Surgeons, Austrian Section, October 3–6.* Vecsei, Vienna: Informatica, 232–236, 1983.

11. Caspar W. Die ventrale interkorporale Stabilisierung mit der HWS-Trapez-Osteosyntheseplatte—indikations, technik, ergebnisse. *Orthopaedische Praxis* 12:981–988, 1984.

12. Caspar W. The trapezial osteosynthetic plate technique: a new technology for anterior cervical fusion and interbody stabilization. Presented at the First Annual Meeting of American Association of Neurological Surgeons and Congress of Neurological Surgeons, Joint Section of Spinal Disorders of AANS and CNS, Grenelefe, Florida, 1984.

13. Caspar W. Anterior stabilization with the trapezial osteosynthetic plate technique in cervical spine injuries. In: *First Common Meeting of the Cervical Spine Research Society and of its European Section, June 20–22.* Strassbourg, Germany: Cervical Spine Research Society, 57, 1985.

14. Caspar W. Anterior stabilization with the trapezial osteosynthetic plate technique in cervical spine injuries. *Cervical Spine* 1:198–204, 1987.

15. Caspar W. Anterior cervical fusion and Caspar plate stabilization for cervical trauma. Presented at the AANS and CNS Joint Section on Spine and Peripheral Nerve, Cancun, Mexico, February 14, 1989.

16. Caspar W. *Anterior cervical fusion and interbody stabilization with the trapezial osteosynthetic plate technique.* Tuttlingen, Germany: Aesculap Scientific Info. 12. 7th Ed., 1989.

17. Caspar W. The trapezial plate osteosynthesis. An advanced technology for anterior internal stabilization in cervical spine injuries and for the treatment of neck instability due to non-traumatic causes. Presented at the Annual Meeting of the American Association Neurological Surgeons, Washington, D.C., April 1, 1989.

18. Caspar W, Barbier DD, Klara PM. Anterior cervical fusion and Caspar plate stabilization for cervical trauma. *Neurosurgery* 25:491–502, 1989.

19. Charnley J. *The closed treatment of common fractures.* London: Livingstone, 1961.

20. Cloward R. The anterior approach for removal of ruptured cervical disks. *J Neurosurg* 15:602–617, 1958.

21. Cloward RD. Treatment of acute fractures and fracture dislo-cation of cervical spine by vertebral body fusion. A report of 11 cases. *J Neurosurg* 18:205–209, 1961.

22. Dereymaker A, Mulier J. Nouvelle cure chirurgicale des discopathies cervicales. La meniscectomie par vioe ventrale, suivie d'arthrodese par greffe intercorporeale. *Neurochirurgie* 2:233–234, 1956.

23. de Oliveira JC. Anterior plate fixation of traumatic lesions of the lower cervical spine. *Spine* 12:324–329, 1987.

24. Ducker TB, Salcman M, Daniell HB. Experimental spinal cord trauma. III: Therapeutic effect of immobilization and pharmacologic agents. *Surg Neurol* 10:71–76, 1978.

25. Goffin J, Plets C, Van den Bergh R. Anterior cervical fusion and osteosynthetic stabilization according to Caspar: a prospective study of 41 patients with fractures and/or dislocations of the cervical spine. *Neurosurgery* 25:865–871, 1989.

26. Gassman J, Seligson D. The anterior cervical plate. *Spine* 8:700–707, 1983.

27. Herrmann HD. Metal plate fixation after anterior fusion of unstable fracture dislocation of the cervical spine. *Acta Neurochir* 32:101–111, 1975.

28. Keblish P, Keggi K. Mechanical problems of the dowel graft in anterior cervical fusion. *J Bone Joint Surg [Am]* 49A:198, 1967.

29. Koranyi E, Bowman EC, Knecht CD, Janssen M. Holding power of orthopedic screws in bone. *Clin Orthop* 72:283–286, 1970.

30. Lesoin F, Cama A, Lozes G, Servato R, Kabbag K, Jomin M. The anterior approach and plates in lower cervical post-traumatic lesions. *Surg Neurol* 21:581–587, 1984.

31. Levin AB. Anterior spinal cord decompression with bone and plate fixation: a 13-year experience. Presented at the Annual Meeting of the American Association Neurological Surgeons, Washington, D.C., April 5, 1989.

32. Muller ME, Allgower M, Willenegger H. *Technique of internal fixation of fractures.* New York: Springer-Verlag, 1965.

33. Orozco R, Llovet TJ. Osteosintesis en las fractures de raquis cervical. *Revista Ortop Traumatol* 14:285–288, 1970.

34. Orozco R, Llovet TJ. Osteosintese en los lesiones traumaticos y degenerativos de los coluvos cervoca. *Rev Traumatologia Cirurgia Rehabil* 1:42–52, 1971.

35. Robinson RA, Smith GW. Anterolateral cervical disc removal and interbody fusion for cervical disc syndrome. *Bull Johns Hopkins Hosp* 96:223–224, 1955.

36. Rosenweig N. "The get up and go" treatment of acute unstable injuries of the middle and lower cervical spine. *J Bone Joint Surg [Br]* 56B:392, 1974.

37. Senegas J, Gauzere JM. Pladoyes pour la chirurgie anterieure dans le traitemant des traumatismes graves des cinq derieres vertebres cervicales. *Rev Chirurg Orthop* 62(suppl II):123–128, 1976.

38. Shoung HM, Lee LS. Anterior metal plate fixation in the treatment of unstable lower cervical spine injuries. *Acta Neurochir* 98:55–59, 1989.

39. Smith GW, Robinson RA. Treatment of certain cervical spine disorders by anterior removal of the intervertebral disc and interbody fusion. *J Bone Joint Surg [Am]* 40A:607, 1958.

40. Tippets RH, Apfelbaum RI. Anterior cervical fusion with the Caspar instrumentation system. *Neurosurgery* 22:1008–1013, 1988.

41. Tscherne H, Hiebler W, Muhr G. Zur operativen Behandlung von Frakturen und Luxationen der Halswirbelsaule. *Hefte Unfallheilk* 108:142–145, 1971.

42. Verviest H. Antero-lateral operation for fractures and dislocations in the middle and lower parts of the cervical spine. *J Bone Joint Surg [Am]* 51A:1489–1530, 1969.

43. White AA, Hirsch C. An experimental study of the immediate load bearing capacity of some commonly used iliac bone grafts. *Acta Orthop Scand* 42:482–488, 1971.

44. White A, Jupiter J, Southwick W, Panjabi M. An experimental study of the immediate load bearing capacity of three surgical constructions for anterior spine fusions. *Clin Orthop* 91:21–28, 1973.

CHAPTER 11

Posterior Microlaminotomy (Keyhole) for Lateral Soft Discs and Spurs

Paul H. Young

The keyhole laminotomy-foraminotomy has been applied extensively for the posterior decompression of individual nerve roots affected by lateral soft disc protrusions or spondylotic spurs projecting into the foramen (1–8). The addition of the operating microscope to this procedure limits the perioperative morbidity associated with the soft tissue and bony opening, and enhances the safety with which this procedure can be performed around sensitive neural structures.

INDICATIONS

Indications (Fig. 1) are as follows: a significant lateral soft disc herniation and associated root compression with appropriate radicular symptoms and signs, osteophytic root compression with appropriate radicular symptoms and signs, and foraminal disc or spur root compression with corresponding radicular symptomatology not relieved by appropriate conservative measures.

EXPOSURE OF THE INTERLAMINAR SPACE

See Chapter 2.

LAMINOTOMY-FORAMINOTOMY

The interlaminar space is carefully identified and cleared of overlying soft tissue particularly at its lateral apex. The medial facet-interlaminar space apex junction is identified. Using the high-speed drill (Midas M-8 or cutting burr), a partial laminotomy-facetotomy

is performed beginning at the junction between the most lateral aspect of the interlaminar space (the apex) and the most medial aspect of the facet joint (Fig. 2). The medial one-third to one-half of the facet is progressively removed, as is a similar amount of the adjoining cranial and caudal laminae. An ~2–3-cm round or oval opening is thus created.

The posterolateral portion of the superior lamina and the medial part of the inferior articular facet are removed first. This enlarges the apex of the interlaminar space, and permits the progressive removal of the medial side of the superior facet and the lateral corner of the inferior lamina flush with the inner aspect of the pedicle. The nerve root is located directly above the pedicle and immediately under the superior facet. A distinct layer of loose fibrous tissue containing epidural veins lies immediately beneath the thin lateral part of the ligamentum flavum, and progressive excision of the ligament carefully in a medial direction will safely expose the lateral portion of the dura. The position of the spinal canal and lateral dural margin is used as an anatomical landmark, establishing a clear plane of dissection along the proximal nerve root and lateral epidural venous structures. Progressive lateral dissection can then proceed along the root as it enters the foramen.

The medial border of the pedicle should be identified early and followed anteriorly to the floor of the spinal canal to establish an epidural plane between the lateral dura and the posterolateral vertebral body below. Staying in this same space, rostral dissection can proceed to identify the plane between the disc space and the anterior surface of the nerve root axilla.

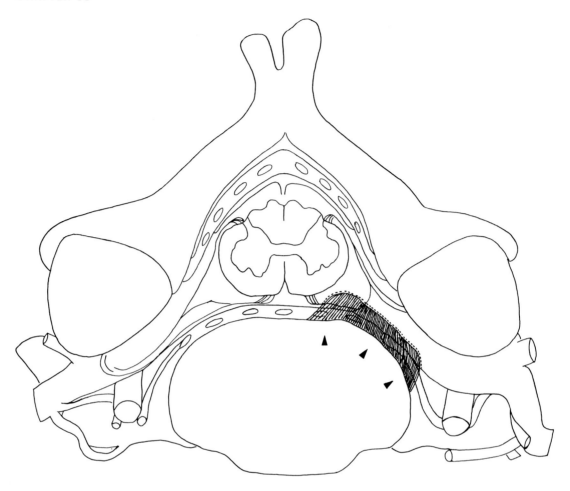

FIG. 1. Indications for a posterior microlaminotomy.

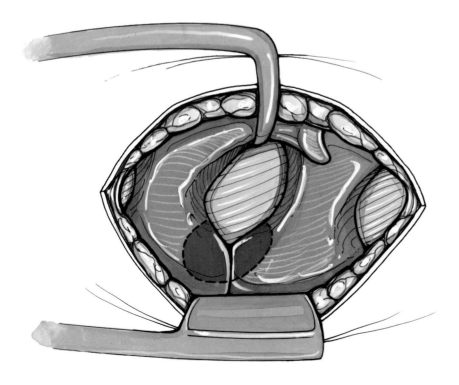

FIG. 2. The location and size of "keyhole" laminotomy-foraminotomy.

Following this initial exposure, the posterior foraminal wall is then removed, utilizing a plane of dissection between the perineural tissue and the bone of the anterior aspect of the superior facet to avoid mechanical pressure on the root. Further removal of inferior facet permits direct visualization of both superior and inferior pedicles, and allows palpation along the first 5 mm of root laterally into the foramen.

One of the most important technical points is the establishment of a plane of dissection in the foramen between the nerve root sleeve and the extradural tissue composed of fat, fibrous tissue, and epidural veins. In spondylotic root compression, dense root sleeve perineural adhesions are a common finding with tethering of the root to the foramen. These must be retracted away from the nerve root against the bony canal and carefully coagulated with the bipolar. This provides better exposure of the nerve root and helps in the identification of the extruded disc or spur beneath it. Using cranial retraction of the nerve root, access to the posterior surface of the vertebral disc is achieved.

In soft disc sequestrations, the disc fragment has most often extruded through the annulus and posterior longitudinal ligament lateral to the dural sac (Fig. 3). When the compressed root has been exposed, it is gently retracted upward and the extruded disc fragments are removed with a small disc rongeur, suction, or small nerve hook. Soft disc sequestered fragments are generally multiple, and present anterior and inferior to the nerve root or in the axilla. Fragments inferior to the root are much more common than those cephalid. Retraction of the nerve root while exploring for sequestered fragments or exposing spurs should be done only with care and restraint (Fig. 4). It is not advisable to enter the disc space from this approach.

If an anomalous bifed root is present with separate ventral and dorsal root dural sleeves (35%), sequestered fragments may be wedged between the roots, generally obscuring the motor root, which lies inferior to the larger sensory root. In addition, the dural covering of the smaller motor root is quite thin. Failure to recognize this situation can easily result in motor root injury when disc fragments are grasped. In muscle, paralyzing agents are avoided; compression, traction, or coagulation of motor roots results in immediate muscle contraction, and this response can be used as

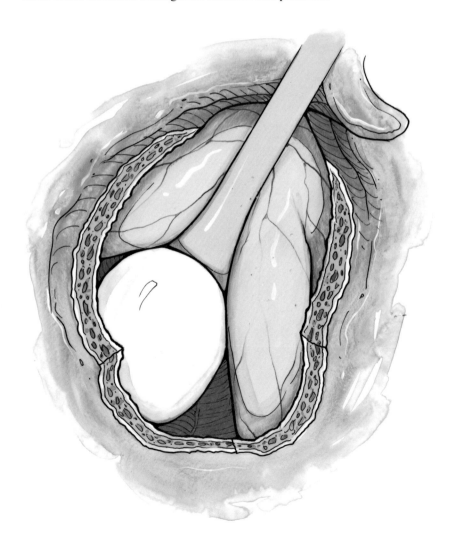

FIG. 3. Retraction of an upper cervical nerve root to identify a lateral focal disc prolapse.

an intraoperative "evoked response" of impending root injury, telling the surgeon to "back off."

When adequately decompressed, the root sleeves fill with cerebrospinal fluid (CSF) and expand with CSF pulsations.

When using a small foramenotomy opening, it may be, on occasion, necessary to further explore the foramen for spurs or sequestered disc fragments. In this situation, the opening should be enlarged inferiorly by removing more of the superior lamina of the vertebra below. Under no circumstances, though, should >50% of the facet be removed. Spurs projecting into the anterior aspect of the foramen from the uncovertebral process of the vertebral bodies are often associated with dense perineural fibrous adhesions that bind the root to the lateral bony canal. Careful separations of these adhesions with a small blunt hook is necessary prior to an attempt at spur removal. The removal of spurs in this region should be done only under direct

visualization. If spurs, particularly anterior spurs, are not readily visualized, one should be content with a posterior decompression alone. It is particularly inadvisable to attempt the removal of hard spurs or ridges located anterior to the dural sac along the disc space.

Hemostasis

Epidural bleeding is frequently encountered from the perineural plexus around the nerve root in the foramen or from the epidural plexus in the lateral spinal canal. This may require the use of bipolar coagulation and the placement of gel-foam. Care must be taken during coagulation around the dural sleeve of the nerve root or directly on the dura overlying the cord as there may be postoperative numbness, paresthesias, pain, or paraesis related to underlying root or cord thermal or electrical injury (Fig. 5). The packing of these ve-

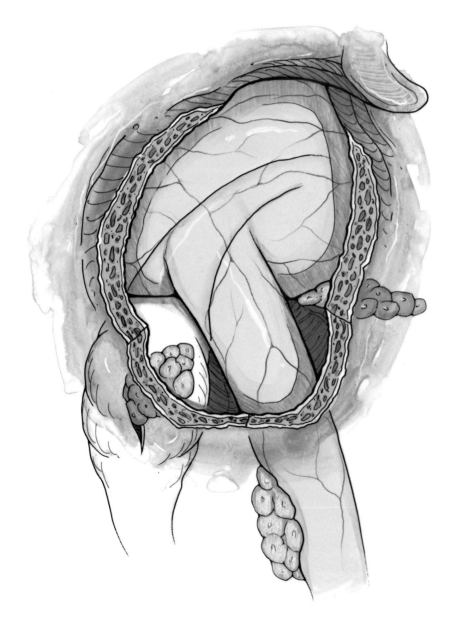

FIG. 4. Upper (C_3 or C_4) disc sequestrations in and around the foramen. The changing relationship between the existing nerve root and disc space as one descends from C_2-T_1 should be noted.

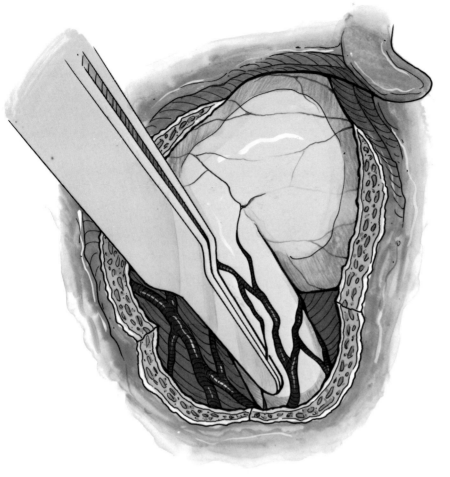

FIG. 5. Bipolar coagulation along the nerve root within the foramen.

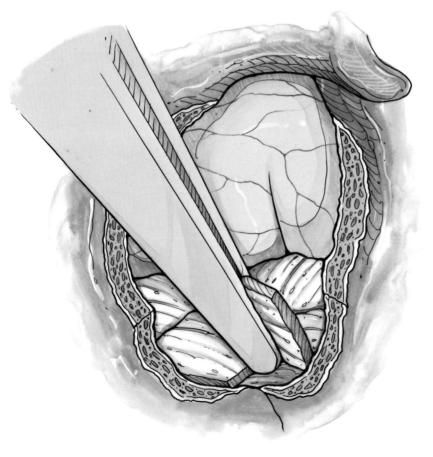

FIG. 6. Gel-foam is placed in the foramen and bony defect covering the nerve root.

nous plexi with gel-foam achieves immediate hemostasis but obscures further exploration.

CLOSURE

Following absolute hemostasis, a small piece of wet gel-foam or fat is placed loosely in the laminotomy defect to take up the dead space (Fig. 6). The wound is closed as described in Chapter 2.

REFERENCES

1. Aldrich F. Posterolateral microdiscectomy for cervical mono-radiculopathy caused by posterolateral soft cervical disc sequestration. *J Neurosurg* 72:370–377, 1990.

2. Epstein JA, Janin Y. Management of cervical spondylotic myelo radiculopathy by the posterior approach. In: *The Cervical Spine*. 1st ed. Philadelphia JB Lippincott, 1983.

3. Henderson CM, Hennessy RG, Shuey HM, Shackelford EG: Posterolateral foraminotomy as an exclusive operative technique for cervical radiculopathy. A review of 846 consecutively operated cases. *Neurosurgery* 13:504–512, 1983.

4. Hudgins WR. Posterior micro-operative treatments of cervical disc disease. In: Youmans, ed. *Neurological surgery*. 3rd ed. Philadelphia: WB Saunders, 2918–2922, 1990.

5. Raynor RB. Anterior or posterior approach to the cervical spine: an anatomical and radiographic evaluation and comparison. *Neurosurgery* 12:7–13, 1983.

6. Raynor RB, Pugh J, Shapiro I. Cervical facetectomy and its effect on stability. In: *Cervical spine I*. New York: Springer-Verlag, 51–54, 1987.

7. Scoville WB, Whitcomb BB, McLauran R. The cervical ruptured disc report of 115 operative cases. *Trans Am Neurol Assoc* 76:222, 1951.

8. Williams RW. Microcervical foraminotomy: a surgical alternative for intractable radicular pain. *Spine* 8:708–716, 1983.

CHAPTER 12

Posterior Cervical Decompressive Techniques

Paul H. Young

The classical neurosurgical exposures of the spinal canal for a wide variety of pathological processes involves a wide decompressive laminectomy, sometimes with an associated decompression tactic (Table 1) (1–14). Recent refinements of these techniques, especially including the use of the operating microscope, have been introduced in an attempt to reduce the postoperative morbidity and long-term complications associated with this approach. Major modifications of the laminectomy include the various laminoplasty techniques, described later in this chapter.

INDICATIONS

Indications are as follows (Fig. 1): multilevel spinal canal stenosis with associated myelopathy when the major compressing lesion is not located anteriorly; congenital or developmental cervical canal narrowing (diameters of <13 mm) with corresponding myelopathic symptomatology (spinal cord diameter of <11 mm); exposure of the spinal canal for surgery involving spinal cord tumors, epidural infection, syringomyelia, or other situations where wide exposure of the spinal canal over multiple segments is necessary; and multilevel ossification of the posterior longitudinal ligament and associated myelopathy.

INITIAL EXPOSURE

A bilateral exposure of the posterior elements and interlaminar spaces extending laterally to the facets is accomplished over the segments of interest, as indicated in Chapter 2 (Fig. 2).

BILATERAL LAMINECTOMY

Using the high-speed drill (Midas M-8 or cutting burr), the laminae of interest are slowly removed from a medial to lateral direction. Each lamina is removed beginning at its inferior margin, identifying the underlying attachments of the ligamentum flavum and then proceeding in a cranial direction. The use of the high-speed drill eliminates the need for separation of the ligament from the overlying laminae for the insertion of footed rongeurs (Fig. 3). The most caudal lamina is removed first, and the procedure is then carried in a cranial direction to include all of the laminae of interest.

TABLE 1. *Traditional approaches for the posterior decompression of spondylotic myelopathy*

Author/year	Procedure
Northfield 1955	Simple bilateral laminectomy extending one segment above and below
Bishara 1971	Addition of medial facetectomies
Rogers 1961	Extensive bilateral laminectomy C1–T1
Scoville 1961	Limited bilateral laminectomy (to symptomatic levels) with bilateral complete facetectomy
Stoops and King 1962	Extensive bilateral laminectomy and complete facetectomy
Schneider 1982	Addition of section dentate ligament
Fox et al. 1972	Addition of duroplasty
Epstein et al. 1982	Addition of spur removal

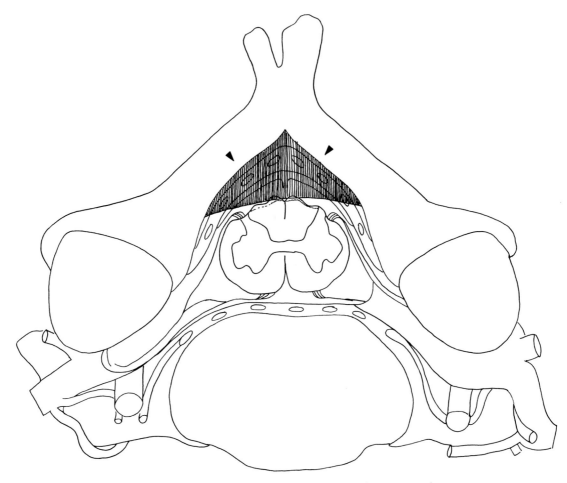

FIG. 1. Indications for posterior decompressive approaches.

The spinous process is thinned along its attachment to the laminae and removed with a large rongeur. As the removal of laminae is accomplished bilaterally, care should be taken to preserve the ligamenta flava as a safety shield, covering the underlying dura and spinal cord and preserving hemostasis in the epidural venous plexus. No downward pressure should be exerted during any bone removal maneuver upon the underlying ligamenta flava and underlying cord. In addition, the use of footed rongeurs placed beneath the

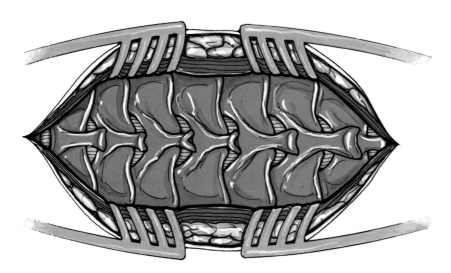

FIG. 2. Posterior exposure for multi-level decompression.

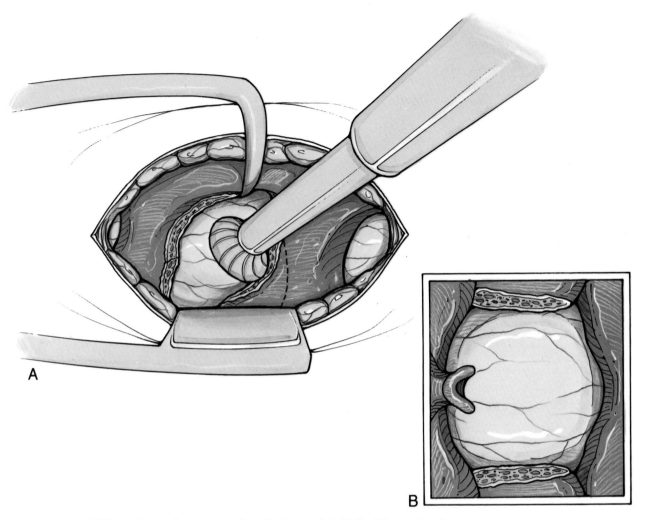

FIG. 3. A: Laminectomy using high-speed drill. **B:** Bilateral laminectomy completed.

bony margins of the lamina should be avoided in patients with very narrow canal diameters (<13 mm) due to the possibility of worsening underlying spinal canal compromise. The bony removal should extend laterally to the most medial margin of the facet joints (Fig. 4).

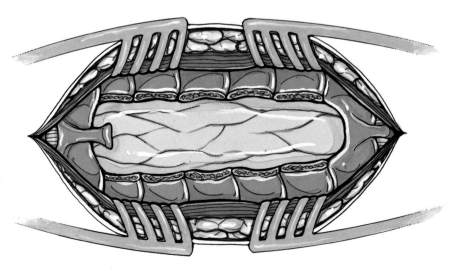

FIG. 4. Exposure following multilevel bilateral laminectomy.

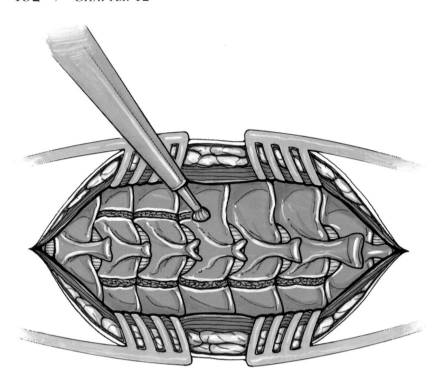

FIG. 5. Bilateral longitudinal gutters created with the high-speed drill at the laminae-facet junction.

MULTISEGMENT ONE PIECE LAMINECTOMY (EN FACE)

Longitudinal channels are cut laterally on the extreme lateral portion of each lamina with the high-speed drill just medial to the facets (Fig. 5). This is accomplished bilaterally, and following incision of the rostral and caudal ligamenta flava the entire posterior element roof is lifted in one piece (Fig. 6). Care is exercised to avoid any kinking of the underlying spinal canal contents.

FORAMINOTOMY

Spondylotic radicular compression requires further lateral decompression. The foraminotomy commences with the removal of the most medial aspect of the facet overlying the proximal nerve root. The high-speed drill (diamond burr) is used to progressively remove a portion of the inferior facet of the superior vertebra in addition to the superior facet of the inferior vertebra (Fig. 7). In general, 50% of the total facet can be removed bilaterally without fear of significant postop-

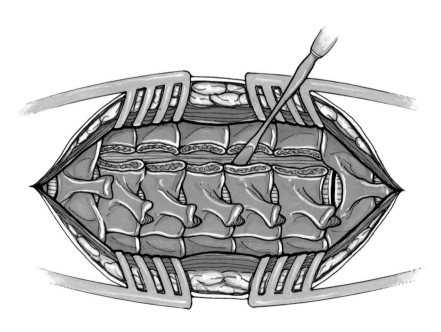

FIG. 6. Elevation of posterior arches en block.

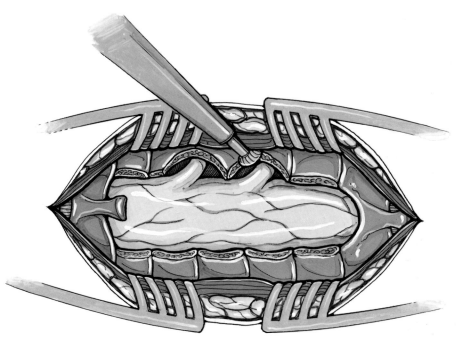

FIG. 7. Multilevel bilateral laminectomy and partial facetectomy.

erative instability. Greater than 50% removal of the facet particularly if bilateral significantly increases the risk of postoperative destabilization (1). Fifty percent facetectomies permit visualization of 5–6 mm of the root. When necessary, further root visualization is accomplished by angled undercutting of the superior facet.

The bony roof of the foramen can be removed entirely using the high-speed drill, or a small sheet of bone can be left behind to be lifted and removed with an angled curette or small Kerrison rongeur (1–2 mm). As the roof of the foramen is elevated, the radicular veins will distend and some oozing may occur. In all instances, this can be controlled well with a combination of bipolar cautery and gel-foam packing. The foraminotomy should not be considered complete until it has extended 1 cm lateral to the most lateral margin of the spinal canal or 5 mm along the proximal nerve root (Fig. 7). Passage of a nerve hook through the foramen should be done only under direct visualization; the use of a small angled mirror may be helpful in this situation.

During performance of the laminectomy and/or foraminotomy, it is imperative not to leave jagged bony spicules along the edges of the bony removal. Exposed bony surfaces should be coated with bone wax using a small dissector to complete hemostasis. Epidural bleeding, especially occurring in the lateral spinal canal, can be easily controlled with the accurate placement of small squares of gel-foam held in position by cotton strips. Pressure upon the gel-foam should be directed only laterally and not downward upon the dura or nerve roots.

The use of a limited foraminotomy and not extending the laminectomy into multiple facet joints prevents postoperative kyphosis and other deformities sometimes seen after multisegment trauma or tumor surgery or in wide exposures in younger patients. The extent of the laminectomy should include the laminae bordering the level of symptomatology and extend one level above and below. Clearly, no attempt should be made from this approach to remove anterior osteophytes (either extra- or transdurally) due to the significant risk of increased neurologic disability. In addition, extensive intradural procedures in patients with myelopathy due to spondylosis clearly do not expand the indications of the posterior approach to include the decompression of large anterior compressive forces. As a result, the use of dentate ligament section or duroplasty for decompression of anterior spondylosis cannot be condoned.

LAMINOPLASTY TECHNIQUES

Advantages of laminoplasty techniques (15–40) include: greater safety than with the conventional total midline laminectomy because the laminae are transected along the lateral border of the spinal canal, where there is more abundant space between the laminae and the compressed spinal cord than there is in the midline; greater stability of the spine after surgery that permits patients to mobilize early; and the prevention of delayed postoperative complications such as kyphosis and swan neck deformities.

Open-Door Laminoplasty

Using the high-speed drill, the spinous processes are cut short and bony gutters are created bilaterally along the medial margins of the facets. Following creation of this trough bilaterally, the ligamenta flava between the laminae at both upper and lower ends are transected. The bony gutter on the hinged side is made slightly more lateral than on the open side. Spinous process sutures are placed through the capsules around the facets on the hinged side to keep the decompression open (Fig. 8). As each lamina is elevated, any remaining yellow ligament and adhesive fibrous bands between the dura and the inner surface of the lamina is carefully divided.

The open-door laminoplasty can also be kept open using laminar bone grafts placed in the opened gutter at several segments (Fig. 9), or a small fixation device screwed into the facets and wired to the spinous processes (Fig. 10).

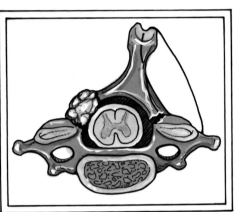

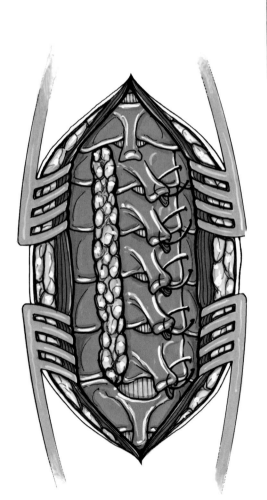

FIG. 8. Open-door laminoplasty fixed with spinous process sutures.

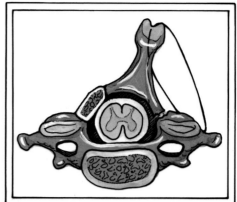

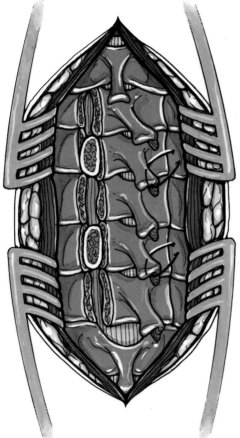

FIG. 9. Open-door laminoplasty fixed with laminar bone grafts.

Bifed Laminoplasty

A midline trans-spinous bony opening is performed through the posterior arch. A bilateral laminotomy is performed at the medial pedicular plane. The two posterior arch halves are then spread apart to open the spinal canal. The hemi-arches are secured in place by a longitudinal bone strut (Fig. 11).

Z-Shaped Laminoplasty

A Z-shaped laminar incision is performed with the high-speed drill cutting successive laminae alternatively. The individual laminae are then elevated, split laterally, and sutured to each other, forming a higher arch to the spinal canal (Fig. 12).

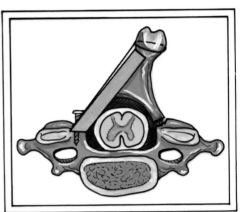

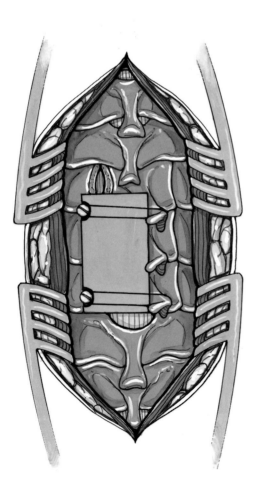

FIG. 10. Open-door laminoplasty fixed with plating.

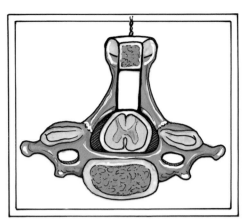

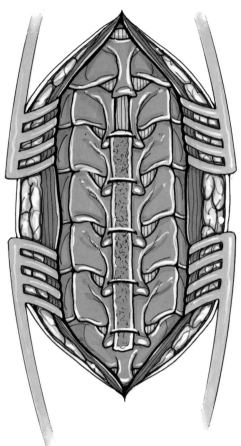

FIG. 11. Bifed laminoplasty fixed with longitudinal bone strut.

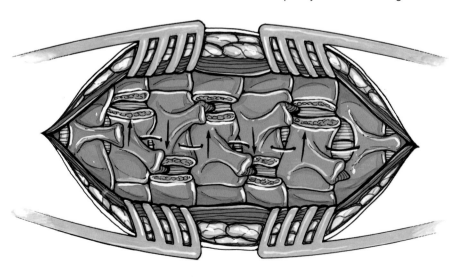

FIG. 12. Z-shaped laminoplasty.

REFERENCES

Posterior Decompression

1. Bishara SN. The posterior operation in treatment of cervical spondylosis with myelopathy: a long-term follow-up study. *J Neurol Neurosurg Psychiatry* 34:393–398, 1971.
2. Cusick JF, Ackmann JJ, Larson J. Mechanical and physiological effects of dentatotomy. *J Neurosurg* 46:767–775, 1977.
3. Epstein JA, Carras R, Lavine LS, Epstein BS. The importance of removing osteophytes as part of the surgical treatment of myeloradiculopathy in cervical spondylosis. *J Neurosurg* 30:219, 1969.
4. Epstein JA, Janin Y, Carras R, et al. A comparative study of the treatment of cervical spondylotic myeloradiculopathy. Experience with 50 cases treated by means of extensive laminectomy, foraminotomy and excision of osteophytes during the past ten years. *Acta Neurochir (Wien)* 61:89–104, 1982.
5. Epstein JA, Janin T. Management of cervical spondylotic myelopathy by the posterior approach. In: *The cervical spine.* 1st ed. Philadelphia: JB Lippincott, 402–410, 1983.
6. Fager CA. Posterior surgical tactics for the neurological syndromes of cervical disc and spondylotic lesions. *Clin Neurosurg* 25:218–244, 1978.
7. Fox JL, Byrd EB, McCullough DC. Results of cervical laminectomy with dural graft for severe spondylosis with narrow canal. *Acta Latinoamer* 18:90–95, 1972.
8. Kahn EA. The role of the dentate ligaments in spinal cord compression in the syndrome of lateral sclerosis. *J Neurosurg* 4:191–199, 1947.
9. Northfield DWC. Diagnosis and treatment of myelopathy due to cervical spondylosis. *Br Med J* 2:1474–1477, 1955.
10. Piepgras DG. Posterior decompression for myelopathy due to cervical spondylosis. Laminectomy alone versus laminectomy with dentate ligament section. *Clin Neurosurg* 24:509–515, 1977.
11. Raynor RB, Pugh J, Shapiro I. Cervical facetectomy and its effect on spine strength. *J Neurosurg* 63:278–282, 1985.
12. Rogers L. The treatment of spondylotic myelopathy by mobilisation of the cervical cord into an enlarged spinal canal. *J Neurosurg* 18:490–492, 1961.
13. Schneider RC. Treatment of cervical spine disease. In: Schneider RC, Kahn EA, Crosby EC, Taren JA, eds. *Correlative neurosurgery.* 3rd ed. Springfield, IL: Charles C Thomas, 1094–1174, 1982.
14. Scoville WB. Cervical spondylosis treated by bilateral facetectomy and laminectomy. *J Neurosurg* 18:423–428, 1961.

Laminoplasty Techniques

15. Arima T. Postlaminectomy malalignments of the cervical spine. *Noh-Shinkei Gaisho* 1:71–78, 1969.
16. Fujiwara K, Yonenobu K, Hiroshima K, et al. An analysis of the factors prognosticating therapeutic results of cervical myelopathy. Presented at the annual meeting of Cervical Spine Research Society, Palm Beach, Florida, December 1986.
17. Hattori S, Miyamoto T, Kawai S, Saiki K, Imagawa T. A comparative study of spinal canal enlargement and laminectomy in the cervical spine. Presented at the annual meeting of Cervical Spine Research Society, Palm Beach, Florida, December 1980.
18. Hirabayashi K, Sasaki T, Takeda T. The posterior and anterior operation in treatment of cervical disc lesions including cervical spondylosis. A long-term follow-up study. *Chubu Scisai-shi* 15:786–788, 1972.
19. Hirabayashi K. Expansive open-door laminoplasty for cervical spondylotic myelopathy. *Shujutsu* 32:1159–1163, 1978.
20. Hirabayashi K, Miyakawa J, Uzawa M. Canal-expansive laminoplasty as a new method of cervical posterior decompression. *Chubu Seisai-shi* 22:417–419, 1979.
21. Hirabayashi K, Satomi K, Wakono K. Operative treatment for cervical spine disc lesions. Presented at the 8th annual meeting of Cervical Spine Research Society, Palm Beach, Florida, December 1980.
22. Hirabayashi K, Miyakawa J, Satomi K, et al. Operative results and postoperative progression of ossification among patients with cervical posterior longitudinal ligament. *Spine* 6:354–364, 1981.
23. Hirabayashi K, et al. Expansive open-door laminoplasty for cervical spinal stenotic myelopathy. *Spine* 8:693–699, 1983.
24. Hirabayashi K. Pre-operative cases of the anterior spinal decompressive surgery for cervical spondylotic myelopathy. In: *The Cervical spine.* 253–296, 1987.
25. Hirabayashi K, Satomi K. Operative procedure and results of expansive open-door laminoplasty. *Spine* 13:870–876, 1988.
26. Itoh T, Tsuji H. Technical improvements and results of laminoplasty for compressive myelopathy in the cervical spine. *Spine* 10:729–736, 1985.
27. Kawai N, Hattori S, Shigetomi Y. Enlargement of the cervical canal indication and the technique. *Seikei Saigai Geka* 23:39–44, 1980.
28. Kimura I, Oh-Hamam M, Shingu H. Cervical myelopathy treated by canal-expansive laminoplasty. *J Bone Joint Surg [Am]* 66A:914–920, 1984.
29. Kurokawa T, et al. Enlargement of spinal canal by the sagittal splitting of spinal processes. *Bessatsu Seikeigeka* 2:234–240, 1982.
30. Kykwai S, Sunago K, Doi K, Saika M, Taguchi T. Cervical laminoplasty (Hattori's method) procedure and follow-up results. *Spine* 13:1245–1250, 1988.
31. Matsuzaki H, Toriyama S, Sugawara T, et al. Cervical canal-expansive laminoplasty with unilateral fusion. *Bessatsu Seikeigeka* 2:249–252, 1982.
32. Miyazaki K, Kirita Y. Extensive simultaneous multisegment laminectomy for myelopathy due to ossification of the posterior longitudinal ligament in the cervical region. *Spine* 11:531–542, 1986.
33. Nakano N, Tomita T. Enlargement of cervical spinal canal for cervical myelopathy. *Seikeigeka* 31:453–461, 1980.
34. Nakano T, Nakano K. Comparison of the results of laminectomy and open-door laminoplasty for cervical spondylotic myeloradiculopathy and ossification of the posterior longitudinal ligament. *Spine* 13:792–794, 1988.
35. Nakano N, Nakano T, Nakano K. Laminectomy versus open-door laminoplasty for cervical spondylotic radiculomyelopathy and OPLL. In: *Cervical spine II.* 179–182, 1989.
36. Oyama M, Hattori S, Moriwaki N. A new method of cervical laminectomy. *Chubu Seisai-shi* 16:792–794, 1973.
37. Tsuji H. Laminoplasty for patients with compressive myelopathy due to so-called spinal stenosis in cervical and thoracic regions. *Spine* 7:28–34, 1982.
38. Tsuyama N. Ossifications of the posterior longitudinal ligament of the spine. *Clin Orthop* 184:71–84, 1984.
39. Watanabe K, Hirabayashi K. Expansive laminoplasty for cervical stenotic myelopathy. *Seikeigeka* 32:357–362, 1981.
40. Watanabe T, et al. Expansive laminoplasty (Chiba) for cervical spondylotic myelopathy. *Shujutsu* 41:519–527, 1987.

CHAPTER 13

Microsurgical Approaches to Cervical Spinal Cord Tumors

Paul C. McCormick and Bennett M. Stein

Tumors of the cervical spine can originate in and/or involve the spinal cord, nerve roots, meninges, epidural venous plexus, bony elements, and supporting soft tissue. Anatomically (and radiographically), tumors of the spinal canal can be divided into extradural, intradural extramedullary, and intramedullary.

Extradural tumors are those located outside of the dura mater yet inside of the spinal canal. Primary extradural tumors may arise from the dura, nerve roots (external to the dura), connective tissue, fat, blood vessels, lymphatic tissues, and other tissues found in the epidural space. Benign extradural tumors include meningiomas, neurinomas, fibromas, lipomas, dermoids, epidermoids, hematomas, and other vascular lesions. In addition, tumors arising from the bony elements may invade the spinal cord. Unfortunately, the vast majority of extradural tumors (particularly in adults) are both malignant and metastatic. A discussion of these lesions can be found in Chapter 14.

The *intradural extramedullary tumors* represent a group of generally benign tumors including meningiomas and neurinomas (which account for 60–70%), neurofibromas, dermoids, epidermoids, and lipomas. Metastatic lesions in this region are unusual.

Intramedullary tumors intimately involve the substance of the spinal cord. Though quite unusual, they are among the most difficult and hazardous tumors to treat surgically, not only of tumors in the cervical spine but of tumors throughout the entire nervous system. The small size, anatomical complexity, and exquisite sensitivity to manipulation characteristic of the cervical spinal cord make the use of operating microscope in approaches to these lesions absolutely essential.

GENERAL CONSIDERATIONS

Incidence

Intramedullary spinal cord tumors (IMSCTS) account for ~20–25% of spinal tumors and 2–4% of all central nervous system neoplasms (11,21,22,49). If primary and metastatic epidural tumors are excluded, IMSCTS represent approximately one-third of all spinal intradural neoplasms in adults and nearly 40–50% in the pediatric population (27,43,52).

Initial reports suggested a proportionate occurrence of IMSCTS throughout the spinal cord. The cervical cord, measuring ~10 cm in length and comprising ~22.5% of spinal cord tissue (40), was reported to harbor 15–27% of IMSCTS (9,49,52,54,57). However, a review of several recent surgical series totaling 282 patients with IMSCTS demonstrates a strikingly disproportionate occurrence within the cervical cord (Table 1) (1,6,8,10,12,14,20,21,28,34,50). Sixty-eight percent of all IMSCTS either arise from or extend into the cervical segments of the spinal cord.

There are several reasons for this apparent disparity between earlier and more recent studies. The inclusion of extramedullary and extradural tumors (including herniated intervertebral discs) and the addition of filum terminale neoplasms and chordomas as intramedullary tumors in earlier studies are at least partly responsible for this disparity. In addition, most early studies relied on histological confirmation obtained at surgery for inclusion (49,54,57). Because many of these patients were not operated upon, they were thereby excluded from review (19,24,49,57,58). Thus, it seems that re-

TABLE 1. *Incidence of cervical cord involvement with intramedullary tumors*

Author, year	Tumor type	Total cases	Cervical cord involvement (%)
Greenwood, 1963	Ependymoma	9	8 (88)
	Teratoma	1	1 (100)
DeSousa, 1979	Ependymoma, astro., misc.	21	9 (43)
Fisher, 1980	Ependymoma	16	9 (56)
Guidetti, 1981	Ependymoma	34	23 (68)
	Astrocytoma	53	32 (60)
	Hemangioblastoma	12	5 (42)
Epstein, 1982	Astrocytoma	19	17 (89)
Alvisi, 1984	Ependymoma	7	5 (71)
	Astrocytoma	16	10 (63)
Cooper, 1985	Ependymoma (14) Astro. (11), misc. (4)	29	26 (90)
Herrmann, 1988	Ependymoma	5	5 (100)
	Astrocytoma	3	3 (100)
	Hemangioblastoma	3	2 (67)
	Misc.	4	3 (75)
Solomon and Stein, 1988	Hemangioblastoma	8	4 (50)
Cohen, 1989	Malignant astro.	19	12 (63)
McCormick and Stein, 1989	Ependymoma	23	17 (74)
Totals		282	191 (68)

Astro., Astrocytoma; misc., miscellaneous tumors (oligodendroglioma, lipoma, dermoid, epidermoid, neruinoma, etc.).

cent studies perhaps more accurately illustrate the yet unexplained tendency for IMSCTS to involve the cervical spine.

Types of Tumors

Primary glial tumors (specifically *astrocytoma* and *epenymoma*) and *hemangioblastoma* represent >90% of cervical intramedullary spinal cord tumors (CIMSCTS) (Table 2) (21,22,49). A variety of other neoplasms account for the remaining 10%. Although these less common tumors will not be considered in any detail, it is important for the surgeon to recognize that many of these neoplasms are histologically benign and potentially amenable to microsurgical removal.

In addition, nonneoplastic pathology, such as vascular and inflammatory processes, may involve the spinal cord and mimic a CIMSCT. Surgery in some of these patients may also prove rewarding (Fig. 1) (36). The authors have recently treated nine patients with myelopathy and magnetic resonance imaging (MRI) evidence of intramedullary pathology in whom surgical exploration revealed only an ill-defined spinal cord

TABLE 2. *Approximate incidence of intramedullary spinal cord tumors*

Tumor type	Approximate incidence	Comments
Astrocytoma	40–45%	Higher in children, 10% malignant
Ependymoma	35–40%	Higher in adults, rarely malignant
Hemangioblastoma	3–11%	May be multiple, 10–23% VHL
Miscellaneous tumors	5–10%	
Glial (oligodendroglioma, ganglioglioma)	1–2%	
Inclusion tumors (cysts): teratoma, dermoid, epidermoid, lipoma, neurenteric	1–5%	1% adults, 1–10% pediatric
Neurinoma	1–2%	May be pigmented
Metastasis	1%	2% of autopsies in cancer patients
Melanoma	<1%	Primary or metastatic
Direct extension from brainstem	<1%	Pediatric; usually ependymoma, astrocytoma, medulloblastastoma
Nontumorous pathology Infectious/inflammatory	1–2%	
Abcess (bacterial/fungal)	<1%	
Sarcoidosis	<1%	
Vascular cavernous malformation	1%	Erroneous diagnosis common

VHL, von Hippel Lindau.

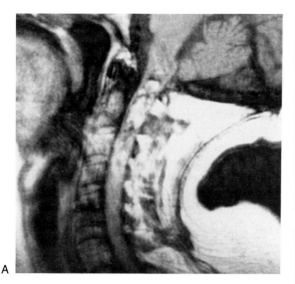

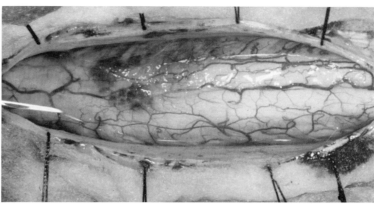

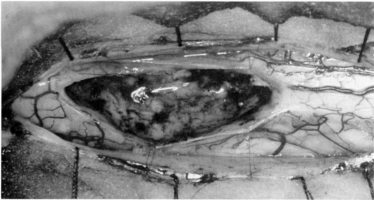

FIG. 1. A: T1-weighted sagittal MRI. Intramedullary mass in the upper cervical cord. The appearance is characteristic of a cavernous malformation (CM). B: Operative photograph. The CM seen through the dorsal cord surface. C: Operative photograph, following complete resection of the CM.

swelling or discoloration (Fig. 2). Multiple sclerosis was suspected in many of these cases but could not be confirmed. Biopsy usually revealed only nonspecific inflammation, gliosis, or mild demyelinization.

Clearly not all imaged pathology is surgical, and the microsurgical exploration of ill-defined lesions for diagnosis should certainly be undertaken with caution. These cases underscore the importance of the correlation of clinical, radiological, and laboratory data in determining appropriate management strategies.

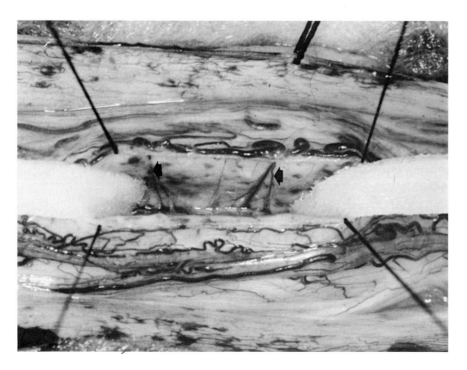

FIG. 2. Operative photograph. Patient with subacute myelopathy and focal signal increase on MRI. Only ill-defined cord swelling and discoloration is evident. No mass is apparent and multiple biopsies revealed only non-specific inflammatory changes. Note the somewhat enlarged longitudinal array of penetrating pial veins which allow maintenance of a midline orientation (*arrows*).

PATHOLOGY OF CIMSCT

Astrocytomas, irrespective of age, are slightly more common than *ependymomas* (21,22,49,54). In children, ependymomas are quite rare, probably three or four times less common than astrocytomas (27,43, 49,52). Cervical astrocytomas, however, particularly those at the cervicomedullary junction, are common in young children (10,12). The predominance of astrocytomas becomes less marked in adolescence and early adult years; by approximately the age of 30, ependymomas become slightly more common than astrocytomas and progress to predominate even more with advancing age (25,49). Despite these trends, it is usually not possible to differentiate astrocytoma from ependymoma preoperatively.

The majority of spinal astrocytomas and ependymomas are histologically benign. All 23 spinal ependymomas in the authors' series were benign (34). Mork (37,38), in a review of 54 spinal ependymomas, noted only one case of anaplastic ependymoma. Malignant astrocytoma and glioblastoma (Kernohan Grade III and IV), however, account for ~10% of intramedullary astrocytomas. These aggressive tumors are characterized by a rapidly progressive clinical course, high incidence of cerebrospinal fluid (CSF) tumor dissemination, and poor survival (mean, 6 months) regardless of treatment (6,21,24,49). Long-term survival is rarely reported with spinal glioblastoma (1).

A number of early authors included the classification of spongioblastoma under the heading of "glial tumors" (1,19,21,24). This term is now rarely used in the typing of astrocytomas. We suspect that these neoplasms represent either the tanacytic variant of ependymoma or a type of juvenile pilocytic astrocytoma, which, like their intracranial counterparts in the hypothalamus and optic pathways, may be more hamartomatous than neoplastic in behavior (15,29,30).

Unlike astrocytomas and ependymomas, *hemangioblastomas* are evenly distributed throughout the spinal cord, although some authors have reported a cervical predominance (23,32). They may arise at any age but are rare in childhood (43). Spinal hemangioblastomas are usually sporadic in occurrence but up to 25% of patients will have evidence of *von Hippel–Lindau (VHL) syndrome* (39). This syndrome is autosomal dominant in inheritance, with variable and incomplete penetrance (4,39). Patients with VHL syndrome tend to become symptomatic at an earlier age than with sporadic forms. Multiplicity also suggests the association with VHL syndrome (39).

CLINICAL FEATURES

The importance of early diagnosis in patients with CIMSCTS cannot be overstated. It is clear that *functional results following microsurgical resection are directly related to the patient's preoperative neurological status.* Not only is operative morbidity reduced, but the capability for functional recovery is greater in patients presenting with minor neurological deficits. Significant or longstanding preoperative deficits are much less likely to be improved by successful surgery.

Unfortunately, the early diagnosis of a CIMSCT remains problematical and elusive. Although the development and availability of contemporary imaging techniques (MRI) have shortened the time from symptom onset to diagnosis, the duration of symptoms for benign CIMSCTS remains characteristically long, with an average of 2–3 years (22,34). The extremely slow growth rate of these tumors and the ability of the spinal cord to tolerate its associated compression are partly responsible.

The "classic" *central cord syndrome* associated with CIMSCTS is infrequent in these patients. The clinical features of CIMSCTS are primarily dependent on both the sagittal and axial relationships of the tumor to the spinal cord as well as the direction and rate of tumor growth. Differential mechanical and perhaps vascular susceptibility of fiber tracts and cell groups may also contribute to symptomatology. In addition, indirect phenomena such as peritumoral edema, cyst formation, and poorly understood vascular derangements can produce clinical effects at a considerable distance from the tumor. All these factors serve to confound the early diagnosis of a CIMSCT and frequently result in a delayed or erroneous initial diagnosis. In the authors' series of 17 patients with cervical intramedullary ependymoma, three patients had undergone previous surgery, including median nerve tenolysis, cervical laminectomy, and cyst aspiration, for an erroneous diagnosis of carpal tunnel syndrome, cervical spondylosis, and syringomyelia, respectively.

Clinically, patients with spinal hemangioblastoma present with a slowly progressive spinal cord syndrome. Rarely is there an ictus due to subarachnoid hemorrhage (39). It would appear that symptoms produced by hemangioblastoma tend to be more lateralized and of shorter duration than with benign glial tumors.

The symptoms of CIMSCTS include pain, sensory abnormalities, motor loss, and autonomic dysfunction.

Pain is the most common presenting symptom of CIMSCTS in the adult population (22,34,49,54,57). It is the initial complaint in 60–70% and occurs eventually in 80–90% of patients. Pain appears to be somewhat less common in the pediatric population, accounting for the initial symptom in ~50% of children (10,12,19,43).

When pain is the initial symptom, it is frequently present for months to years before the onset of objective neurological complaints. In our series, the duration of pain averaged 16 months, with one patient having an 8-year history of severe neck pain prior to the development of objective neurological dysfunction. Pain associated with CIMSCTS is usually a poorly described ache of variable intensity localized to the neck and often roughly corresponding to the level of the tumor; it is rarely radicular. The pain is often constant and may or may not progress in severity. It is generally unaffected by activity, head position, pressure, or Valsalva maneuvers. Extension to the medial scapulae is common, and, although radiation into the arm may occur, it is ill-defined and cannot be considered radicular. Occasionally, a dysesthetic or electric-like quality to the pain may exist.

Sensory or motor complaints are the initial symptom in 30–40% of patients (22,34,49,54). Sensory disturbances were generally more common than motor, either as an initial symptom or following pain in the authors' series (34), but motor complaints may predominate (22), or both may be seen with equal frequency (54). Regardless of whether the initial objective neurological complaint is sensory or motor, it usually begins, and is most marked by the time of diagnosis, in the *upper extremities*. An exception to this is the sensory disturbance produced by tumors arising at the cervicothoracic junction, which may occasionally present with unusual dysesthetic complaints in the lower extremities.

Sensory abnormalities often begin distally in the arm or hand, tend to progress proximally, and may ultimately spread into the opposite arm. They are often described as paresthesiae or dysesthesiae, and are usually constant in nature. Complaints of numbness are unusual. A *dissociated suspended sensory loss* has not been a constant feature in the authors' experience, and when present it is usually subtle and somewhat irregular in distribution. A well-defined sensory level is usually apparent only late in the clinical course of CIMSCTS.

Motor disturbances are initially likely to involve one arm. Unlike sensory abnormalities, patients are more apt to complain of *proximal limb weakness.* Curiously, mild or moderate atrophy of the intrinsic muscles of one or both hands was identified in eight of 17 patients in our series, but this was generally not noted to be of functional consequence by the patients. Complaints related to upper limb spasticity are unusual.

Lower extremity and sphincter dysfunction generally occur at variable periods following the onset of upper extremity symptoms. The disturbance is often subtle initially, with the patient describing increasing stiffness, fatigue, diminished exercise tolerance, or minor difficulties walking on inclined surfaces. Sphincter dysfunction appears relatively late and is heralded by the onset of urinary frequency and urgency.

Autonomic dysfunction, such as Horner's syndrome, and pilomotor or sudomotor abnormalities, is a relatively late finding and is unlikely to be present by the time of diagnosis in the author's experience.

By the time of diagnosis, patients with a CIMSCT will invariably demonstrate objective neurological deficits. The pattern and severity of the deficits can be quite variable. Deficits are usually bilateral but often predominate on one side. Two patients with cervical intramedullary ependymoma in the authors' series had an incomplete Brown-Sequard syndrome when examined. Reflex changes, often with a mixed pattern of hypoactive and hyperactive responses in the upper limbs and hyperactive lower limb reflexes, may be the only objective abnormality on exam. They are the most sensitive indicator of spinal cord dsyfunction, as sensory deficits are often difficult to interpret and unreliable unless a dissociated suspended pattern is present. Weakness, usually bilateral, is often more apparent in one arm.

RADIOLOGICAL EVALUATION

MRI is the procedure of choice for diagnosis of a CIMSCT. Sagittal T1-weighted images usually identify and accurately localize an intramedullary neoplasm and demonstrate the presence of associated peritumoral edema or cysts (Fig. 3). Occasionally, there may be only an ill-defined spinal cord swelling, and the administration of a paramagnetic contrast agent is necessary to identify the location of the tumor (Fig. 3B). With the exception of vascular lesions, it is generally not possible to determine tumor type on the basis of MRI appearance (Figs. 1 and 6B).

In cases where clinical and MRI data do not establish the presence of a CIMSCT, we have found it useful to perform *myelography* followed by *computerized tomography* (*myelo/CT*). If these studies do not demonstrate clear evidence of focal spinal cord enlargement, it is advisable to defer operative management and follow the patient conservatively.

If the lesion appears vascular on MRI or myelo/CT, *selective spinal angiography* is performed.

SURGICAL CONSIDERATIONS

A number of aspects concerning the surgical management of cervical intramedullary spinal cord tumors must be stressed. The surgeon should assume that the majority of all intramedullary tumors are benign and potentially resectable. In the face of a conflicting frozen tissue diagnosis, intraoperative decisions should be made according to the gross rather than histological tumor characteristics, since, like ependymomas, some low-grade astrocytomas are also well circumscribed and amenable to complete resection.

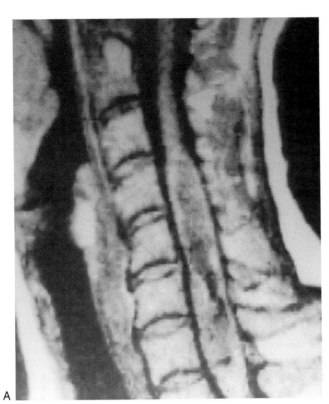

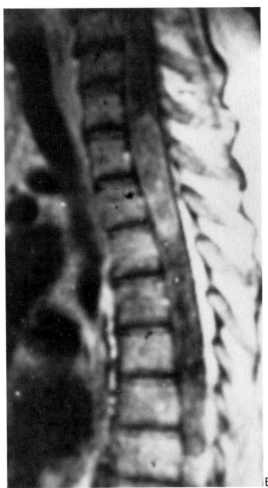

FIG. 3. A: T1-weighted sagittal MRI. Cervical intramedullary ependymoma. This solid tumor has irregular margins and is located at the C6–T1 vertebrae with an associated rostral cyst. **B:** T1-weighted gadolinium (Gd-DPTA) enhanced sagittal MRI. The focal nature and location of the tumor is clearly defined. A rostral cyst is obvious.

If histological examination clearly demonstrates a benign ependymoma, then microsurgical removal should occur. This is particularly important for large tumors that initially may seem infiltrative or that severely compress the surrounding spinal cord into an almost unrecognizable configuration. It is remarkable how a thin ribbon-like appearing spinal cord may not only function reasonably well but also have the capacity for a certain amount of recovery following tumor removal. Thus, even extremely large or extensive ependymomas should not detour the surgeon from a complete removal.

Finally, reoperation for recurrent tumor is extremely difficult, particularly if the patient has received previous radiation therapy. Dissection planes are obscured by gliosis, spinal cord plasticity is more tenuous, and complications of wound healing are frequent. Considering that patients with recurrent tumors usually present at a lower clinical grade (Table 3) and that recovery is poorer in patients with more severe preoperative deficits (Table 4), it seems logical that complete removal should be performed at the initial operation whenever possible.

MICROSURGICAL TECHNIQUES

Positioning

Following routine anesthetic induction and oropharyngeal intubation, the patient is placed prone and positioned to maintain a perpendicular orientation between the entire extent of the tumor and the surgeon. The prone position is preferred because it comfortably allows the assistance of a second surgeon which facilitates tumor removal. Movement of the spinal cord secondary to respiratory excursions with the patient in the prone position does not present a significant technical problem since the enlarged spinal cord is minimally affected by CSF pulsations and the use of

TABLE 3. *Clinical/functional classification scheme*

Grade	Definition
I	Neurologically normal; mild focal deficit not significantly affecting function of involved limb; mild spasticity or reflex abnormality; normal gait
II	Presence of sensorimotor deficit affecting function of involved limb; mild to moderate gait difficulty; severe pain or dysesthetic syndrome impairing patient's quality of life; still functions and ambulates independently
III	More severe neurological deficit; requires cane/brace for ambulation or significant bilateral upper extremity impairment; may or may not function independently
IV	Severe deficit; requires wheelchair or cane/brace with bilateral upper extremity impairment; usually not independent

pial sutures further restricts spinal cord movement. Peri-operative steroids and antistaphylcoccal antibiotics are administered. Somatosensory evoked potential monitoring during tumor removal has been of limited practical value and is employed primarily for investigative purposes.

Exposure

A standard midline incision and subperiosteal reflection of the paraspinal muscles is performed as described in Chapter 2. The laminectomy should include the medial facet joint only in the thoracic spine (if the exposure also involves this area) to minimize the risk of delayed cervical instability (particularly in extensive exposures in children).

Finding the Tumor

A midline dural incision is made leaving the arachnoid intact to prevent inadvertent injury to the underlying vessels. The spinal cord is inspected and the dorsal midline is grossly estimated by noting the dorsal root entry zones bilaterally. Occasionally the tumor may appear to have totally replaced the dorsal surface of the spinal cord (Fig. 4A). This should be differentiated from compression or thinning of the posterior columns which frequently occurs with benign tumors (Fig. 4B). When replacement of cord tissue by tumor is encountered, this represents an ominous sign and is usually indicative of a malignant astrocytoma (6). Astrocytomas are more likely to be exophytic than ependymomas (Fig. 4C).

TABLE 4. *Clinical summary of 17 patients with cervical intramedullary ependymoma*

Case number	Age (years), sex[a]	Initial symptom	Duration of symptoms[b] (months)	Cord enlargement (tumor level)		Clinical/functional grade		
						Initial preoperative (most recent preoperative[c])	Recent follow-up (length[d]) (months)	Net grade change
1	50, M	Paresthesiae, hand	23	C1–T1	(C2–C7)	I (III)	III (159)	0
2	19, M	Pain, back	16	C2–T1	(C3–T1)	I (III)	IV (159)	−1
3	35, F	Pain, neck	86	C2–C7	(C3–C7)	I (III)	II (156)	+1
4	46, M	Pain, neck, arm	38	C2–C7	(C4–C7)	I	I (146)	0
5	41, F	Pain, neck	13	C2–T2	(C3–T1)	I	I (121)	0
6	36, M	Pain, neck	96	C1–T3	(C3–C7)	I (IV)	IV (89)	0
7	43, F	Pain, neck	24	C2–T3	(C5–C7)	III	I (66)	+2
8	32, F	Pain, back	35	C4–T1	(C7)	II	I (59)	+1
9	32, M	Gait difficulty	7	C4–T9	(C5–T2)	III	II (43)	+1
10	49, F	Pain, neck, back	17	C3–T1	(C5–C7)	II	I (42)	+1
11	64, F	Numbness, hands	30	C2–C5	(C4–C5)	I	II (39)	−1
12	70, F	Numbness, hands	37	C3–C7	(C5–C7)	II	II (36)	0
13	52, F	Pain, neck	46	C4–T1	(C4–C7)	I	I (33)	0
14	42, M	Paresthesiae, arms	30	C3–T1	(C5–C6)	I (II)	I (23)	+1
15	48, M	Weakness, arm	14	C3–C7	(C4–C7)	I (III)	II (21)	+2
16	61, F	Pain, arm	26	C4–T1	(C5–C7)	III	II (14)	+1
17	35, F	Pain, back	10	C3–T1	(C4–C7)	I	I (6)	0

[a] Age at time of initial diagnosis.
[b] Duration of symptoms prior to initial diagnosis.
[c] Cases 1, 2, 3, 6, 8, 10, 18, and 19 had previous operation ± radiation therapy. Clinical grade in parentheses indicates clinical status prior to most recent treatment.
[d] Length of follow-up following completion of most recent treatment.
C, cervical; T, thoracic; L, lumbar.

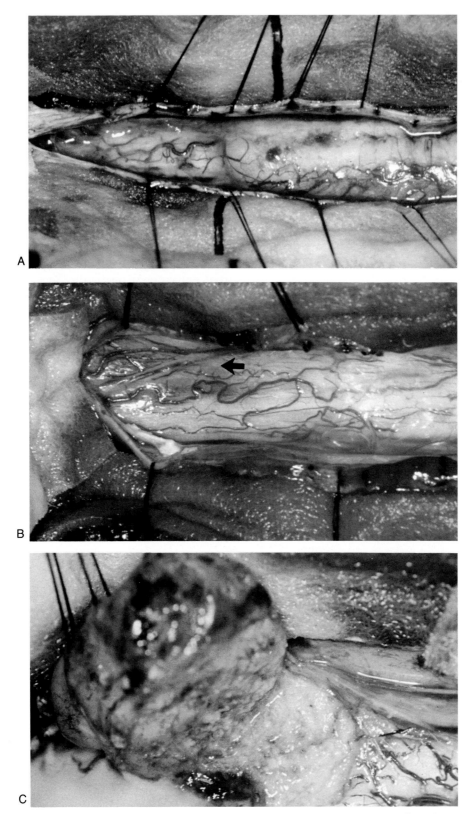

FIG. 4. A: Operative photograph. Replacement of the dorsolateral cord surface by tumor in a patient with malignant astrocytoma. **B:** Operative photograph. A thinned almost transparent dorsal cord surface (*arrow*) from a rostral cyst in a patient with a benign intramedullary ependymoma. **C:** Operative photograph. Dorsal cord replacement and exophytic component of a glioblastoma.

Using the operating microscope, the arachnoid is then opened with a small knife. A relatively constant fold, the septum posterius, that attaches to the pia in the posterior median septum, helps define the dorsal cord midline. The midline pia is bipolar cauterized and cut beginning in the region of maximum cord swelling and carried rostrally and caudally as far as necessary to expose the polar regions of the tumor (Fig. 5). Small crossing pial vessels are coagulated and cut but larger longitudinally oriented vessels are dissected, if possible, and displaced laterally.

Tumor Removal

The myelotomy is deepened by gentle spreading of the posterior columns using microforceps or microdissectors. Identification of a vertical array of penetrating pial vessels on the medial surface of each posterior column assures that the midline orientation has been maintained (Fig. 2). The tumor will usually be encountered at a depth of ~2 mm. Gentle but constant superior and lateral traction on each dorsal hemicord is achieved with fine pial sutures.

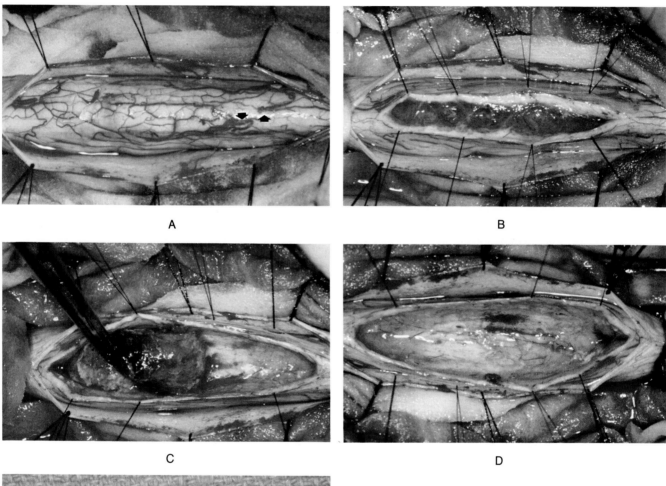

A

B

C

D

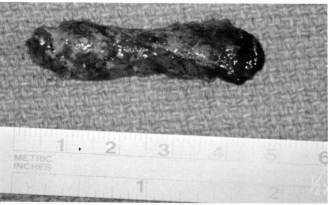

E

FIG. 5. Operative photographs demonstrating sequence of tumor removal. **A:** Initial exposure shows enlarged spinal cord. Note the enlarged veins (*arrows*) that frequently identify the caudal margin of the tumor. **B:** Exposure of dorsal tumor surface following midline myelotomy. **C:** Dissection of the ventral tumor plane is facilitated by gentle superior traction on the tumor. **D:** Cavity remaining following tumor removal. The pia is not closed. **E:** Photograph of tumor specimen. The circumscribed nature of spinal ependymomas.

It is at this point that determinations of the gross and histological characteristics of the tumor are made. If no clear demarcation exists between tumor and spinal cord and frozen section identifies the tumor as an astrocytoma, aggressive removal should not be attempted. A generous but limited internal decompression is performed in these cases primarily to ensure adequate tissue for histological examination. A more radical (99%) tumor removal (until the tumor-cord interface is established) does not appear to alter the clinical course in patients with astrocytoma in the authors' experience. If, however, there appears to be a plane between tumor and spinal cord, regardless of tumor histology, operative removal should continue until the plane definitely disappears.

The myelotomy is lengthened and deepened to fully expose the entire rostro-caudal extent of the tumor and should actually continue a few millimeters above and below the tumor margins to permit greater lateral retraction and visibility while minimizing tension on the spinal cord.

Ependymomas appear as a soft red or grayish mass with a variable number of vessels crossing the tumor surface. Although these tumors are somewhat friable, ependymomas are sharply circumscribed and gentle blunt manipulation will not violate the tumor surface. The rostral tumor is frequently rounded and often projects into the cyst, which aids dissection. The caudal pole is usually more tapered since inferior cysts are less common. Often there is a tough fibrous connection between the caudal tumor and the central canal.

Astrocytomas are more grayish red and may give the appearance of circumscription, particularly on the dorsal cord-tumor interface. This demarcation is rarely as well defined as that seen with ependymomas and usually the infiltrative nature of these tumors becomes evident with further dissection.

The dorsal and lateral tumor margins are established by gentle traction on the tumor against the counter-traction provided by the pial sutures. Spreading with microforceps parallel to the long axis of the tumor easily develops the dissection plane owing to the differences in texture and consistency between the tumor surface and the surrounding gliotic margin of the spinal cord. Feeding vessels and the more fibrous attachments are cauterized and divided close to the tumor. The decision to internal debulk the tumor is usually made once the dorsal half of the tumor is exposed. It is generally preferable to maintain the tumor intact during the entire dissection but in some cases the bulk of the tumor hinders precise visualization of the dissection plane, thereby requiring a prohibitive amount of spinal cord retraction. In these cases the dorsal tumor surface is incised and internal decompression of the tumor is performed with the ultrasonic aspirator. Too much internal tumor removal, however, may cause fragmentation of the tumor surface and obscuration of the correct dissection plane resulting in an undesirable piecemeal removal.

Dissection of the ventral plane is the most difficult aspect of tumor removal for several reasons. Less advantage can be taken of the difference in texture between tumor and spinal cord because the pial sutures do not transmit effective counter-traction to the ventral cord-tumor interface. Thus, the tumor margin appears less distinct and requires sharp dissection techniques. In addition the anterior median fissure extends almost to the central canal and the tumor is frequently in close approximation to the anterior spinal artery and branches. The major vascular supply to the tumor is derived from penetrating branches of the anterior spinal artery. Nonetheless, with superior traction on the tumor directed perpendicular to the long axis of the spinal cord, the tumor can be carefully separated from the anterior spinal vessels that are easily identified, systematically coagulated and divided.

Closure

Following tumor removal the resecton bed is inspected. Any bleeding is controlled with warm saline irrigation or the application of oxidized cotton. As the pial traction sutures are removed, the cord assumes its normal position. No attempt is made to reapproximate the dorsal hemicords with pial sutures. The dura is closed primarily, if possible, since dural substitute patch grafts increase the risk of postoperative cerebrospinal fluid leak. A dural patch is utilized for decompression if little tumor has been removed. The remainder of the wound is closed in a standard fashion (see Chapter 2).

Hemangioblastoma

The techniques of surgical removal for a hemangioblastoma are similar to those employed for the resection of an intramedullary spinal arteriovenous malformation (AVM) (5). These are formidable appearing lesions both angiographically and intraoperatively and may simulate an AVM with respect to vascularity and AV shunting (Fig. 6A). Most present on the dorsal or dorsolateral pial surface, thus obviating the need for myelotomy (Fig. 6C and D). Purely intramedullary hemangioblastoma or those tumors with a ventral pial surface presentation should be approached through a standard midline myelotomy. They are well encapsulated and separate easily from the surrounding neural tissue. All dissection and manipulation should be performed on the surface of the tumor. Entry into the tumor for decompression is not an option because of significant bleeding which is difficult to control and will

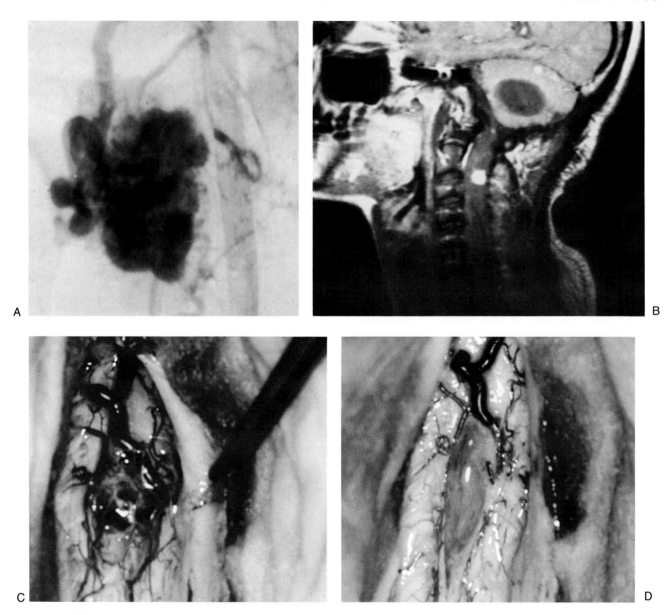

FIG. 6. A: Lateral view of vertebral arteriogram. Vascular nature of an intramedullary hemangioblastoma. The presence of feeding arteries and early draining vein make it difficult to differentiate from an AVM. **B:** T1-weighted gadolinium (Gd-DPTA) enhanced sagittal MRI. Intense enhancement of a focal intramedullary nodule suggestive of hemangioblastoma. The presence of multiple cerebellar nodules and a cystic cerebellar mass virtually assures the diagnosis of hemangioblastoma. **C:** Operative photograph. A hemangioblastoma presenting on the dorsal pial surface. The vascular nature of the tumor is obvious. **D:** Operative photograph. Total removal.

obscure dissection planes. Dissection should proceed systematically around the tumor surface with ligation of feeding arteries and cauterization of the tumor capsule. Draining veins should be preserved, if possible, but if they hinder visualization they can be safely coagulated and divided.

Using this approach even large tumors will become less turgid with the ultimate delivery of an initially non-visualized tumor capsule into the operative field allowing en bloc removal. Preservation of at least one venous pedicle until all feeding arteries are divided is advisable. A curious phenomenon associated with intramedullary spinal hemangioblastoma is surrounding spinal cord swelling, which may extend a considerable distance both above and below the tumor (50). The etiology of the cord swelling remains obscure but we suspect a vasogenic edema factor secreted by the tumor. The edema resolves following removal of the tumor. We have occasionally witnessed a similar phenomenon with ependymomas.

SURGICAL OUTCOME

Early

In the immediate postoperative period, the majority of patients will demonstrate some degree of increased neurological deficit. Careful testing will almost invariably reveal new posterior column deficits (34). Worsening of an existing motor deficit is also common, but most patients return to their preoperative motor status within three months postoperatively. Posterior column dysfunction resulting from surgery also tends to improve but generally does not return to the preoperative level. Fortunately, these persistent sensory deficits are relatively minor and rarely of any functional consequence. Significant and persistent operative neurological morbidity is now a rare occurrence and is usually associated with the aggressive removal of malignant tumors (6). Advances in perioperative management and adherence to microsurgical techniques have all but eliminated operative mortality for CIMSCTS.

Complications related to the wound deserve mention. Dehiscence, infection, and CSF leak are frequent in patients who have undergone previous surgery and radiation therapy. It has been our experience that these problems rarely resolve with conservative management and frequently lead to potentially serious morbidity. Early return to the operating room for debridement and reclosure, often with muscle or musculofascial flaps, is imperative (47,59).

A frequent phenomenon following surgery for CIMSCTS is the appearance of a dysesthetic syndrome. While subjective complaints of numbness, out of proportion to objective sensory deficit, are also common (and usually of little functional significance), dysesthetic complaints may be perceived as particularly annoying and often debilitating to the patient because of their constancy. The severity of the dysesthesiae, and the patient's emotional response, are quite variable ranging from intermittent and clinically insignificant "pins and needles" sensations to persistent distressing, often causalgia-like, complaints of "itching," "crawling," or "burning" dysesthesiae.

This syndrome generally appears early in the postoperative period and frequently seems to follow a posterior column or radicular distribution. Patients with preoperative dysesthesiae seem especially prone to develop this syndrome postoperatively, but no other predictive factors have been identified. The dysesthesiae are generally refractory to various forms of medical therapy but are usually self-limited with resolution or amelioration of complaints several months following surgery. The physiological basis of this syndrome is unclear but the anatomical distribution of the dysesthesiae suggests injury to the posterior columns or dorsal root entry zone.

Objective neurological recovery from preoperative deficits is difficult to assess (Tables 3 and 4) (35). Functional improvement relative to the patient's pre-operative status is commonly due to adaptive strategies gained through physical and occupational therapy rather than true neurological recovery. Thus, the value of early enrollment into long-term and aggressive physical medicine programs cannot be overstated. Clearly, however, return of neurological function does occur. Unlike extramedullary neoplasms, however, recovery is rarely dramatically witnessed in the early postoperative period (except occasionally following the removal of a hemangioblastoma). More commonly recovery is slow and may subtly progress over a period of many months to years. As already stated, recovery is more apt to occur in patients with mild or moderate deficits of short duration.

Long-Term Outcome

The long-term outcome following removal of a CIMSCT seems most dependent on tumor histology. Benign encapsulated neoplasms such as hemangioblastoma or intramedullary neurinoma are amenable to complete removal and will rarely recur. If, however,

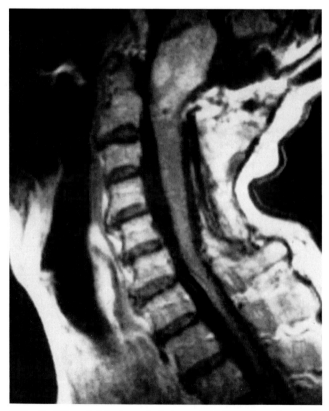

FIG. 7. T1-weighted gadolinium (Gd-DPTA) enhanced sagittal MRI. Huge recurrence of a cervicomedullary pigmented neurinoma three years following apparent total resection.

there is doubt in the surgeon's mind about the completeness of resection or histological benignity of the tumor periodic clinical and MRI evaluation should be performed. One of our patients recently died from recurrence of an intramedullary pigmented neurinoma at the cervicomedullary junction 3 years following what was believed to be a total resection (Fig. 7). Review of the initial pathological specimen demonstrated microscopic foci of malignancy.

The management of ependymomas is a bit less clear. Although these are benign, noninvasive neoplasms, their glial derivation, lack of capsulation, and friable nature pose a continued risk of recurrence regardless of treatment. The overall treatment goal in these patients should be viewed, therefore, as long-term management aimed at optimal preservation of neurological function. The evidence is now overwhelming that this is best achieved through complete removal alone at the initial operation (3,14,18,24,32,34,41,42,51). Total removal utilizing microsurgical techniques can be performed with acceptable morbidity and a low incidence of recurrence. These results are clearly superior to subtotal resection followed by radiation therapy (3,24, 34,37,49). In our series of 23 patients with intramedullary ependymoma treated by surgical removal alone, there has been no definite clinical or radiological evidence of tumor recurrence at follow-up of 6–159 months (mean, 62 months). Seven patients have been followed a minimum of 10 years following surgery (34).

Radiation Therapy

The use of radiation therapy (RT) following subtotal removal of spinal ependymomas is prevalent. Studies that support the efficacy of RT for incompletely resected ependymomas, however, are difficult to interpret because of small patient populations, inclusion of patients without tissue diagnoses, limited follow-ups, inadequate or no matched cohorts treated without RT, survivals as the only evaluation, and the limited or absent discussion of surgery and clinical follow-up (3,16,17,31,33,44–46,48,53,55). The favorable results ascribed to RT may reflect the extremely slow growth rate and natural history of these tumors. Despite these limitations, the accumulated data in these series seem to suggest that RT may be beneficial following subtotal removal of an intramedullary ependymoma. We recommend adjuvant RT for patients with malignant ependymoma or the rare benign tumor that can not be totally resected. Extension of unresectable tumor into the brain stem (28) or an exophytic tumor are examples of benign intramedullary ependymomas that potentially cannot be safely resected. No benefit of RT following grossly complete removal of a spinal ependymoma has ever been demonstrated, and, considering the risk of RT, its use to theoretically sterilize or control residual microscopic tumor foci following complete removal cannot be supported.

All patients must be followed long-term postopera-

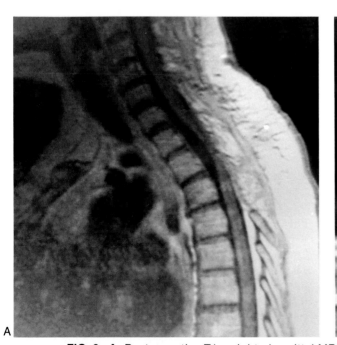
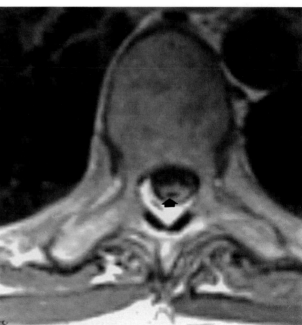

A   B

FIG. 8. A: Postoperative T1-weighted sagittal MRI. Spinal cord atrophy most marked at the level of tumor resection. There is dorsal tethering of the spinal cord and a large ventral subarachnoid space at this level. Persistence of both rostral and caudal cysts can be seen. **B:** T1-weighted axial MRI. Performed three spinal segments below the level of tumor resection. A persistent intramedullary cyst (*arrow*).

tively with periodic clinical and MRI evaluation because of the potential risk of tumor recurrence. Although not much is known about the postoperative MRI characteristics following removal of CIMSCTS, it has been our experience, based on 14 patients, that spinal cord atrophy (extending varying degrees above and below the level of tumor resection), dorsal tethering of the spinal cord to the posterior dura (with a large ventral subarachnoid space), and diminution, but persistence of intramedullary cysts, are the most common MRI findings (Fig. 8). In the case of suspected tumor recurrence, the recommendation for reoperation should be based on both clinical and MRI evidence of tumor recurrence.

It is extremely difficult to evaluate the effects of surgical resection on the long-term outcome of patients with intramedullary astrocytomas. The natural history of these tumors is quite variable and somewhat age related. In pediatric patients many intramedullary astrocytomas exhibit an almost hamartomatous behavior with perhaps up to 50% of patients demonstrating long-term, disease-free, and functional survival, irrespec-

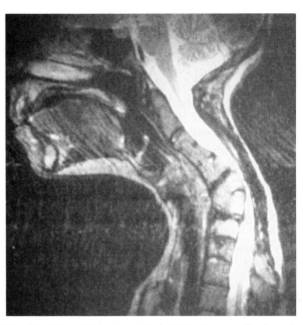

FIG. 10. T2-weighted sagittal MRI. Severe flexion deformity with cord compression in a 30-year-old woman treated with surgery and RT for an intramedullary tumor at the age of 16 years.

tive of the extent of surgical resection or receipt of RT (Fig. 9) (10,27). These are also the tumors that are most likely circumscribed and amenable to grossly complete or nearly complete resection. Thus, it may be that the biological nature of spinal astrocytomas not only determines prognosis but surgical resectability rather than the reverse. Malignant astrocytomas, however, also appear to be more common in younger age groups (6,49).

Recent reports of complete (99%) removal of intramedullary astrocytomas have established only that aggressive surgery may be performed with acceptable neurological morbidity but have not, as yet, been shown to alter the natural history of this neoplasm in the ~50% of pediatric patients whose tumors exhibit a progressive course (12,13). In addition, there is potentially serious morbidity attendant to aggressive surgical removal which include delayed cervical flexion deformity (''swan neck''), progression of scoliosis, and CSF tumor dissemination (Fig. 10) (10,52). Ironically, because of their delayed appearance, these complications are more likely to affect patients with the most benign clinical course who are least likely to have benefited from aggressive removal. Because it is difficult to preoperatively determine the natural history of astrocytomas in pediatric patients we have adopted a more conservative approach to treatment. If the tumor appears well circumscribed, we will continue with removal. If an infiltrating tumor is encountered, only myelotomy and limited internal resection is performed. RT is not given postoperatively, and the

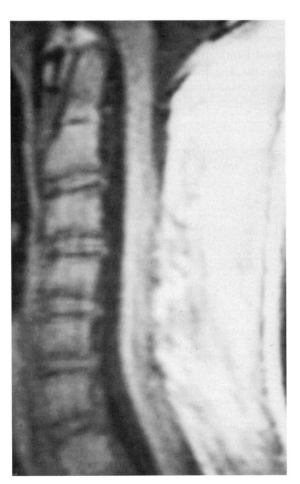

FIG. 9. T1-weighted sagittal MRI. Ten years following radical but subtotal resection of a high cervical astrocytoma without RT in a 9-year-old boy. No evidence of tumor recurrence.

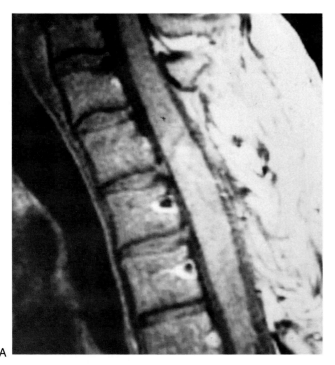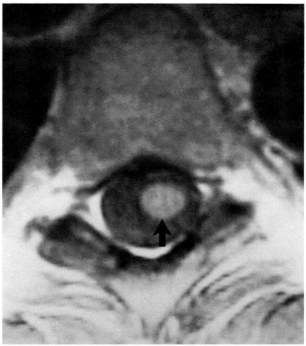

A   B

FIG. 11. A: T1-weighted sagittal MRI. A 36-year-old man 2 years after radical subtotal removal of an intramedullary astrocytoma. The increased signal intensity and cord enlargement are indicative of tumor recurrence. **B:** T1-weighted gadolinium (Gd-DPTA) enhanced axial MRI. Clearly defines the recurrent tumor (*arrow*). The patient, however, has not become clinically symptomatic from this recurrence.

patient is followed. If the patient becomes symptomatic from tumor recurrence, the reoperation with more aggressive removal is performed, followed by RT.

In adults, astrocytomas most frequently pursue a progressive course. Only a very tenuous correlation has been made between aggressiveness of removal and disease-free survival (1,21). Cooper (7,8), however, noted no correlation between extent of removal and survival. Thus, it seems unlikely that radicular tumor removal significantly affects survival in the majority of patients. Our approach to adults with an intramedullary astrocytoma is similar to that for pediatric patients although we are somewhat more aggressive with initial tumor removal because it can be performed safely and may prolong the disease-free interval. Almost all tumors will ultimately recur; MRI will demonstrate the recurrence usually well before symptoms arise (Fig. 11). The authors currently defer reoperation until the patient becomes clinically symptomatic because the interval between MRI and clinical evidence of recurrence may extend up to a few years.

Surgery for malignant astrocytoma is more limited. Biopsy only is performed followed by RT and chemotherapy. Reoperation is only considered if there is an exophytic component in a deteriorating but neurologically functional patient.

REFERENCES

1. Alvisi C, Cerisoli M, Guilioni M. Intramedullary spinal gliomas: long-term results of surgical treatments. *Acta Neurochir* 70:169–179, 1984.
2. Austin G. The nature and significance of pain of the spinal cord. *Surg Forum* 10:782–785, 1959.
3. Barone BM, Elvidge AR. Ependymomas. A clinical survey. *J Neurosurg* 33:428–438, 1970.
4. Christoferson LA, Gustafson MB, Petersen AG. Von Hippel-Lindau's disease. *JAMA* 178:280–282, 1961.
5. Cogen P, Stein BM. Spinal cord arteriovenous malformations with significant intramedullary components. *J Neurosurg* 59:471–476, 1983.
6. Cohen AR, Wisoff JH, Allen JC, et al. Malignant astrocytomas of the spinal cord. *J Neurosurg* 70:50–54, 1989.
7. Cooper PR, Epstein F. Outcome after operative treatment of intramedullary spinal cord tumors in adults [Abstract]. Presented at the 4th Annual Joint Section on Disorders of the Spine and Peripheral Nerves, Phoenix, Arizona, February 16–20, 1988.
8. Cooper PR, Epstein F. Radical resection of intramedullary spinal cord tumors in adults. *J Neurosurg* 63:492–499, 1985.
9. Craig WM, Shelden CH. Tumors of the cervical portion of the spinal cord. *Arch Neurol Psychiatry* 44:1–16, 1940.
10. DeSousa AL, Kalsbeck JE, Mealey J, et al. Instraspinal tumors in children. *J Neurosurg* 51:437–445, 1979.
11. Elsberg CA. *Surgical disease of the spinal cord, membranes and nerve roots.* New York: Paul B. Hueber, 1941.
12. Epstein F, Epstein N. Surgical treatment of spinal cord astrocytomas in childhood. *J Neurosurg* 57:685–689, 1982.
13. Epstein F, Epstein N. Surgical management of holocord intramedullary spinal cord astrocytomas in children. *J Neurosurg* 54:829–832, 1981.
14. Fisher G, Mansuy L. Total removal of intramedullary ependy-

momas: follow-up study of 16 cases. *Surg Neurol* 14:243–249, 1980.

15. Friede RL, Pollack A. The cytogenetic basis for classifying ependymomas. *J Neuropathol Exp Neurol* 37:103–118, 1978.

16. Garcia DM. Primary spinal cord tumors treated with surgery and post-operative irradiation. *Int J Radiat Oncol Biol Phys* 11:1133–1139, 1985.

17. Garrett PG, Simpson WJK. Ependymomas: results of radiation treatment. *Int J Radiat Oncol Biol Phys* 9:1121–1124, 1983.

18. Garrido E, Stein BM. Microsurgical removal of intramedullary spinal cord tumors. *Surg Neurol* 7:215–219, 1977.

19. Grant FC, Austin GM. The diagnosis, treatment and prognosis of tumors affecting the spinal cord in children. *J Neurosurg* 13:535–545, 1956.

20. Greenwood J. Intramedullary tumors of the spinal cord. A follow-up study after total surgical removal. *J Neurosurg* 20:665–668, 1963.

21. Guidetti B, Mercuri S, Vagnozzi R. Long-term results of the surgical treatment of 129 intramedullary spinal gliomas. *J Neurosurg* 54:323–330, 1981.

22. Guidetti B, Fortuna A. Differential diagnosis of intramedullary and extramedullary tumors. In: Vinken PJ, Bruyn GW, eds. *Handbook of clinical neurology.* Vol. 19. Amsterdam: North-Holland, 51–75, 1975.

23. Guidetti B, Fortuna A. Surgical treatment of intramedullary hemangioblastoma of the spinal cord. *J Neurosurg* 27:530–540, 1967.

24. Guidetti B. Intramedullary tumors of the spinal cord. *Acta Neurochir (Wien)* 17:7–23, 1967.

25. Guidetti B, Fortuna A, Moscatelli G, et al. I tumori intramidollari. *Lav Neuropsichiat* 35:1–409, 1964.

26. Guidetti B. Mielopatie da spondilosi cervicale. *Bologna Med* 1958.

27. Hendrick EB. Spinal cord tumors in children. In: Youmans JR, ed. *Neurological surgery. Vol. 5.* 2nd ed. Philadelphia: WB Saunders, 3215–3221, 1982.

28. Herrmann HD, Neuss M, Winkler D. Intramedullary spinal cord tumors resected with CO$_2$ laser microsurgical technique: Recent experience in 15 patients. *Neurosurgery* 22:518–522, 1988.

29. Hoffman HJ, Hendrick EB, Humphreys RP. Management of optic pathway gliomas [Abstract]. Presented at the Annual Meeting AANS, Toronto, Ontario, April 24–28, 1988.

30. Hoffman HJ. Supratentorial brain tumors in children. In: Youmans JR, ed. *Neurological surgery. Vol. 5.* 2nd ed. Philadelphia: WB Saunders, 2702–2732, 1982.

31. Ilgren EB, Stiller CA, Hughes JT, et al. Ependymomas: A clinical and pathological study. Part II—survival features. *Clin Neuropathol* 3:122–127, 1984.

32. Malis LI. Intramedullary spinal cord tumors. *Clin Neurosurg* 25:512–539, 1978.

33. Marks JE, Adler SJ. A comparative study of ependymomas by site of origin. *Int J Radiat Oncol Biol Phys* 8:37–43, 1982.

34. McCormick PC, Torres R, Post KD, Stein BM. Intramedullary ependymoma of the spinal cord. *J Neurosurg* 72:523–533 1990.

35. McCormick PC, Stein BM. Spinal ependymoma: Evaluation of recovery following complete removal. In: Holtzman, Stein, eds. *Surgery of the spinal cord: potential for regeneration and recovery.* New York: Plenum Press, 1991 (in press).

36. McCormick PC, Michelsen WJ, Post KD, et al. Cavernous malformation of the spinal cord. *Neurosurgery* 23:459–463, 1988.

37. Mork SJ, Loken AC. Ependymoma. A follow-up study of 101 cases. *Cancer* 40:907–915, 1977.

38. Mork SJ, Risberg G, Krogness K. Anaplastic ependymomas of the spinal cord. *Neuropathol Appl Neurobiol* 6:307–311, 1980.

39. Neumann HPH, Eggert HR, Weigel K, et al. Hemangioblastomas of the central nervous system: a 10-year study with special reference to von Hippel-Lindau syndrome. *J Neurosurg* 70:24–30, 1989.

40. Piersol GA. Anatomy of the spine and spinal cord. In: Frazier CH, ed. *Surgery of the spine and spinal cord.* New York: D. Appleton, 1–97, 1918.

41. Post KD, Stein BM. Surgical management of spinal cord tumors and arteriovenous malformations. In: Schmidek HH, Sweet WH, eds. *Operative neurosurgical techniques. Vol 2.* New York: Grunne and Stratton, 1487–1507, 1987.

42. Rawlings CE, Giangaspero F, Burger PC, et al. Ependymomas: a clinicopathologic study. *Surg Neurol* 29:271–281, 1988.

43. Ross AT, Bailey OT. Tumors arising within the spinal canal in children. *Neurology* 3:922–930, 1953.

44. Sagerman RH, Bagshaw MA, Hanbery J. Considerations in the treatment of ependymoma. *Radiology* 84:401–408, 1965.

45. Salazar OM, Rubin R, Bassano D, et al. Improved survival of patients with intracranial ependymomas by irradiation: dose selection and field extension. *Cancer* 35:1563–1573, 1975.

46. Schwade JG, Wara WM, Sheline GE. Management of primary spinal cord tumors. *Int J Radiat Oncol Biol Phys* 4:389–393, 1978.

47. Seyfer AE, Joseph AS. Use of trapezius muscle for closure of complicated upper spinal defects. *Neurosurgery* 14:341–345, 1984.

48. Shaw EG, Evans RG, Scheithauer BW, et al. Radiotherapeutic management of adult intraspinal ependymomas. *Int J Radiat Oncol Biol Phys* 12:323–327, 1986.

49. Sloof JL, Kernohan JW, MacCarthy CS. *Primary intramedullary tumors of the spinal cord and filum terminale.* New York: WB Saunders, 1964.

50. Solomon RA, Stein BM. Unusual spinal cord enlargement related to intramedullary hemangioblastoma. *J Neurosurg* 68:550–553, 1988.

51. Stein BM. Surgery of intramedullary spinal cord tumors. *Clin Neurosurg* 26:529–542, 1979.

52. Tachdjian MO, Matson DD. Orthopaedic aspects of intraspinal tumors in infants and children. *J Bone Joint Surg [Am]* 47A:223–248, 1965.

53. Wara WM, Phillips TL, Sheline GE. Radiation tolerance of the spinal cord. *Cancer* 35:1558–1562, 1975.

54. Webb JH, Craig WM, Kernohan JW. Intraspinal neoplasms in the cervical region. *J Neurosurg* 10:360–366, 1953.

55. West CR, Bruce DA, Duffner PK. Ependymomas. Factors in clinical and diagnostic staging. *Cancer* 56:1812–1816, 1985.

56. Wisoff JH, Epstein FJ. Spinal cord astrocytoma of children and young adults. In: Long DL, ed. *Current therapy in neurological surgery. vol. 2.* Philadelphia: BC Decker, 240–242, 1989.

57. Woltman HW, Kernohan JW, Adson AW, et al. Intramedullary tumors of the spinal cord and gliomas of intradural portion of filum terminale: fate of patients who have these tumors. *Arch Neurol Psychiatry* 65:378–393, 1951.

58. Wood EH, Berne AS, Taveras JM. The value of radiation therapy in the management of intrinsic tumors of the spinal cord. *Radiology* 63:11–24, 1954.

59. Zide BM, Wisoff JH, Epstein FJ. Closure of extensive and complicated laminectomy wounds. *J Neurosurg* 67:59–64, 1987.

CHAPTER 14

Approaches to Cervical Spine Infections and Bone Tumors

Paul H. Young

INFECTIONS OF THE CERVICAL SPINE

Though less common than in years past, infectious processes involving the cervical spine can still present a diagnostic dilemma (1–23). Classical tuberculous vertebral involvement involves destruction of the cervical vertebral body(s) leading to eventual collapse and the production of a kyphotic deformity. Tuberculosis is now rarely seen in the United States except in migrant populations.

Pathogenesis

Infectious agents primarily spread to the cervical spine via a hematogenous route related to the abundant vascular supply of the vertebral body and cancellous bone. Extension into the disc space frequently occurs with narrowing or collapse of the disc space in addition to the development of subchondral sclerosis and surface irregularity. Eventual anterior vertebral body collapse can lead to a significant kyphotic deformity.

Signs and Symptoms

Patients with vertebral body or disc space infections present with stiffness in the neck, malaise, easy fatigueability, loss of appetite, lethargy, fever and night sweats, pain in the neck with radiation into the shoulders, headache, and radiculopathic or myelopathic signs and symptoms. Clinical findings include marked local tenderness, paraspinous spasm and rigidity, local curvature abnormality, and neurological deficits.

Acute osteomyelitis may lead to acute or chronic compression of the spinal cord or roots due to epidural purulent protrusions or pathological subluxation. Rapid evaluation, recognition, and treatment is essential, particularly in patients presenting with marked neurologic disturbances such as quadriplegia.

Diagnosis

The correct diagnosis is based on a high index of suspicion in conjunction with blood test abnormalities (elevated sedimentation rate and white blood cell abnormalities consistent with indoluent infection) and radiographic findings. Magnetic resonance imaging (MRI) is the imaging procedure of choice, being as sensitive as radionucleid bone scanning to the presence of an infectious nucleus. Computed tomography (CT) myelography may be necessary in isolated instances to precisely identify the effects of the infectious process of the spinal canal and foramen.

Sequelae

Sequelae of inadequately treated vertebral or disc space infectious processes are spontaneous fusion, increased root or cord symptoms, menigitis or epidural abscess, osteomyelitis, septicemia with distal spread of infections (SBE etc.), and vertebral malalignment and deformity.

Treatment

The hallmark of treatment for infectious processes affecting the cervical spine remains intravenous drug therapy dictated by the appropriate organisms' sensitivity. It is clear, particularly in the tuberculous varieties, that drugs and not surgery are the most important weapons. In fact, with many infectious processes, eventual ossification and bony ankylosis will occur due to spontaneous fusion of the affected bony margins and posterior facet joints without the need for a surgical procedure.

Indications for Surgery

It is important that surgical intervention in this setting not worsen the instability of the spine. Most patients respond well to an adequate nonsurgical program consisting of immobilization and antibiotics. Surgical intervention, however, may tend to shorten the patient's recuperation through the evacuation of purulent material thereby creating a better bed for bone fusion. The following principles for surgical management should be kept in mind: evidence of nerve root or spinal cord compression with appropriate signs and symptoms, failure to respond over an adequate time to appropriate antibiotics, severe unrelenting pain, and vertebral body distraction or other bony-ligamentous involvement with resultant instability.

Goals of Management

Goals of management are specific localization of organism by the least invasive technique possible (needle biopsy, open biopsy, exploration, etc.), minimization of instability and deformity, adequate decompression to improve neurological deficits, drainage of purulent material or abscess, and an adequate orthodesis to improve instability.

Surgical Treatment

Since the vast majority of infectious processes occur ventral to the cord, the anterior or anterolateral approaches are most indicated in this setting.

Bone grafting in a septic bed generally presents a serious problem, but in the cervical spine the presence of abundant vascularity makes grafting safe and effective. Despite that satisfactory performance of a grafting procedure, appropriate antibiotic treatment throughout the postoperative period remain important.

Cortical-cancellous grafts from the ilium or a combination of fibula, rib, and iliac crest are the best choice. The grafts should be positioned in good beds of bleeding cancellous bone and should be surrounded by viable vascular soft tissue.

CERVICAL SPINE BONE TUMORS

Primary tumors arising from the bony elements of the cervical spine are indeed rare (24–70). Approximately 15% of all primary bone tumors occur in the spinal column, and only a fraction of these are found in the neck.

Tumor Types

The primary cervical spine tumors can be divided into benign and malignant categories.

Primary benign tumors in order of decreasing frequency include neurofibroma, aneurysmal bone cyst, benign giant cell tumor, benign osteoblastoma, solitary eosinophilic granuloma, solitary plasmacytoma, chondromixoid fibroma, desmoid tumor, hemangioma, and osteocartilaginous exostosis.

Primary *malignant tumors* of the cervical spine in order of decreasing frequency include chordoma, myeloma, lymphoma, mesenchymal chondrosarcoma, chondrosarcoma, osteosarcoma, Ewing sarcoma, Paget's sarcoma, postradiation sarcoma, fibrosarcoma, aggressive solitary plasmacytoma, fibrous histocytoma, hemangioendothelioma, and hemangioparacytoma.

In children, the more common benign tumors include osteoid osteoma, osteoblastoma, and aneurysmal bone cyst, whereas the malignant varieties include neuroblastoma, Ewing's sarcoma, and histiocytosis.

Metastatic lesions are most frequently found in the elderly patient. These lesions are found most frequently invading the vertebral body and pedicle and less frequently in the posterior elements, which is the reverse of that seen with benign lesions.

Signs and Symptoms

The diagnosis of a spinal cord tumor requires a high index of suspicion. The most frequent initial symptom is pain. If root or cord compression is not present, appropriate radicular or myelopathic signs and symptoms may be delayed.

Radiographic Evaluation

The evaluation of patients with primary spine tumors is similar to that for patients with cervical spondylosis (see Chapter 4).

Operative Treatment

The principle treatment of primary bone tumors in the cervical spine revolves around surgery, which attempts to totally remove the tumor mass, relieve the patient's pain and/or neurological syndrome, relieve or prevent a neurological deficit, and restore mechanical spine stability.

Contraindications to Surgery

Contraindications to surgery are elderly debilitated patients with metastatic lesions; patients with tumors that are associated with a very poor prognosis; patients undergoing high-dose irradiation; patients with significant medical difficulties, especially cardiac, pulmonary, or renal failure; and patients with unresectable lesions.

OPERATIVE APPROACHES

Reconstruction of the cervical spine with bone struts of fibula, ribs, iliac crest, etc. can be achieved anteriorly, whereas stabilization can be obtained posteriorly. The standard anterolateral approach can be used to replace single or multiple vertebral bodies and adjacent discs. Multiple levels require the anterior placement of long struts using ribs or fibula. The use of methyl methacrylate as a stabilizing technique should be avoided whenever possible (see Chapter 10).

Approaches

Indications for the posterior approach are tumors involving the spinous processes or laminae, intraspinal tumor extending from the laminae into the articular facets, and instability requiring a posterior fusion.

Indications for an anterolateral approach are medial tumors of the vertebral body with or without subligamentous extension.

Indications for the antero-lateral approach are tumor extending into the transverse processes, pedicles, and posterolateral joints; and tumor involving the costal horn of the foramen transversarium and the anterior tubercles (provides lateral exposure to the bony wall) around the spinal nerves and vertebral artery.

Anterior Approach

The anterolateral approach permits extensive exposures for tumor removal and bone fusion extending all the way from the base of the occiput to the upper thoracic region (1). Combined anterior and anterolateral procedures permit total corpectomies from C3 to C7 (see Chapters 2 and 7).

Posterior Approach

In metastatic lesions or benign lesions localized to posterior elements, the posterior approach is preferred. Surgery is rarely indicated for decompression alone, so along with a decompression a surgical stabilization procedure should be performed to provide immediate stability. From the posterior approach, this generally involves using a wire technique augmented with autologous bone grafts.

On occasion, combinations of anterior and posterior procedures may be necessary to provide satisfactory access and stability. As previously noted, decompressive laminectomy alone as sole treatment is rarely indicated.

REFERENCES

Infection

1. Abramovitz JN, Batson RA, and Yablon JS. Vertebral osteomyelitis: the surgical management of neurologic complications. *Spine* 11:418–420, 1986.
2. Baker AS, Ojemann RG, Swartz MN, et al. Spinal epidural abscess. *N Engl J Med* 293:463–468, 1975.
3. Browder J, Meyers R. Infections of the spinal epidural space: an aspect of vertebral osteomyelitis. *Am J Surg* 37:4–26, 1937.
4. Cloward RB. Metastatic disc infection and osteomyelitis of the cervical spine. *Spine* 3:194–201, 1978.
5. Digby JM, Kersley JB. Pyogenic non-tuberculous spinal infection: an analysis of thirty cases. *J Bone Joint Surg* 61B:47–55, 1979.
6. Forsythe M, Rothman RH. New concepts in the diagnosis and treatment of infections of the cervical spine. *Orthop Clin North Am* 9:1039–1051, 1978.
7. Ghormley RK, Bickel WH, and Dickson DD. A study of acute infectious lesions of the intervertebral discs. *South Med J* 33:347–353, 1940.
8. Hodgson AR, Stock FE. Anterior spine fusion for the treatment of tuberculosis of the spine: the operative findings and results of treatment in the first one hundred cases. *J Bone Joint Surg* 42:295–310, 1960.
9. Hodgson AR, Stock FE, Fang HS, Ong, GB. Anterior spinal fusion. The operative approach and pathological finding in 412 patients with Pott's disease of the spine. *Br J Surg* 48:172–178, 1960.
10. Hughes JE, Vigiacinto GV, Sundaresan N. Osteomyelitis of the cervical spine: surgical series. In: *Cervical spine II*. New York: Spinger-Verlag, 160–167, 1989.
11. Kemp HBS, Jackson JW, Jeremiah JD, et al. Pyogenic infections occurring primarily in intervertebral discs. *J Bone Joint Surg [Br]* 55B:698–714, 1973.
12. Kemp HBS, Jackson JW, Jeremiah JD, et al. Anterior fusion of the spine for infective lesions in adults. *J Bone Joint Surg [Br]* 55B:715–734, 1973.
13. LaRocca H. Spinal sepsis. In: *The Spine*. Rothman RH, Simeone FA, eds. Philadelphia: WB Sanders, 757–774, 1975.
14. Louis R. Surgery for tuberculosis of the cervical spine with reduction of deformity. In: *Cervical spine II*. New York: Springer-Verlag, 149–154, 1985.
15. Messer HD, Litvinoff J. Pyogenic cervical osteomyelitis of the cervical spine associated with parenteral drug use. *Arch Neurol* 33:571–576, 1976.
16. Rodegerdts U, Rao DR, Weidner A. The cervical spine infected after surgery. In: *Cervical spine II*. New York: Springer-Verlag, 139–142, 1989.
17. Savini R, Gargiulo G, DiSilvestre M, Gualdrini G. The treatment

of cervical spine infections. In: *Cervical spine II*. New York: Springer-Verlag, 143–148, 1989.

18. Smith TK, Cotler JM, Cotler HB. *Fusion technique for spinal infections in spinal fusion*. New York: Springer-Verlag, 1990.

19. Stauffer RN. Pyogenic vertebral osteomyelitis. *Orthop Clin North Am* 6:1015–1027, 1975.

20. Stone DB, Bonfiglio M. Pyogenic vertebral osteomyelitis, a pitfall for the internist. *Arch Intern Med* 112:491–500, 1963.

21. Stone JL, Cybulski GR, Rodriquez J, Gryfinski ME, Kant R. Anterior cervical debridement and strut grafting for osteomyelitis of the cervical spine. *J Neurosurg* 70:879–883, 1989.

Tumors

22. Barcena A, Lobato RD, Rivas JJ, et al. Spinal metastatic disease: analysis of factors determining functional prognosis and the choice of treatment. *Neurosurgery* 15:820–827, 1984.

23. Barron KD, Hirano A, Araki S, Terry RD. Experiences with metastatic neoplasms involving the spinal cord. *Neurology* 9:91–106, 1959.

24. Batson OV. The function of the vertebral veins and their role in the spread of metastases. *Ann Surg* 112:138–149, 1940.

25. Boland PJ, Lane JM, Sundaresan N. Metastatic disease of the spine. *Clin Orthop* 169:95–102, 1982.

26. Caldicott W. Diagnosis of spinal osteoid osteoma. *Radiology* 92:1192–1195, 1969.

27. Capanna R, Albisinni U, Picci P, Calderoni P, Campanacci M, Spingfield DS. Aneurysmal bone cyst of the spine. *J Bone Joint Surg [Am]* 67A:527–531, 1985.

28. Chadduck WM, Boop WC Jr. Acrylic stabilization of the cervical spine for neoplastic disease. Evolution of a technique for vertebral body replacement. *Neurosurgery* 13:23–29, 1983.

29. Dahlin DC, Unni KK. *Bone tumors: general aspects and data on 8,542 cases*. 4th ed. Springfield, IL. Charles C Thomas, 552, 1986.

30. Fielding J, Pyle R, Fiette V. Anterior cervical vertebral body resection and bone grafting for benign and malignant tumors. *J Bone Joint Surg [Am]* 61A:251–253, 1979.

31. Fidler MW. Pathologic fractures of the cervical spine: palliative surgical treatment. *J Bone Joint Surg [Br]* 67B:352–357, 1985.

32. Fornasier VL, Horne JG. Metastases to the vertebral column. *Cancer* 36:590–594, 1975.

33. Green NE, Robertson WW, Kilroy AW. Eosinophilic granuloma of the spine with associated neural deficit. *J Bone Joint Surg [Am]* 62A:1198–1202, 1980.

34. Harrington KD. The use of methylmethacrylate for vertebral-body replacement and anterior stabilization of pathological fracture-dislocations of the spine due to metastatic malignant disease. *J Bone Joint Surg [Am]* 63A:36–46, 1981.

35. Harrington KD. Anterior cord decompression and spinal stabilization for patients with metastatic lesions of the spine. *J Neurosurg* 61:107–117, 1984.

36. Harrington KD. Metastatic disease of the spine. *J Bone Joint Surg [Am]* 68A:1110–1115, 1986.

37. Harrington KD. Current concepts review: metastatic disease of the spine. *J Bone Joint Surg [Am]* 68A:1110, 1986.

38. Hershman E, Bjorkengren J, Fielding J, Allen S. Osteoid osteoma in a cervical pedicle. *Clin Orthop* 213:116–117, 1986.

39. Higanbotham NL, Phillips RF, Farr HW, Hustu HO. Chordoma: thirty-five year study at Memorial Hospital. *Cancer* 20:1841–1850, 1967.

40. Jackson RP, Reckling FW, Mants FA. Osteoid osteoma and osteoblastoma: similar histologic lesions with different natural histories. *Clin Orthop* 128:303–313, 1977.

41. Keplinger JE, Bucy PC. Giant cell tumors of the spine. *Ann Surg* 154:648–661, 1961.

42. Lee CK, Rosa R, Fernand R. Surgical treatment of tumors of the spine. *Spine* 11:201–208, 1986.

43. Livingston KE, Perrin RG. The neurosurgical management of spinal metastases causing cord compression. *J Neurosurg* 49:839–843, 1978.

44. Luck J, and Monsen D. Bone tumors and tumor-like lesions of vertebrae in spinal disorders. Diagnosis and treatment. In: Ruge D, Wiltse L, eds. *Spinal disorders: diagnosis and treatment*. Philadelphia: Lea and Febiger, 274–286, 1977.

45. McAllister Vl, Kendall BE, Bull JW. Symptomatic vertebral hemangiomas. *Brain* 98:71–80, 1975.

46. McLeod RA, Dahlin DC, Beabout JW. The spectrum of osteoblastoma. *Am J Roentgenol* 126:321–325, 1976.

47. Mac Lelland D, Wilson F. Osteoid osteoma of the spine. *J Bone Joint Surg [Am]* 49A:111–121, 1967.

48. Nay M, Paterson D, Taylor T. Aneurysmal bone cysts of the spine. *J Bone Joint Surg [Br]* 60B:406–411, 1978.

49. Ono K, Yonenobu K, Ebara S, Fujiwara K, Yashamita K, Fuji T, Dun E. Prosthetic replacement surgery for cervical spine metastases. *Spine* 13:817–822, 1988.

50. Parrish F, Pevy J. Surgical management of aneurysmal bone cyst. *J Bone Joint Surg* 49:1597–1604, 1967.

51. Perrin RG, McBroom RJ. Spine fixation after anterior decompression for symptomatic spinal metastases. *Neurosurgery* 22:324–327, 1988.

52. Pettine K, Klassen RA. Osteoid osteoma and osteoblastoma of the spine. *J Bone Joint Surg [Am]* 68A:354–361, 1986.

53. Phillips E, Levine An. Metastatic lesions of the upper cervical spine. *Spine* 14:1071–1077, 1989.

54. Prete P, Thorne R. Low cervical chordoma: Report of two cases. *Orthopedics* 3:643, 1980.

55. Raycroft J, Hockman R, Southwick W. Metastatic tumors involving the cervical vertebrae: surgical palliation. *J Bone Joint Surg [Am]* 60A:763–768, 1978.

56. Scoville WB, Patmer AH, Samra A. The use of acrylic plastic for vertebral replacement or fixation in metastatic disease of the spine. Technical note. *J Neurosurg* 27:274–279, 1967.

57. Shives TC, Dahlin DC, Sim FH, Pritchard DJ, Earle JD. Osteosarcoma of the spine. *J Bone Joint Surg [Am]* 68A:660–668, 1986.

58. Siegel T, Tiqva P, Siegal T. Vertebral body resection for epidural compression by malignant tumors: results of forty-seven consecutive operative procedures. *J Bone Joint Surgery [Am]* 67A:375, 1985.

59. Southwick WO, Robinson RA. Surgical approaches to the vertebral bodies in the cervical and lumbar regions. *J Bone Joint Surg [Am]* 39A:631, 1957.

60. Stener B, Johnson OE. Complete removal of three vertebrae for giant-cell tumour. *J Bone Joint Surg [Br]* 53B:278–287, 1971.

61. Stener B. Total spondylectomy in chondrosarcoma arising from the seventh thoracic vertebra. *J'Bone Joint Surg [Br]* 53B:288–295, 1971.

62. Verbiest H. Giant cell tumors and aneurysmal bone cysts of the spine. *J Bone Joint Surg [Br]* 47B:691, 1965.

63. Verbiest H. Tumors involving the cervical spine. In: Bailey RW, Sherk HH, eds. *The cervical spine*. Philadelphia: J B Lippincott, 430, 1984.

64. Villas C, Lopez R, Arrien A, Zubieta T. Osteoid osteoma affecting articular process at the cervical spine: infrequent localization and difficult diagnosis. In: *cervical spine II*. New York: Springer-Verlag, 216–224, 1989.

65. Weatherly CR, O'Brian TP, Oswestry VK. Simultaneous combined anterior and posterior approach to the cervical spine for resection of an osteoblastoma. In: *Cervical spine II*. New York: Springer-Verlag, 263–268, 1989.

66. Weinstein JN, McLain RF. Primary tumors of the spine. *Spine* 12:843–851, 1987.

67. Yong-Hing K, Kalamchi A, MacEwen G. Cervical spine abnormalities in neurofibromatosis. *J Bone Joint Surg [Am]* 61A:695–699, 1979.

CHAPTER 15

Perioperative Care for Cervical Spine Patients

Paul H. Young

The perioperative care of cervical spine patients includes the use of conservative treatment modalities either pre- or postoperatively, the routine preoperative evaluation, and standard postoperative care.

CONSERVATIVE PRE- AND POSTOPERATIVE TREATMENT

The conservative treatment options for cervical spine patients is similar to that available for patients with lumbar spine difficulties and other pain syndromes in general. These measures include rest, immobilization, analgesics, transcutaneous stimulator (TENS) unit, muscle relaxants, anti-inflamatory medications, heat, massage and chiropractic manipulation, ultrasound, traction, and exercise.

Rest

Bed rest alone, although frequently a mainstay of treatment for lumbar spine disorders, is seldom helpful in cervical spine abnormalities. Frequently, the pain of spondylotic radicular compression is exacerbated by the supine position. Patients with the most severe cervical pain syndromes frequently resort to the semi-sitting position (as in a recliner chair) for relief, abandoning any attempt to lie in bed even to sleep. The use of specially designed cervical pillows and other devices to restore and maintain better cervical curvature and posture are of some benefit in selected cases.

Immobilization

Cervical orthoses are routinely used to obtain some measure of external support and immobilization pre-operatively in cervical spine patients (1–3,5). Commonly, this immobilization or support is crucial during a period of bone graft healing or ligamentous repair. The commonly used cervical immobilization devices or orthosis include soft collar, Philadelphia collar, Somi brace, rigid cervical–thoracic brace, and halo vest.

Soft Cervical Collar

The soft cervical collar is the least restrictive of the cervical devices and as a result is the least effective in controlling cervical motion. Cervical flexion and extension is reduced by only 25%, lateral bending by 10%, and rotation by 20%. The soft collar generally consists of a Stockinet-type material covering foam rubber. The soft collar is by far and away the most easily tolerated orthoses, but, conversely, its use is limited by an inability to restrict cervical motion to any significant degree. In many situations, the role of the collar is that it serves as a reminder to the patient that it is important to restrict activities that involve excessive cervical motion. Patients undergoing single-level anterior (interbody) and posterior procedures are placed in a soft cervical collar for 2–4 weeks.

Philadelphia Collar

The Philadelphia collar is more effective than the soft collar in limiting cervical motion. Flexion and extension is limited by up to 70%, lateral bending by 35%, and rotation by nearly 50%. The Philadelphia collar consists of a molded styrofoam support with anterior and posterior plastic struts fastened with velcro. It also has molded mandibular and occipital supports that extend to the upper thoracic region. As noted above, the Philadelphia collar is most effective in limiting flexion and extension motions, and for this reason it is widely applied as routine postoperative care following cervical disc procedures, where limiting these particular cervical motions is routinely necessary. Patients undergoing multilevel anterior (interbody) or posterior approaches are placed in a Philadelphia collar for 6–10 weeks pending radiographic confirmation of stability.

Somi Brace

"Somi" is an acronym for sterno-occipito-mandibular immobilizer. The Somi brace is more effective than the Philadelphia collar in limiting rotation. Cervical flexion and extension is similarly limited by up to 70%, lateral bending by 35%, but rotation is restricted by 65%. The Somi brace has a rigid anterior plastic chest piece, onto which mandibular and occipital struts are connected. In addition to effectively immobilizing the upper cervical spine in flexion and rotation, it restricts rotation frequently important in C1–C2 abnormalities. Also, it is an easy brace to apply, and it can be put on in the supine position. For immobilization following upper cervical spine procedures, the Somi brace can be substituted for the Philadelphia collar.

Rigid Cervical-Thoracic Brace

This more rigid orthosis is better than either the Philadelphia collar or the Somi brace in preventing cervical flexion and extension. Cervical flexion and extension with this device is reduced by at least 80%, lateral bending by 65%, and rotation by 75%. The rigid cervical-thoracic brace has molded mandibular and occipital supports attached by adjustable struts to anterior and posterior plates. This device is more effective than the other devices in restricting all types of neck motion and is indicated in those instances when greater stabilization is necessary than that obtained with the less restrictive devices. The rigid cervical-thoracic brace is used for most multilevel anterior strut graft patients for 12–20 weeks.

Halo Vest

The most stabilizing yet unfortunately most uncomfortable cervical orthosis is the halo vest. This device limits cervical flexion and extension and lateral bending by >95% and rotation by >99%. The halo vest consists of a molded plastic vest attached to a metal ring. The ring is rigidly affixed via pins to the skull.

Due to its more invasive properties, the halo vest is restricted in use to situations where strict immobilization is required in the face of significant, demonstrable instability. Multilevel anterior corpectomy patients undergoing strut fusions may require 10–16 weeks of halo immobilization.

The need for external immobilization is tailored to the individual case. In addition to the need for short-term stabilization, the risk factors associated with immobilization are taken into account in terms of choosing the appropriate orthosis. These added risks include age, obesity, diabetes, the amount of pulmonary or cardiac insufficiency, presence of osteoporosis or other systemic disorders, alcoholism, heavy smoking, etc.

Analgesic Medication

Analgesics are prescribed to a degree consistent with the level of pain. Perioperative injectable or oral narcotic medications are routinely used, whereas routine oral narcotics for home use are generally denied. Clearly, the patient's psychological status and propensity for disability are factors in the determination of analgesic strengths.

TENS Unit

TENS can be useful as an adjunctive analgesic device, particularly in patients with chronic pain of several months' duration.

Muscle Relaxants

Muscle relaxants are prescribed when significant paracervical muscle spasm contributes to the pain syndrome. Intravenous muscle relaxants may be necessary in isolated situations of severe muscle spasm but require hospitalization. The cumulative effects of analgesics and muscle relaxants should be taken into account, particularly in the elderly or debilitated patient.

Antiinflammatory Medications

The use of antiinflammatory medications is a routine part of the perioperative care of cervical spine patients. Nonsteroidal antiinflammatory regimens are based on the patient's response to previous drugs, individual sensitivities, and the need for continuous versus intermittent antiinflammatory activity. Cortisone and its derivatives are prescribed sparingly in situations unresponsive to other antiinflammatory agents.

Heat

Dry, moist, or deep heat treatments are commonly administered as part of a physical therapy protocol for patients with cervical degenerative disease. Frequent associated muscle spasm is particularly responsive to this modality.

Massage and Manipulation

Cervical massage and mild manipulation are helpful in reducing the inflammatory component of cervical degenerative disc disease and restoring normal relaxation to paracervical musculature. Forced chiropractic manipulation in the face of cervical spondylosis should be avoided due to the risk of sudden worsening or catastrophic spinal cord, root, or vertebral artery injury.

Ultrasound

Ultrasound has been proven beneficial in the treatment of inflammatory disorders particularly along the spinal axis. Routinely, it permits a rapid improvement in symptomatology including muscle relaxation.

Traction

Holter-type cervical traction is routinely administered to patients with cervical spondylosis using 6–8 lb of traction for 20–30-min periods (4). Larger amounts of weight are avoided due to the increasing incidence of mandibular, occipital, neck, or shoulder pain related to the presence of the device. Response weights of 50% in spondylotic radiculopathy patients can be expected over the short term, whereas fewer long-term responses are seen.

Exercise

Exercise has only a limited role of play in the preoperative care of patients with cervical spondylosis, particularly in the face of significant root pain. Range of motion activities and mild exercise against force are used postoperatively to restore normal neck range of motion and paraspinous muscle function.

PREOPERATIVE EVALUATION

The routine preoperative evaluation of patients scheduled to undergo cervical spine procedures should include a general medical evaluation with particular emphasis on the cardiopulmonary system. This should include the use of blood gas analysis and pulmonary function tests in patients suspected of less than normal respiratory functions. The cardiovascular system evaluation if symptomatic should include an electrocardiogram, stress test, 24-hr Holter monitor, or even a coronary angiogram depending on the individual situation.

Patients should be evaluated for the presence of a coagulopathy with PT, PTT, and platelet count determinations and when necessary other bleeding and clotting studies.

POSTOPERATIVE NEUROSURGICAL CARE

Patients following cervical spine surgery are at risk to suffer a number of potential postoperative complications. The recognition of these complications may make admission to the intensive care unit for constant nursing care and intensive monitoring necessary (6,7).

Postanesthetic effects include confusion and drowsiness. It should be noted that the pupillary response to light is the first reflex to return to normal, generally at about the time the patient awakes from anesthesia. Other objective indicators such as the biceps and quadriceps reflex, muscle tone, or Babinski may be affected by the anesthetic, particularly the volatile inhalation anesthetics. Generally, these abnormalities disappear as the patient fully awakens from anesthesia. However, positive Babinski signs and spasticity or clonus can be seen up to 2 hr postoperatively.

Those patients who have worsened postoperative weakness after the administration of a nondepolarizing neural-muscular blocker should be suspected of having myesthenia gravis or pseudocholinesterase deficiency.

On the other hand, it should be noted that increasing headache (especially with vomitting), progressive drowsiness, and evolving monoparesis or hemiparesis, worsening paresthesias, etc. all suggest a neurological complication and should not be blamed on the anesthesia.

RESPIRATORY INSUFFICIENCIES

In the immediate postoperative care of patients following upper cervical spine surgery and particularly patients with preexisting spinal cord injury or myelopathy above C5, particular attention should be directed at the possible development of impaired muscular efforts due to the presence of the motor nuclei to the diaphragm in the upper cervical cord. Patients undergoing the removal of intramedullary tumors may actually require postoperative respiratory assistance. In addition, patients undergoing anterior cervical fusion may develop prevertebral edema or hematoma formation, which can compromise the patient's respiratory pathway or impede the function of respiratory muscles leading to diminished respiratory function.

With high cervical myelopathies, slowly progressive worsening of the respiratory status may occur with increasing edema of the respiratory nuclei. Routine postoperative pulmonary care in most instances should include one or more of the following: physiotherapy, humidification, intermittent positive pressure, and bedside spirometer, etc. Antibiotics should be avoided unless positive cultures have identified pulmonary infection.

The syndrome of hypoventilation or sleep apnea can be seen particularly in patients with mandibular anomalies and heavy set individuals with short-stocky necks. It may begin early in the postanesthetic period, with a vague subjective sensation of air hunger. The patient then becomes progressively drowsy with sighing respirations. When tested, he or she appears anxious and confused. These symptoms should not be misinterpreted as anxiety, and the patient should certainly not be sedated. The pathophysiology seems to be a decreased sensitivity of the respiratory drive for carbon dioxide compounded by mechanical factors such as cervical immobilization and an enlarged prevertebral space causing obstructive apnea. Oxygen should be administered carefully in these patients as their only respiratory drive is hypoxia. Mechanical ventilation may be necessary for a while at night.

POSTOPERATIVE BLOOD PRESSURE CONTROL

Postoperative blood pressure control is important following cervical spine procedures, particularly those in which an extradural clot can accumulate. Short-term control can be obtained by intravenous hypertensive agents such as Arfonade (a ganglionic blocker), Nitroprusside, and Hydrolyzine or Labetalol. Temporary control should be inforced by the patient's previous oral hypertensive medication as soon as feasible. Bed rest and sedation often reduce the hypertensive requirements of postoperative patients. Significant variations in blood pressure and heart rate may be triggered by tracheal sectioning or position changes, requiring constant cardiac and arterial line-monitoring.

Prophyaxis for Gastrointestinal Bleeding

The use of antacids or H2 histamine blockers such as Cimetidine or Zantac should be considered as part of the routine postoperative care for cervical spine patients.

Pulmonary Embolism

Pulmonary embolism is a constant threat to the bedridden, paraplegic, or quadriplegic patient. It requires the use of minidose heparin prophylaxis, 5,000 U subcutaneously twice daily and pneumatic airboots.

Gastrointestinal Distulance

Gastrointestinal atony and reflex paralytic ilious should be looked for in all cervical spine patients.

Metabolic Imbalance

Negative nitrogen balance due to exaggerated catabolic state and immobilization can lead to hypoproteinemia and hypocalcemia. The other electrolyte abnormality most frequently encountered is hyponatremia related to inappropriate secretion of ADH.

POSTSURGICAL BLEEDING

One must determine whether postsurgical bleeding is a result of the surgery with poor hemostasis or is a manifestation of an underlying coagulopathy.

Postoperative anemia may be due to blood loss from surgery, marrow decompression, phlebotomy, volume overload, etc.

Autonomic Dysfunction

A "cholinergic crisis" can occur with reflex bradycardia, sweating, pilomotor erection, and headaches. This can be precipitated by bladder fullness, tracheal suctioning, and other painful sensations below the level of the myelopathy. Treatment involves the use of anticholinergic drugs.

Urinary Atony

The continuous use of an indwelling catheter beyond the first 2 or 3 days should be avoided. In patients with a severe myelopathy, a definitive program of bladder care should be established.

Decubitus Prevention

The prevention of decubitus ulcers involve rotation every 2 hr, the early care of pressure sensitive areas, and the use of special beds.

Routine Postoperative Instructions for Interbody Fusions

Depending on the nature of the fusion, the patient is placed in a soft cervical collar or other more rigid device immediately after surgery and permitted to ambulate as soon as her or his postanesthesia recovery permits. Antiinflammatory medications, mild muscle relaxants, and analgesics are prescribed in the immediate postoperative period. Depending on the type of fusion and number of spaces involved, the soft collar is progressively removed at 2–10 weeks after surgery and the patient instructed to begin gentle neck motion. Normal mobility is restored by 1–3 months postoperative with a mild progressive neck exercise program.

Long-Term Myelopathy Concerns

Psychological factors and philosophical considerations in severely myelopathic patients demand a coordinated and unified approach, dealing with both patient and family through the physicians, nurses, physical therapists, social workers, and others involved. The overall approach must be positive. Rehabilitation involves the realistic establishment of short-term goals.

REFERENCES

1. Fisher SV, Bowar JF, Awad EA, et al. Cervical orthoses effect on cervical spine motion: roentgenographic and goniometric method of study. *Arch Phys Med Rehabil* 58:109–115, 1977.
2. Johnson RM, Hart DL, Simmons EF, et al. Cervical orthoses: a study comparing their effectiveness in restricting cervical motion in normal subjects. *J Bone Joint Surg [Am]* 59A:332–339, 1977.
3. Johnson RM, Owen JR, Hart DL, Callahan RA. Cervical orthoses: a guide to their selection and use. *Clin Orthop* 154:34–45, 1981.
4. Rath WW. Cervical traction, a clinical perspective. *Orthop Rev* 13:430, 1984.
5. Roberts AH. Myelopathy due to cervical spondylosis treated by collar immobilization. *Neurology* 16:951–954, 1966.
6. Ropper AH, Kennedy SF. *Neurological and neurosurgical intensive care.* 2nd ed. Aspen Publications, 1988.
7. Schneider RC. Treatment of cervical spine disease. In: Schneider RC, Kahn EA, Crosby EC, Taren JA, eds. *Correlative neurosurgery.* 3rd ed. Springfield, IL: Charles C Thomas, 1094–1174, 1982.

CHAPTER 16

Complications of Cervical Spine Microsurgery

Paul H. Young

The complications of cervical spine surgery can be divided into the following five categories: (a) errors in preoperative planning, (b) intraoperative catastrophes and avoidable occurrences, (c) accepted postoperative complications, (d) problems associated with bone fusion, and (e) progression in cervical spine degenerative disc disease.

ERRORS IN PREOPERATIVE PLANNING

Incorrect Diagnosis

Cervical spine procedures performed in patients for neck and arm pain but based on an inaccurate diagnosis (i.e., carcinoma of the lung apex) usually fail to produce good clinical results.

Poor Choice of Therapy

Patients with headache and/or neck pain alone should be subjected to surgical intervention only when the strictest indications for surgery are met.

Wrong Operative Approach

Attempts to remove large midline anterior spurs through a posterior approach may not only produce catastrophic results but usually fail to accomplish adequate decompression.

Operations in the Face of Psychoneuroses or Compensation-Disability Disorders

Careful selection in this group of patients is essential to ensure good clinical results.

INTRAOPERATIVE CATASTROPHES

Anterior Approaches

Spinal Cord Injury

Spinal cord injury with resultant quadriplegia, tetraplegia, or paraplegia can occur due to compression, traction, or laceration of the spinal cord (0.1%). Spinal cord injury or worsening of a preexisting myelopathy is clearly the most devastating complication of operations on the cervical spine. Two-thirds of these result in tetraplegia, one-third in a Brown-Sequard syndrome. Special care to avoid unintentional spinal canal intrusion and spinal cord compression is paramount in the prevention of these dire consequences. The use of the operating microscope increases the safety margin of working near the cord by increasing the surgeon's awareness of the affects of each movement on the spinal canal and secondarily the spinal cord.

Major Vascular Injury

Hemorrhage due to perforation or laceration of the carotid sheath structures including the carotid artery and internal jugular vein or the vertebral artery and paravertebral plexus may occur or an AV fistula may be produced. Nothing produces more excitement in the operating room than inadvertent vertebral artery laceration during cervical disc surgery. The position of the vertebral artery in relation to the uncovertebral and facet joints should be instilled in the surgeon's anatomic memory to prevent this catastrophic event. Should this complication occur, immediate packing and counter-pressure will control the bleeding while thought is given towards radiographic tests of vertebral artery anatomy to permit vertebral artery ligation.

Nerve Injury

The following nerve injuries may occur:

(a) Laceration, transection, or avulsion of a nerve root: This nearly always results in postoperative sensory and/or motor loss. Nerve root injury or contusion can occur with too vigorous manipulation of roots. It is important to be constantly aware of the ever-changing posterior to anterior direction of the roots as they proceed from a medial to lateral direction. In addition, the frequent multiplicity of cervical roots dural sheath endangers them to inadvertent injury. Nerve injury can also occur due to slipped drills, curettes, chisels, or rongeurs.
(b) Laceration of the sympathetic plexus or superior cervical ganglion with resultant Horner's syndrome.
(c) Injury to the brachial plexus with monoparesis or sensory abnormalities (including causalgia).
(d) Transection of the superior laryngeal nerve with resultant thyrocricoid muscle paralysis and permanent fatiguing of the voice or hoarseness.
(e) Transection of the inferior laryngeal nerve, particularly a nonrecurrent inferior laryngeal nerve, with resultant permanent postoperative hoarseness (0.8%): The possibility of an aberrant recurrent laryngeal nerve should be always foremost in the surgeon's mind. Following vocal cord paralysis postoperatively, functional return should be anticipated over 3–5 weeks, although nerve regeneration may take 4–6 months. If necessary, 80% are improved by the injection of Teflon.
(f) Transection of cranial nerves 9, 10, 11, or 12 with significant resultant postoperative deficits especially involving phonation and swallowing.

Avoidable Intraoperative Occurrences

These include (a) perforation of the pharynx, larynx, trachea, or espohagus, either recognized immediately or diagnosed following the development of infectious signs; (b) acute graft expulsion or retropulsion with esophageal or spinal cord injury; (c) failure to completely remove a sequestered disc fragment with significant continued root or spinal cord compression; (d) exploration of the wrong intervertebral level, (although this should be entirely preventable by intraoperative radiographic confirmation; proper preoperative radiographic testing and intraoperative confirmation of radiographic abnormalities are essential in preventing this embarrassment); (e) cerebral infarction due to carotid or vertebral artery embolization or occlusion due to associated but unrecognized atheromatous vessel disease; (f) cerebrospinal fluid (CSF) leak (inadvertent or intended dural laceration, unrepaired or inadequately repaired may result in a postoperative CSF leak; before embarking on cervical spine procedures, the microsurgeon should be familiar with the techniques of opening and closing the dural sack and nerve root sheaths; a fibrin adhesive sealant is available for a watertight closure; it contains a freeze-dried concentrate of human clotting factors that are mixed with thrombin and calcium; this fibrin glue should be used instead of cyanoacrylate glue due to the latter's known neurotoxicity); (g) formation of a postoperative meningocele or pseudomeningocele due to inadequate dural repair; (h) a significant worsened radiculopathy due to a partial root injury during the decompressive procedure; (i) laceration or inadvertent ligation of the thoracic duct; (j) Pneumothorax due to inadvertent perforation of the pleura; (k) formation of postoperative epidural hematoma; (l) development of epidural abscess or meningitis due to unrecognized or poorly treated superficial or deep wound infections; and (m) uilateral blindness produced by pressure of an assistant's hand resting on the globe.

Posterior Approach

This approach involves (a) spinal cord injury with resultant quadriplegia, tetraplegia, or paraplegia due to unwarranted attempts at the removal of disc fragments or spurs located along the anterior aspect of the spinal canal and nerve roots or from aggressive attempts at dentate ligament section; (b) spinal cord injury resulting from too vigorous spinal cord retraction during intramedullary or other intradural procedures; (c) spinal cord injury due to spinal cord compression or contusion resulting from inadvertent penetration of an instrument into the spinal canal; (d) spinal cord injury from rigorous placement of instruments into the spinal canal or performing bony removal such as laminectomy (0.4%); (e) reflex sympathetic dystrophy following partial nerve root or cord injury; (f) inadequate removal of sequestered disc or spondylotic bars with persistent spinal cord or radicular compression; (g) increase in myelopathic findings following inadequate stabilization in turning the patient from the supine to the prone position for positioning at surgery; (h) spinal cord injury due to loosening of the head immobilization device intraoperatively; (i) intraoperative ischemia due to blockage or expulsion of the endotracheal tube; (j) instability as a result of a wider than necessary laminectomy with total facet removal (particularly in the young patient); (k) leakage of cerebrospinal fluid due to inadvertent dural laceration or faulty dural repair; (l) formation of postoperative meningocele due to inadvertent dural laceration or inadequate dural repair; (m) excessive intraoperative blood loss due to compression of the abdomen; (n) laceration of the vertebral artery as it ascends over the lateral portions of C1; (o) postoperative compressive hematoma in the subdural or epidural space following closure with poor hemostasis; (p) deep paraspinous or epidural wound infection; (q) air embolism or cerebral ischemia from procedures performed in the sitting position; (r) corneal damage due to compression on the orbits while positioning; and (s) compression of the peripheral nerves while on the operating table in the prone position.

ACCEPTED POSTOPERATIVE COMPLICATIONS

Accepted postoperative complications are described here (36–41).

Anterior Approach

These include (a) retropharyngeal or prevertebral edema and/or hematoma formation with compression of the trachea and esophagus and postoperative hoarseness or dysphagia; (b) postoperative hoarseness due to stretching of the superior laryngeal or recurrent laryngeal nerves with nerve contusion or edema; (c) retraction related problems resulting in hoarseness, dysphagia or sensation of a lump in the throat with permanent swallowing abnormalities (0.08%); (d) immediate and subacute postoperative discomfort with nagging neck, shoulder, and interscapular pain often lasting several months (worse without bone graft); (e) persistent chronic postoperative pain due to perineural inflammation; (f) postoperative inflammatory discitis; and (g) subcutaneous wound infection (1%).

Posterior Approach

These include (a) superficial wound infection (2%); (b) subcutaneous wound dehiscence (0.4%); (c) excessive blood loss from the paraspinous muscle mass;

(d) instability following decompression with resultant abnormal mobility or subluxation and associated neurological deficits; (e) cervical lordosis, kyphosis, and/or subluxation due to facet injury following wide decompression (particularly in children); (f) unintended superior or inferior extension of the fusion past the area of interest; (g) late closure of an adequate laminectomy decompression due to extradural fibrosis or laminoplasty due to reclosure of the laminar door; (h) breakage of wires with ongoing instability; (i) diminished range of motion (particularly in laminoplasty); (j) paresthesiae secondary to sublaminal wire passage; (k) opacification of the posterior longitudinal ligament; and (l) sleep apnea or respiratory failure.

PROBLEMS ASSOCIATED WITH BONE FUSION

Problems associated with bone fusion are as follows (42–52): (a) progressive degenerative changes occurring at the levels above and below a fused segment; (b) graft extrusion (1–13%), with dysphasia, kyphotic instability, or persistent neurologic symptoms; (c) graft collapse (autograft 16%, allograft 28%); (d) failure of fusion with resultant spondylolisthesis, and nonunion and lack of graft incorporation with pseudoarthrosis (5–26%) (Figs. 1 and 2) (higher rate of pseudoarthrosis with multiple level fusions); (e) infections of the fusion site with the potential for infection with hepatitis or

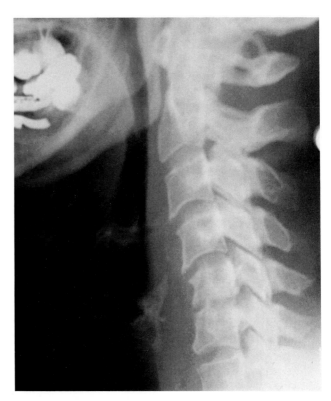

FIG. 1. Pseudoarthrosis at C5–C6 6 months following Cloward fusion in an asymptomatic patient.

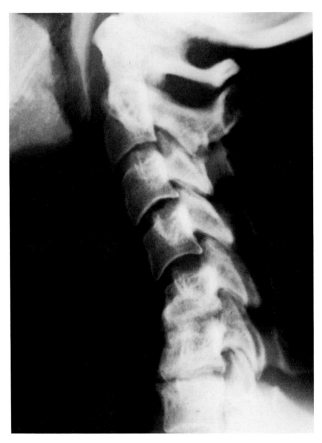

FIG. 2. Two level pseudoarthrosis (C5–C6 and C6–C7) 8 months following Smith-Robinson fusion in a symptom-free patient.

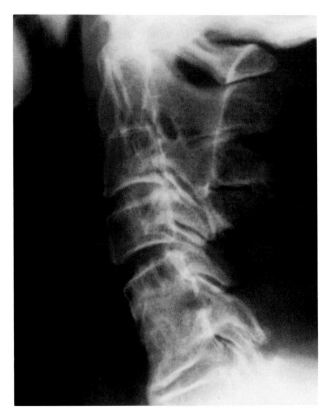

FIG. 3. Spondylosis developing at the level below a previous C4–C5 procedure 3 years after successful Cloward fusion.

AIDS virus; (f) esophageal perforation due to graft expulsion, and (g) problems related to the harvesting of the bone graft, including (53–57) hematoma (15%), vascular and peritoneal injury, graft site infection (7%), long-term pain at the graft site (25%), and nerve injury affecting the lateral femoral cutaneous, iliohypogastric, ilioinguinal, genital femoral, or cluneal nerves (12%).

COMPLICATIONS RELATED TO THE NATURAL HISTORY OF DEGENERATIVE CERVICAL DISC DISEASE

These include (a) recurrent disc protrusion at the operative level or contralaterally after settling; (b) new disc protrusion or progressive spondylosis occurring at adjoining motion segments due to increased stress and strain imposed by the loss of the operative disc space (Fig. 3); (c) late recurrence of symptoms after initial success of excision of a disc prolapse due to progressive spondylosis of the nerve root canal secondary to degenerative changes; (d) progressive os-

sification of the ligamentum flavum following fusion; and (e) atrophy of the ligamentum flavum following fusion with adherence of the ligament to the nerve root sleeves.

REFERENCES

Neural Injury

1. Bulger RF, Rejowski JE, Beatty RA. Vocal cord paralysis associated with anterior cervical fusion: considerations for prevention and treatment. *J Neurosurg* 62:657–661, 1985.
2. Crandall PH, Batzdorf U. Cervical spondylotic myelopathy. *J Neurosurg* 25:57–66, 1966.
3. Flynn TB. The neurologic complications of anterior cervical interbody fusions. *Spine* 7:536–539, 1982.
4. Heeneman H. Vocal cord paralysis following approaches to the anterior cervical spine. *Laryngoscope* 83:17–21, 1973.
5. Jan M. Guaze A, Santini JJ, et al. Thrombose d'une artere radiculaire apres exerese discoosteophytique parvoie anterieure pour nervalgie cervicobrachiale. *Neurochirurgie* 24:351–353, 1978.
6. Kraus DR, Stauffer ES. Spinal cord injury as a complication of elective anterior cervical fusion. *Clin Orthop Rel Res* 112:130–141, 1975.
7. Horwitz NH, Rizzoli HV. *Post-operative complications of extracranial neurological surgery.* Williams & Wilkins, 76–84, 1987.
8. Krieger AJ, Rosomoff HL. Sleep-induced apnea. Part 2. Res-

piratory failure after anterior spinal surgery. *J Neurosurg* 39:181–185, 1974.

9. Levy WJ, Dohn DF, Hardy RW. Central cord syndrome as a delayed postoperative complication of decompressive laminectomy. *Neurosurgery* 11:491–495, 1982.

10. Murphey F, Simmons JCH, Brunson B. Surgical treatment of laterally ruptured cervical disc. Review of 648 cases, 1939 to 1972. *J Neurosurg* 38:679–683, 1973.

11. Mayfield FH. Complications of laminectomy. *Clin Neurosurg* 23:435–439, 1976.

12. Phillips DG. Surgical treatment of myelopathy with cervical spondylosis. *J Neurol Neurosurg Psychiatry* 36:879–884, 1973.

13. Sang UH, Wilson CB. Postoperative epidural hematoma as a complication of anterior cervical discectomy. *J Neurosurg* 49:288–291, 1978.

14. Scoville WB. Posterior keyhole laminotomy: complications. In: Dunsker SB, ed. *Cervical spondylosis.* New York: Raven Press, 169–171, 1981.

15. Stauffer ES, Kraus FR. Spinal cord injury as a complication of elective anterior cervical fusion. *Clin Orthop* 112:130, 1975.

16. Sugar O. Spinal cord malfunction after anterior cervical discectomy. *Surg Neurol* 15:4–8, 1982.

17. Tew JM Jr, Mayfield FH. Surgery of the anterior cervical spine: prevention of complications. In: Dunsker SB, ed. *Cervical spondylosis.* New York: Raven Press, 191–208, 1981.

18. West CGH. Bilateral brachial paresis following anterior decompression for cervical spondylosis. *Spine* 11:176–178, 1986.

19. Williams JL, Allen MB, Harkess JW. Late results of cervical discectomy and interbody fusion. Some factors influencing the results. *J Bone Joint Surg [Am]* 50A:277–286, 1968.

20. Yonenobu K, Okada K, Fuji T, Fujiwara K, Yamashita K, Ono K. Causes of neurologic deterioration following surgical treatment of cervical myelopathy. *Spine* 11:818–823, 1986.

Death

21. Aronson NI. The management of soft cervical disc protrusion using the Smith-Robinson approach. *Clin Neurosurg* 20:253–258, 1973.

22. Espersen JO, Buhl M, Eriksen EF, et al. Treatment of cervical disc disease using Cloward's technique. 1. General results, effect of different operative methods and complications in 1106 patients. *Acta Neurochir (Wien)* 70:97–114, 1984.

23. Fager CA. Management of cervical disc lesions and spondylosis by posterior approaches. *Clin Neurosurg* 24:488–507, 1977.

24. Lesoin F, Bouasakao N, Clarisse J, et al. Results of surgical treatment of radiculomyelopathy caused by cervical arthrosis based on 1000 operations. *Surg Neurol* 23:350–355, 1985.

25. Mosdal C. Cervical osteochondrosis and disc herniation. Eighteen years' use of interbody fusion by Cloward's technique in 755 cases. *Acta Neurochir (Wien)* 70:207–225, 1984.

26. Nurick S. The natural history and the results of surgical treatment of the spinal cord disorder associated with cervical spondylosis. *Brain* 95:101–108, 1972.

27. Scoville WB, Whitcomb BB. Lateral rupture of cervical intervertebral disks. *Postgrad Med* 39:174–180, 1966.

28. Tew JM Jr, Mayfield FH. Complications of surgery of the anterior cervical spine. *Clin Neurosurg* 23:424–434, 1976.

Visceral Injury

29. Clark K. Anterior operative approach for benign extradural cervical lesions. In: Youmans JR, eds. *Neurological surgery. Vol. 4.* 2nd ed. 2613–2628, 1982.

30. Connolly ES, Seymour RJ, Adams JE. Clinical evaluation of anterior cervical fusion for degenerative cervical disc disease. *J Neurosurg* 23:431–437, 1965.

31. Esperson JO, Buhle M, Eriksen EF, et al. Treatment of cervical disc disease using Cloward's Technique. *Acta Neurochir (Wien)* 70:57–114, 1984.

32. Epstein JA, Epstein NE. Complications of cervical laminectomy, how to avoid them, diagnosis and treatment. In: *Cervical spine II.* New York: Springer-Verlag, 171–178, 1985.

33. Newhouse KE, Lindsey RW, Clark CR, Lieponis J, Murphy MJ. Esophageal perforation following anterior cervical spine surgery. *Spine* 14:1051–1056, 1989.

34. Smith GW, Robinson RA. The treatment of certain cervical spine disorders by anterior removal of the intervertebral disc and interbody fusion. *J Bone Joint Surg [Am]* 40A:607–624, 1958.

35. Stewart DY. Anterior approach to degenerative disk disease of the cervical spine. *NY State J Med* 61:3083–3096, 1961.

Infection

36. Cloward RB. Complications of anterior cervical disc operations and their treatment. *Surgery* 69:175–182, 1971.

37. Henderson CM, Hennessy RG, Shuey HM Jr, et al. Posterior-lateral foraminotomy as an exclusive operative technique for cervical radiculopathy: a review of 846 consecutively operated cases. *Neurosurgery* 13:504–512, 1983.

38. Odom GL, Finney W, Woodhall B. Cervical disk lesions. *JAMA* 166:23–28, 1958.

39. Raaf JE. Surgical treatment of patients with cervical disk lesions. *J Trauma* 9:327–338, 1969.

40. Tew Jm Jr, Mayfield FH. Complications of surgery of the anterior cervical spine. *Clin NSG* 23:424–434, 1976.

41. Tomford WW, Starkweather RJ, Goldman MH. A study of the incidence of infection in the use of banked allograft bone. *J Bone Joint Surg* 63:244–248, 1981.

Stabilization

42. Braunstin EM, Hunter LY, Baily RW. Long term radiographic changes following anterior cervical fusion. *Clin Radiol* 38:121–126,1986.

43. Brown MD, Malinin TI, Davis PB. A roentgenographic evaluation of frozen allografts versus autografts in anterior cervical spine fusions. *Clin Orthop* 119:231, 1976.

44. Cattell HS, Clark GL Jr. Cervical hyphosis and instability following multiple laminectomies in children. *J Bone Joint Surg [Am]* 49A:713–720, 1967.

45. Ishida Y, Suzuki K, Ohmori K, Kikata Y, Hattori Y. Critical analysis of extensive cervical laminectomy. *Neurosurgery* 24:215–222, 1989.

46. Fager CA. Failed neck syndrome: an ounce of prevention. *Clin Neurosurg* 27:450–465, 1980.

47. Mestdagh H, Debroucker R, Letendart J, Delcour JP, Reyford H. Functional results of anterior interbody fusion in injuries to the lower cervical spine. In: *Cervical spine.* 195–197, 1987.

48. Mikawa Y, Shikata J, Yamamuro T. Spinal deformity and instability after multilevel cervical laminectomy. *Spine* 12:6–11, 1987.

49. Sim FH, Svien HJ, Bickel WH, et al. Swan neck deformity. A review of twenty one cases. *J Bone Joint Surg [Am]* 56A:564–580, 1974.

50. Simons EH, Bhalla SK. Anterior cervical discectomy and fusion—a clinical and biomechanical study with 8 year follow-up. *J Bone Joint Surg [Br]* 51B:227–237, 1969.

51. Stabler CL, Eismont FJ, Brown MD, Green BA, et al. Failure of posterior cervical fusions using cadaveric bone graft in children. *J Bone Joint Surg [Am]* 67A:371, 1985.

52. Yasuoka S, Peterson HA, Laws ER Jr, MacCarty CS. Pathogenesis and prophylaxis of postlaminectomy deformity of the spine after multiple level laminectomy: difference between children and adults. *Neurosurgery* 9:145–152, 1981.

Graft Site

53. Abbott KH. Anterior cervical disc removal and interbody fusion. A preliminary review of 101 patients followed for one to three years. *Bull Los Angeles Neurol Soc* 28:251–259, 1963.
54. Connolly ES, Seymour RJ, Adams JE. Clinical evaluation of anterior cervical fusion for degenerative cervical disc disease. *J Neurosurg* 23:431–437, 1965.
55. Dohn DF. Anterior interbody fusion for treatment of cervical-disk conditions. *JAMA* 197:897–900, 1966.
56. Jacobs B, Krueger EG, Leivy DM. Cervical spondylosis with radiculopathy. Results of anterior diskectomy and interbody fusion. *JAMA* 211:2135–2139, 1970.
57. Schneider RC. Treatment of cervical spine disease. In: Schneider RC, Kahn EA, Crosby EC, Taren JA, eds. *Correlative neurosurgery*. 3rd ed. Springfield, IL: Charles C Thomas, 1094–1174, 1982.

Subject Index